Assessment of Chronic Pain Patients with the MMPI-2

MMPI-2 Monographs

Assessment of Chronic Pain Patients with the MMPI-2

Laura S. Keller and
James N. Butcher

MMPI-2 Monographs
Volume 2

University of Minnesota Press • Minneapolis • Oxford

Published by the University of Minnesota Press
2037 University Avenue Southeast, Minneapolis, MN 55414
Printed in the United States of America on acid-free paper

Keller, Laura Sue.
    Assessment of chronic pain patient with the MMPI-2 / Laura S.
Keller and James N. Butcher.
        p.   cm. — (MMPI-2 monograph series ; v.2)
    Includes bibliographical references and index.
    ISBN 0-8166-1861-5 (hc)
    1. Intractable pain—Diagnosis.   2. Minnesota Multiphasic
Personality Inventory.   I. Butcher, James Neal, 1933–
II. Title.   III. Series.
    [DNLM: 1.   Chronic Disease—psychology.   2. MMPI.   3. Pain—
psychology.   WM 145 K285a]
RB127.K38   1991
616'.0472—dc20
DNLM/DLC
for Library of Congress   90–11333
                                                                                 CIP

A CIP catalog record for this book is available from the British Library

The University of Minnesota is an
equal-opportunity educator and employer

Contents

Tables

Figures

Foreword

This monograph reports a monumental piece of work. The research reported here had two major aims: (1) to examine the comparability of MMPI-2 with the original MMPI; and (2) to collect and study clinical data on chronic pain patients, both for its own sake and as a way of assessing the clinical relevance of MMPI-2 in the important domain of chronic pain. Both aims were achieved with thoroughness and distinction.

The book contains a comprehensive and penetratingly analyzed review of the literature of chronic pain and, more particularly, of work done with the MMPI in regard to pain. It then goes on to describe in rich detail Dr. Keller's study. She collected MMPI protocols on the AX, experimental MMPI booklet, which permitted a direct comparison of MMPI and MMPI-2 items, scale scores, codetypes, and profile clusters. The subjects were 463 chronic pain patients undergoing the multidisciplinary pain treatment program at the Sister Kenny Institute in Minneapolis. This data set made possible meaningful comparisons of original MMPI and MMPI-2 data and a host of demographic and psychosocial variables accumulated concomitantly. Circumstances limited "medical" data to data that could be derived from clinic-patient chart review. Such data are notoriously unreliable, but Dr. Keller's management of that problem was careful, cautious, and procedurally sound. The analysis of those data provided a highly productive assay of the clinical relevance of MMPI-2, as well as of the original MMPI.

The monograph also contains a thoughtful discussion of strategies for item analysis, codetyping of test profiles, and cluster analyses. The monograph then reports the use of the application of these analyses to the chronic pain patient data. The caution displayed in interpreting these findings—which will have important implications for choosing research strategies in regard to codetyping vs. cluster analyses—is exemplary. An extensive set of clinical case applications is also provided, which should prove very helpful to clinicians.

My enthusiasm for this work is obvious. I believe that Drs. Keller and Butcher have made a very important contribution to our knowledge, as well as providing a sound basis for applying the MMPI-2.

Wilbert E. Fordyce, Ph.D.
Professor Emeritus
University of Washington School of Medicine
Seattle, Washington

Preface

In recent years a multidimensional model of chronic pain has emerged, taking into account affective, cognitive, behavioral, social, and somatosensory aspects of the pain experience. This model requires detailed assessment of other areas of a patient's functioning in addition to the traditional medical examination. Currently, the Minnesota Multiphasic Personality Inventory (MMPI) is the most widely used standardized personality test with chronic pain patients. However, the MMPI has recently been revised, resulting in publication of the MMPI-2 in August 1989. Major changes include rewording and replacement of some items, a new normative population, a new method of computing T-score transformations, and a new set of content scales.

This monograph is intended to help clinicians and researchers interested in the chronic pain patient population to learn about the usefulness of the MMPI with this patient group and begin to make the transition from the MMPI to the MMPI-2. It is largely based on the doctoral dissertation of the first author under the advisorship of the second author at the University of Minnesota Department of Psychology. The monograph begins with an overview of the problem of chronic pain, continues with a review of the history of MMPI applications with pain patients, discusses the revision of the MMPI, and then reports the first large research study using the MMPI-2 with this clinical population. General goals of the research study were to provide normative data on the MMPI-2 for pain patients, to discover similarities and differences between the MMPI and the MMPI-2 that clinicians and researchers will need to know when using the revised test with this sample, and to provide some initial data on demographic and clinical correlates of MMPI-2 patterns and scales in the chronic pain patient population. We conclude with a discussion of interpretive suggestions, some case examples, and recommendations for future research directions.

We wish to acknowledge the contributions of numerous individuals to this monograph. The first author's interest in focusing on chronic pain patients developed during her internship under the guidance of Drs. Wilbert Fordyce, Kelly Egan, Joan Romano, and Judith Turner of the University of Washington Pain Service. Their enthusiasm about working with the complex problems presented by pain patients was contagious, and their commitment to improving the assessment and treatment of these clients provided inspiration for this work.

The insightful comments and suggestions of the other members of Dr. Keller's dissertation committee, Professors Richard Depue, Glenn Gullickson, Gloria Leon, and Carolyn Williams are acknowledged with gratitude. We also thank the two anonymous reviewers who provided valuable editorial comments on this manuscript, and are indebted to Beverly Kaemmer of the University of Minnesota Press for editorial assistance.

We deeply appreciate the cooperation and assistance of the Sister Kenny Institute Chronic Pain Program in allowing access to their patient population and charts. Program director David Jones and medical director Dr. Matthew Monsein were extremely helpful and cordial. Particular thanks are due program staff Mary Mulvehill, Mary Corlette, Kim Young, and Ginger St. John for going out of their way to make sure testing procedures ran smoothly, for providing access to patient charts, and for providing coders with room to work. It was a pleasure to work with them.

Karen Gayda assisted at all phases of this project with secretarial and organizational help, as well as serving as a chart reviewer. Without her, we believe most of the MMPI restandardization projects would never have been completed! The long and tedious process of reviewing patient charts was speeded up tremendously by the many hours Karen, along with Troy Witta, Janet Chang, and Jay Butcher, contributed to this project. Janet, Karen, and Kyunghee Han are also to be thanked for their accurate and rapid data entry.

We appreciate the comments Drs. Norman Cohen and Yossef Ben-Porath gave on an early draft of the chart review form. Yossef, along with Wendy Slutske and Nathan Weed, provided invaluable suggestions on data analysis and computer programming. Kirsten Hostetler's assistance with graphing profiles and figures was greatly appreciated, as was Chris Elwell's help with numerous secretarial tasks.

Funding for this research came from a variety of sources. The University of Minnesota Press and the University of Minnesota Department of Conferences supported some of the salaries of personnel who worked on this project. National Computer Systems provided scoring of the experimental MMPI forms. Data analysis was funded through University of Minnesota Computer Center grants.

Finally, we wish to particularly acknowledge the generosity of the more than 400 chronic pain patients at Sister Kenny Institute who agreed to share their personal experiences with others through this project. This volume is dedicated to them, in the hope that it and future research will eventually help to alleviate the suffering associated with the problem of chronic pain.

L. S. K.
J. N. B.

Assessment of Chronic Pain Patients with the MMPI-2

Chapter 1
The Problem Of Chronic Pain

Chronic, intractable pain is not only an enormously frustrating clinical problem, but it also exacts a huge cost in personal suffering, productivity, and financial losses to society at large. In the United States, one-third to one-half the population will seek medical attention for a persistent pain problem at some time in their lives (Chapman & Bonica, 1985; Strang, 1985). Low back pain is the principal diagnosis in 10% of all chronic health conditions, and painful musculoskeletal conditions are the leading cause of activity limitation in patients of working age (Andersson, Pope, & Frymoyer, 1984; Kelsey, White, Pastides, & Bisbee, 1979; Steinberg, 1982).

Although most individuals experiencing back pain do not seek medical attention or make major alterations in their activities (Crook, Rideout, & Brown, 1984; Reisbord & Greenland, 1985), the number of persons annually who are partially or totally disabled by back pain may run as high as 8 million (Bonica, 1980). A review of studies from the 1970s and earlier concluded that chronic back disorders caused the loss of 240 million workdays annually (Chapman & Bonica, 1985). Each year, about 2% of all U.S. employees have compensable back injuries (Kelsey et al., 1979). The cost in productivity is particularly evident when considering that the incidence of back pain is highest in working-age adults between 25 and 55 years old (Cypress, 1983; Harkins, Kwentus, & Price, 1984; Steinberg, 1982).

The financial costs of health care and compensation are astronomical: a recent congressionally mandated Institute of Medicine (IOM) report on pain and disability found that "between 1970 and 1982, estimated total disability expenditures from all sources for members of the population age 18 to 64 years old more than doubled, from $60.2 billion to $121.5 billion in real 1982 dollars" (1987, p. 91). The Social Security Disability Insurance program has expanded rapidly over the past quarter-century: "between 1960 and 1985, the number of beneficiaries increased by 480 percent and the total annual benefits paid under the program increased by 778 percent. This growth far outstripped the increase in the U.S. adult population, which grew by only 51 percent during that period, and that of the working population insured for disability under SSA, which increased by 135 percent" (p. 38). Back injuries account for 20-30% of all Workers' Compensation costs (Edwards, 1983; Snook & Jensen, 1984), and the frequency of claims for back injury has risen more rapidly than for any other injury (Fordyce, 1984; Steinberg, 1982).

On the positive side, most cases of back pain are self-limited; 80-90% of patients recover within two months of seeking medical attention and only 2 to 4% suffer for more than six months with any given episode (Steinberg, 1982; Strang, 1985). However, given the high prevalence of back pain and its high recurrence rate, this is still a significant and costly subgroup of the U.S. labor force. As the duration of the problem increases, the chance of returning to work drops drastically (Beals & Hickman, 1972) and the costs in disability payments, litigation, and medical expenses rise: about 25% of back injury cases account for about 90% of the compensation costs (Snook & Jensen, 1984; Strang, 1985).

These statistics certainly suggest that medical science has not developed a simple, effective treatment for intractable pain. To understand the reasons for this, it is necessary to understand the complexity of the problem. Pain is most commonly thought of as a warning signal of tissue injury or disease. This specificity definition assumes that the amount of pain experienced is roughly proportional to the amount of tissue damage sustained. However, such a purely physiological, dualistic model of pain ("real" = clearly related to tissue damage, "imaginary" = suffering with no clear organic base) is relatively new in the history of pain concepts (Chapman & Bonica, 1985; Ford, 1983; Fordyce, 1976; Pennebaker, 1982). Aristotle and Plato regarded pain as a passion and an emotion, and Biblical references recognize that "pain felt in the body may well arise from misery, sadness or unhappiness" (Merskey, 1980, p. 4). Even our daily language retains an affective conception of pain: "you really hurt me by saying that"; "he's really a pain in the neck."

The past two decades have witnessed a move away from the dichotomous, Cartesian model of pain and a return to a multidimensional definition that recognizes affective, cognitive, behavioral, and social components as well as somatosensory aspects (Chapman & Bonica, 1985; Eisenberg, 1977; Ford, 1983; Fordyce, 1976, 1978; Melzack & Wall, 1965, 1983; Pennebaker, 1982; Turk & Flor, 1984). The specificity model was unable to account for the observed absence of pain in certain injury states or for the persistence of pain complaints in the absence of sufficient organic findings. The International Association for the Study of Pain has defined pain as "an unpleasant sensory and emotional experience associated with actual or potential tissue damage, or described in terms of such damage" (1986, p. s217). This definition removes the direct tie between tissue damage and pain, instead emphasizing that pain is a subjective psychological experience which, although the patient must associate it with a somatic sensation, does not necessarily have to result from a physiological stimulus.

This multi-component definition of pain helps in understanding the complexities of chronic pain problems. Definitions of chronic pain vary, but the term itself implies extended duration: these are persistent problems that are refractory to traditional medical treatment. Six months' duration is the usual figure used in studies, as this is well beyond the expected healing time for injuries. Studies vary as to the types of pain problems included in the lump category of chronic pain, but most exclude patients with degenerative diseases or cancer which could cause continuing sensory input from progressive tissue or nerve damage. Thus, implied in the definition is that the patient's experience or complaints of pain go beyond what might be expected from the known extent of organic involvement. Psychosocial factors must be considered in addition to whatever physiological factors may be contributing to the pain complaints. Pain problems of extended duration involve and affect all aspects of patients' lives.

Complexity and Heterogeneity of Chronic Pain

Just as the inadequacies of the specificity model led to the development of a multi-component definition of pain, the inadequacies of traditional medical treatment have led to treatment programs aimed at the multiplicity of physical and psychosocial factors thought to contribute to chronic pain problems. Any assessment or treatment approach must take into consideration the wide variety of factors that have been proposed as influencing pain. For a particular patient, one perspective may be more useful than another in understanding the specific factors causing his or her difficulties. Overall, however, current approaches to the management of chronic pain tend to assume that effective treatment programs need to incorporate to some degree several or all of the conceptual frameworks described below. The particular classification of approaches used here is not meant to be exhaustive or to encompass all organizational schemes presented elsewhere. It is provided as background to the complicated assessment issues to be addressed later in this monograph through one particular multidimensional measure, the Minnesota Multiphasic Personality Inventory (MMPI and MMPI-2).

Medical/Physiological Approach

The traditional medical approach to pain views it as a symptom of an underlying pathological process, with the assumption that treating the underlying physical pathology will cause the pain to disappear. This model of pain is comparable to a telephone communication system: the intensity of the transmitted pain signal and reported location of its source are assumed to be directly related to the extent and location of tissue pathology (Fordyce, 1976; Melzack & Wall, 1965, 1983; Pennebaker, 1982). Medical procedures based on this approach include those designed to eliminate the cause of pain by treating the pathology (such as disc surgeries), those designed to eliminate or reduce the sensitivity of peripheral receptors (such as via anesthetics), those designed to intercept the transmission lines (such as "nerve blocks," surgical cordotomies and rhizotomies), and those designed to eliminate or reduce central receptor sensitivity (such as anesthesia and centrally acting analgesics) (Chapman & Bonica, 1985; Ford, 1983; Wall & Melzack, 1984).

While the traditional medical approach often provides an adequate framework for treatment of acute pain problems, this somatosensory model fails to account for observed variation in individual responses to similar injuries, does not explain documented absence of pain even with severe injury, and does not address the persistence of pain complaints despite lack of discernible tissue damage. For example, although it was often assumed that pain in the presence of pathology such as degenerative disc or cartilage changes was attributable to that pathology, studies now show these same degenerative changes occur naturally and asymptomatically in the majority of the population as part of normal aging (Flor & Turk, 1984). In addition, a sizable number of patients' pain complaints are refractory to conservative medical treatment, few patients remain pain-free with more invasive procedures such as nerve blocks or chemonucleolysis (Flor & Turk, 1984), and less than 50% of back pain surgeries result in complete and permanent relief (Chapman & Bonica, 1985). Indeed, continuing to apply these traditional approaches to a chronic, refractory problem can cause iatrogenic complications: long-term use of narcotic pain medications can lead to tolerance and withdrawal symptoms, even including pain, and surgeries can cause scarring and nerve damage that add to pain problems.

Melzack and Wall (1965) provided a new theory of pain transmission and perception, the "gate control" theory, which addressed some of the observed individual differences in the reporting of pain. They presented a much more complicated physiological model than the traditional specificity theory, demonstrating a complex system of inhibitory and excitatory nerve pathways which "gate" the transmission of pain impulses to the cortex. Activation of some systems may modulate the influence of others: for example, pressure, vibration, and temperature changes can reduce the experience of pain. Acupuncture and transcutaneous electrical nerve stimulation (TENS) are presumed to derive some of their effectiveness from activating inhibitory pathways or competing for input to the spinal column (Flor & Turk, 1984).

This complicated network of interconnected, intermodulating systems helps to explain individual differences in experiencing pain, but it greatly complicates the question of whether an organic basis for an individual's pain exists. Particularly with chronic pain problems, subtle changes in nerve pathways or the balance of sympathetic, sensory, and motor nerve relationships can lead to continuing sensory input. Indeed, the gate control theory suggests it may be fallacious to think of any pain problem as purely "organic" or purely "functional." By placing central importance on cognitive, motivational, and affective activity in the cerebral cortex and its potential to modify perception of peripheral input, the gate control theory necessitates examining the influence of psychosocial factors on the thinking, processing, reacting human being.

Psychodynamic and Psychiatric Traditions

The psychodynamic approach to chronic pain is similar to the traditional medical model in assuming that pain is a symptom of an underlying problem and that treatment should address the underlying pathology. However, the underlying problem is conceptualized as an emotional one, learned in childhood through the association of pain with important formative emotional experiences, particularly with parents. "The key comes through understanding how pain may yield pleasure. . . . Both as a warning system and as a mechanism of defense, pain helps to avoid or ward off even more unpleasant feeling states or experiences and may even offer the means whereby certain gratifications can be achieved, albeit at a price" (Engel, 1959, p. 902). Pain becomes a compromise, a way of reconciling inner drives and needs with external reality (Aronoff & Rutrick, 1985; Pilowsky, 1978).

Psychoanalytic theorists have often described pain patients in terms of three personality patterns: hysteria, hypochondriasis, or depressive equivalent (Engel, 1959; Merskey, 1978; Sternbach, 1974a; Turk & Flor, 1984). Hysteria has been poorly defined, but is often understood as a conversion of mental conflict into somatic symptoms, associated with apparent complacency in the face of disability, concrete focus on symptoms with little ability to take an objective, self-monitoring approach, craving for attention and intimacy with little ability to maintain close relationships, a suggestible, dependent, even manipulative interpersonal style, emotional lability, proneness to chemical dependency, low socioeconomic status, and often clear secondary gains from disability as well as the primary gain of a compromise between impulse and defense. For such patients, somatic symptoms can serve a communicative function: they seem to have little language for psychological or emotional experiences, instead unconsciously communicating distress and seeking gratification of needs through somatic symptoms (Abse, 1974; Chodoff, 1974; Lazare, 1971; Miller, 1987). The current interest in "alexithymia" (literally "no language for feelings") as a trait of patients with psychosomatic illnesses has been reflected in some of the pain literature, with several investigators suggesting that chronic pain populations tend to show high frequencies of alexithymic characteristics (Catchlove, Cohen, Braha, & Demers-Desrosiers, 1985; Mendelson, 1982; Postone, 1986).

The definition of hypochondriasis has also been rather fuzzy through the years. Generally, rather than denoting a psychiatric diagnosis, it has been used as a term to describe characteristics that may cross diagnostic categories. A representative description is "morbid preoccupation with one's body or state of health, either mental or physical, with the further implication that this is the subject of complaints to others" (Kenyon, 1976, p. 1). Principal factors in hypochondriasis have been described as somatic preoccupation, disease phobia, disease conviction with non-response to reassurance, disabled life-style, and multiple somatic complaints disproportionate to organic pathology (Barsky et al., 1986; Pilowsky, 1967). Hypochondriasis has repeatedly been found to correlate highly with various measures of neuroticism, defined as "a broad dimension of normal personality that encompasses a variety of specific traits, including self-consciousness, inability to inhibit cravings, and vulnerability to stress as well as the tendency to experience anxiety, hostility, and depression" (Costa & McRae, 1985, p. 21).

Compared to hysteria, hypochondriasis is generally thought to be characterized by more anxious, depressed somatic preoccupation instead of the seeming complacency of the conversion reaction. Indeed, Kenyon (1976) suggests that some of the hypochondriac's conviction of being ill may stem from focusing on the autonomic correlates of anxiety. Both syndromes are conceptualized as distractions from stressful life situations and uncomfortable emotions, and both may serve to meet dependency needs, express anger, and avoid performance demands in a socially acceptable manner (Chrzanowski, 1974; Kenyon, 1976; Smith, Snyder, & Perkins, 1983). Denial of psychological problems in spite of conflict-ridden developmental histories and current life difficulties is described as a salient feature of the somatizing patient (Bouckoms, Litman, & Baer, 1985; Merskey, 1978).

Engel (1959) provided a psychodynamic formulation that included these features, but emphasized the role of pain as a depressive equivalent. He described pain patients as characterized by developmental histories in which pain, punishment, and affection became linked; pain serves as expiation for guilt and is reinforced by forgiveness and attention from the family. Such patients "unconsciously do not believe that they deserve success or happiness, and feel that they must pay a price for it" (p. 905). Success is difficult to tolerate, whereas withdrawing from life to the shelter of "pain as an old friend" (Penman, 1954) is more comfortable. An alternative developmental history includes familial models of pain, which by the process of identification become incorporated into the child's self-image (Engel, 1959; Pilowsky, 1978). Several researchers have suggested that pain is more likely to serve as a depressive equivalent in families where illness models are present and the family does not define distress in psychological terms (Katon, Kleinman, & Rosen, 1982a, 1982b; Maruta, Swanson, & Swenson, 1976; Pilowsky & Bassett, 1982). The suffering of pain provides an alternative to psychological suffering (Merskey, 1978). Pain is most likely to develop in situations that threaten the loss of a loved one, when too much success is experienced, or when unacceptable aggressive or dependent impulses are aroused.

Blumer and Heilbronn (1981, 1982, 1984) have expanded this model to describe the "pain-prone disorder" characterized by denial of emotional and interpersonal problems, inactivity, anhedonia, depressed mood, guilt, inability to deal with anger and hostility, insomnia, craving for affection and dependency, lack of initiative, and a family history of depression, alcoholism, and chronic pain. Such patients are described as relentless workers premorbidly, becoming infantile in their dependency needs after injury: "the bane of relentless work is replaced by the torture of continuous pain in atonement for the unacceptable infantile needs . . . these patients are compelled to see themselves as solid citizens . . . and the somatization of the psychic conflict helps them to save face" (1981, p. 401). The authors suggest that this is a homogeneous and diagnostically unique group that can be considered part of the "depressive spectrum."

Other researchers have supported the validity of the pain-depression connection in subsets of the chronic pain population, but have also pointed out great heterogeneity in psychiatric status (Gupta, 1986; Roy, Thomas, & Matas, 1984; Turk & Salovey, 1984). In some cases, depression may be a reaction to the pain problem itself and its associated losses. For others, depression may precede the pain: "individuals with affective disorders seek medical care more often than individuals without psychiatric disorders, they often seek care for medical or somatic symptoms (including pain) rather than for psychiatric symptoms, and they often are only seen in the general medical care sector" (IOM, 1987, p. 166). Investigators have suggested identifying a subgroup of pain patients with premorbid and family histories of depression and alcoholism and biological markers of endogenous depression, since this may be a group exhibiting a common pain-depression neurochemical substrate best treated with antidepressant medications (Blumer & Heilbronn, 1982; France, Krishnan, & Trainor, 1986; Katon, Egan, & Miller, 1985; Lindsay & Wyckoff, 1981; Romano & Turner, 1985). Tricyclic antidepressants have been shown to reduce perception of pain for some patients while simultaneously improving mood (Feinmann, 1985; Hendler, 1984). Indeed, "it is often observed clinically that when pain occurs as a symptom of a primary psychiatric disorder, successful pharmacological treatment directed at the disorder itself is accompanied by the alleviation of the pain" (IOM, 1987, p. 175).

Frequency of psychiatric diagnoses and symptoms in chronic pain populations supports the prediction from psychodynamic theory that this group would have a high incidence of hysterical, hypochondriacal, and depressive syndromes and histories of family conflict, abuse, and prior psychiatric problems. Neurotic disorders tend to be much more common than psychotic disorders, although this may be partially the result of patient selection: overtly psychotic pain patients are likely to be sent directly for psychiatric treatment rather than being treated for pain (Aronoff, 1985; Fishbain et al., 1986).

The most frequently diagnosed disorders among pain patients are depression and anxiety syndromes, with frequency estimates varying greatly. Estimates of the incidence of major affective disorder, for example, range from 10% to 100%, and anxiety disorders (including post-traumatic stress disorder) from 7% to 63% (Fishbain et al., 1986; Gupta, 1986; Katon et al., 1985; Kramlinger, Swanson, & Maruta, 1983; Large, 1986; Reich, Tupin, & Abramowitz, 1983; Reich & Thompson, 1987; Romano & Turner, 1985; Roy et al., 1984; Turner & Romano, 1984b). Substance abuse, both of alcohol and of prescription medications such as narcotics and sedative/hypnotics, has been found in up to half of clinical samples, predominantly among the men (Fishbain et al., 1986; Katon et al., 1985; Maruta, Swanson, & Finlayson, 1979; Reich et al., 1983; Reich & Thompson, 1987). Somatoform disorders are also commonly diagnosed, although frequencies vary widely, probably owing to inconsistencies in physicians' assessments of whether there are organic contributors to a patient's difficulties. In addition, from one-third to one-half of pain patient populations have been reported to meet criteria for personality disorder diagnoses, particularly of the dependent, passive-aggressive, histrionic, or narcissistic types (Blazer, 1980-81; Fishbain et al., 1986; Reich et al., 1983; Reich & Thompson, 1987; Van Houdenhove, 1986). All of these figures are limited by inconsistent diagnostic criteria and by differences in patient characteristics across treatment settings.

Interestingly, despite this correlational support for psychodynamic models of chronic pain, most of the clinical literature does not advocate treating pain patients by traditional psychodynamic methods. Instead of engaging in long-term individual therapy to free repressed affect and translate "body language" into "word language" (Abse, 1974), most advocate a multidisciplinary, supportive but behaviorally oriented treatment package aimed at addressing the patient's problems in living (Aronoff & Rutrick, 1985). Although the psychodynamic literature does not directly address matching treatment to personality type, a few speculations might be made. Shipman, Greene, and Laskin (1974) have provided some evidence that response to treatments based on suggestion, such as placebos or hypnosis, may vary with personality type: "the people who responded [best] tended to be psychoneurotic, hysterical, and very unaware of their impulses and feelings" (p. 482). Utilizing suggestions and meeting dependency needs through group therapy might be particularly appropriate for these patients, providing a new set of socially acceptable, non-pain-oriented standards and some peer pressure to conform to these for attention and approval. The more somatically preoccupied and depressed patients might need more activity and exercise (possibly combined with antidepressant medication) than other patients to reduce their symptoms. However, psychodynamic theory would suggest that the main focus would need to be on understanding the meaning of pain for the particular client and the secondary gains supporting illness, so that treatment can explore other avenues for meeting these needs: "alternatives to the pain career" (Sternbach & Rusk, 1973).

Learning Theories

The medical and psychodynamic models assume that pain problems are caused by underlying pathology and that this underlying causative agent must be located and addressed for a treatment to be useful. However, a wealth of research now shows "it has proved practical in a wide variety of situations to approach interpersonal, social, behavioral, or so-called mental illness problems by the direct modification of behavior, without recourse first to modifying alleged underlying personality mechanisms or motivational patterns" (Fordyce, 1976, p. 35). Learning theorists study the systematic relationships of pain behaviors to environmental cues and responses, and seek to treat pain problems through manipulation of these relationships.

Classical conditioning. Pain behaviors can be classified as respondent (re-flexive, elicited by antecedent stimuli) or operant (voluntary, controlled by their consequences). In acute pain states, pain behavior is usually respondent, elicited by sensory input from tissue injury. However, through conditioning processes this pain behavior can come to be elicited by other stimuli associated with the experience of pain. A pain-tension cycle can develop: injury results in pain resulting in muscle tension, muscle tension leads to increased pain eliciting more tension in response, etc. Thus, pain becomes both an antecedent and a consequence of muscular hypertension (Gentry & Bernal, 1977).

Caldwell and Chase (1977) noted that acute pain elicits an autonomic alarm reaction in the individual; this fear and arousal can become associated with whatever was occurring at the time of the initial pain-fear experience. For example, a worker injured in a fall from a building might have a recurrence of pain and fear when trying to return to another job requiring work high above the ground. Investigators such as Muse (1985, 1986) have applied diagnostic criteria for post-traumatic stress disorder to pain patient populations, suggesting that a subgroup may be suffering from phobic overguarding and anxiety reactions brought on by traumatic events. Within 64 consecutive referrals to a pain clinic, 10% met Muse's diagnostic criteria including duration of pain six months or more, existence of a sudden fear-inducing stressor associated with the onset of the pain, intrusive re-experiencing of the initial traumatic experience, reduced in-volvement and responsiveness to the external world, and other symptoms such as hyperalertness, guilt, sleep disturbance, impairment of concen-tration, avoidance of activities arousing recollection of the trauma, and intensification of symptoms by events resembling the initial trauma. The majority of these patients experienced pain in the back and neck, and were diagnosed as having pain related to muscle spasm. Similarly, Benedikt and Kolb (1986) also found 10% of a VA pain clinic sample met criteria for post-traumatic stress disorder. Pain was always localized at the site of a former combat or accident-related injury.

The same conditioning process may occur with a less extreme but repetitive pain problem, such as chronic low back pain. Each twinge elicits renewed fear of worse pain to come, leading to muscle tension and preoccupation with guarding the body from injury. This may lead to increasing disability as the patient uses more protective behaviors, loses strength and flexibility, and reflexively reacts to the resulting pain with further avoidance, guarding, and tension (Caldwell & Chase, 1977; Weisenberg, 1987). "Avoiding stimulation plays an active part in reducing the sufferer's sense of control over pain, and in increasing his or her expectation that exposure will increase pain. These cognitive changes encourage further withdrawal from normal activities and a growing intolerance of stimulation" (Philips, 1987, p. 273). Although research support for the relationship between muscular tension and back pain is equivocal (Turk & Flor, 1984), there is some clinical support for the importance of autonomic conditioning processes in at least a subsample of pain patients. For example, Flor, Turk, and Birbaumer (1985) found that chronic pain patients had greater back muscle reactivity to personal stressors and greater delay in returning to baseline than general pain patients or normal controls.

Treatment of pain following a classical conditioning model usually consists of extinction or counterconditioning. Caldwell and Chase (1977) and Philips (1987) suggest gradually controlled increases in exercise can serve as an extinction procedure, by presenting the conditioned stimulus (exercise) in the absence of the unconditioned stimulus (pain and fear). Since in most cases some pain will persist, making complete extinction of the conditioned response unlikely, Caldwell and Chase suggest the goal should be to help the patient "personally master pain . . . if he initiates his own pain, then he can control it rather than being controlled by it" (p. 149). Muse (1985, 1986) suggests using relaxation and desensitization to provide a competing response (relaxation) which is incompatible with muscle tension, then to repeatedly pair this with the stimuli that previously evoked fear, tension, and pain.

Research is unclear as to the effectiveness of these procedures: it may depend on the site of pain and the selection of patients with evidence of respondent pain. The mechanism of relief may be related to placing the response under operant control or changing cognitive evaluation of self-efficacy rather than a pure classical conditioning paradigm (Philips, 1987; Turk & Flor, 1984; Turner & Chapman, 1982a). It might be hypothesized that patients showing high levels of anxiety would be the group best suited to extinction and counterconditioning treatments.

Operant conditioning. Probably the greatest influence on chronic pain treatment has been the application of operant conditioning to the control of pain behavior (Fordyce, 1976, 1978, 1983; Fordyce, Roberts, & Sternbach, 1985; Sternbach, 1984). Chronic pain provides months or years of opportunities for learning processes to influence the experience and expression of pain. Even as soon as six months after the injury, pain behaviors may be occurring for reasons totally different from when they were first emitted. Rather than being respondent to a sensory stimulus, they may be partially or totally under the control of environmental reinforcers. Three major ways in which operant processes can influence pain behaviors are through direct reinforcement, through indirect reinforcement (avoidance learning), or through an inadequate repertoire or inadequate reinforcement of "well behaviors."

Direct reinforcement of pain behaviors occurs when they are followed by positive consequences. Such a contingency increases the likelihood that pain behaviors will be repeated. Examples of such reinforcement are solicitous attention from family members or medical personnel, rest, medication, and financial compensation. Intensity of pain report has been found to be higher and treatment response poorer among patients whose family members respond solicitously to their complaints (Anderson & Rehm, 1984; Block, Kremer, & Gaylor, 1980; Tarsh & Royston, 1985). Fordyce, Brockway, Bergman, and Spengler (1986) demonstrated that traditional medical approaches, which make rest and medication contingent on pain, result in more claims of continued impairment than strategies which make rest contingent on exercise quotas and medication contingent on passage of time. In some cases, Workers' Compensation payments and ongoing litigation requiring demonstration of disability can reinforce continued illness behavior as well (Butcher & Harlow, 1987; Carron, DeGood, & Tait, 1985; Edwards, 1983; Fordyce, 1984; Strang, 1985).

Pain behaviors can be indirectly reinforced when their occurrence leads to avoidance or reduction of unpleasant events. Classically conditioned responses can eventually come under operant control through their effectiveness in reducing anxiety. For example, guarding behavior may be reinforced because the patient feels less fearful than when engaged in more vigorous movement. Pain behaviors may be reinforced by reducing conflict in the home, by avoiding unwanted sexual activity, or by avoiding unpleasant chores or work. Indirect reinforcement may be particularly powerful for those patients who feel inadequate to perform the social or vocational roles expected of healthy adults. The poorly educated or psychiatrically impaired patient may find it less aversive to be bedridden than to try to compete in the job market. The elderly patient experiencing some cognitive loss may avoid revealing failing memory skills by pleading illness and staying at home (Fordyce, 1978; Harkins, Kwentus, & Price, 1984).

Finally, pain behaviors may be maintained if the client does not receive sufficient reinforcement of "well behaviors," those activities that are incompatible with the sick role and are necessary for the person to function successfully in educational, vocational, and social roles. Examples would be the family who consistently responds to the patient's activities with admonitions to do less, or the patient who would suffer a loss of income by returning to a low-paying job rather than staying on disability payments. In many cases the patient may be handicapped by a deficient repertoire of well behaviors, such as the poorly educated, psychotic, or demented patient. Lack of skills necessary to perform in non-heavy-labor positions can be particularly limiting.

Treatment based on the operant model attempts to lessen the patient's functional disability (not necessarily the subjective experience of pain) by modifying the reinforcement contingencies maintaining pain behavior, and, when necessary, filling gaps in the well behavior repertoire. Typical procedures include making rest contingent on completion of gradually increasing exercise quotas, and gradually weaning patients off pain medications after making them available only on a time-contingent basis rather than being contingent on pain complaints. Staff are taught to reinforce well behaviors with their attention and to ignore pain behaviors as much as possible. Gaps in well behavior repertoires may be addressed through vocational counseling and occupational therapy.

Such programs have generally proven effective in increasing activity level and decreasing medication consumption during treatment, and a subset of patients appear to maintain these gains over time (Fordyce, Roberts, & Sternbach, 1985; Keefe, Gil, & Rose, 1986; Latimer, 1982; Linton, 1986; Roberts & Reinhardt, 1980; Turner & Chapman, 1982b). Fordyce (1983) suggests that one very important factor determining long-term efficacy of such programs is the amount of emphasis placed on maximizing the generalization of treatment gains to the patient's life outside the program. Attempts to ensure that health-compatible reinforcement contingencies will be maintained include working with the patient's family and friends, personal physician or health-care provider, and educational or employment system to teach them to support the gains made in the treatment program.

The effect of operant programs on the patient's subjective experience of pain remains unclear (Turner & Chapman, 1982b), and it is also unclear whether this is an important variable in long-term outcome as measured by behavioral criteria. Most behavioral treatment programs are intensive, multimodal inpatient packages: it has not yet been possible to define which are the active treatment components and whether these vary systematically with patient characteristics. Finally, it is possible that some behavioral techniques owe their effectiveness to changes in the patient's internal experience, a possibility which research on purely operant approaches does not address. Even Fordyce (1983) has suggested that generalization of results might be achieved through the patient learning to use cognitive cues to elicit learned behavioral sequences, a possibility that will be explored further under cognitive approaches.

Social learning and modeling. The ability to learn through observation has particular adaptive value in the area of pain and illness; "vicarious experience can substitute for direct experience without the observer suffering the intense or longterm distress" (Craig, 1978, p. 75). Bandura (1977b) described the crucial importance of observational learning in acquiring new patterns of behavior, particularly interpersonal behaviors. While knowing how to communicate distress and elicit appropriate help from others certainly has adaptive value, social modeling can also result in learning maladaptive patterns such as inappropriate pain complaints, maintenance of sick role behavior when more functional behavior is possible, and avoidance of treatment (such as psychotherapy) that may be in the individual's best interest.

Studies of cultural differences in pain expression strongly support the influence of social learning on at least the public aspects of the pain experience. Patterns of pain behavior vary with ethnic background and, within immigrant populations, increasingly resemble their host culture in succeeding generations (Craig, 1978; Escobar et al., 1987; Katon, Kleinman, & Rosen, 1982a, 1982b; Lipton & Marbach, 1984; Mechanic, 1972; Merskey, 1978). Operant conditioning can occur when cultural and familial models demonstrate the contingencies that may be expected to apply to pain behaviors, influencing the likelihood that the patient will emit those behaviors. Classical conditioning can also occur through observation: children have strong affective and physiological responses to seeing their parents suffer, and thus may learn to associate pain and fear with the stimuli which seemed to be associated with their parents' distress (Craig, 1978, 1983)

From this model, data indicating that chronic pain patients tend to have many relatives with pain problems are interpreted as support for the influence of modeling on the patient's subsequent illness behavior (Edwards, Zeichner, Kuczmeirczyk, & Boczkowki, 1985; Violon & Giurgea, 1984). "In general, the evidence that chronic pain patients have family histories replete with somatic complaints and preoccupation with health concerns suggests important roles for empathetic communication of parental distress about bodily functions . . . intensive instruction in identifying somatic states and symptoms, and acquisition of skills in engaging care from clinicians and health agencies" (Craig, 1983, p. 819).

Treatment based on social learning teaches the client alternative modes of responding to pain and alternative ways of interacting other than through somatic symptoms. The client observes the behaviors and coping strategies modeled by others, including other patients. Research suggests that social learning affects not only the public expression of pain, but also physiological arousal and subjective response to somatic sensations, as well as selectivity of attention to internal vs. external stimulation (Craig, 1978, 1983; Pennebaker, 1982). The importance of these private processes in the development and maintenance of chronic pain will be discussed later under cognitive theories.

Systems Theory

Systems theory shares with psychodynamic and learning models the assumption that pain problems persist because they serve a purpose. In systems theory, this purpose is the maintenance of homeostasis within a system of interdependent components. Pain may be viewed as a symptom of stress within the system, and/or a regulating mechanism that serves to maintain stability. This transactional model emphasizes the reciprocal feedback effect of the patient's behavior on others and others' behavior on the patient (Goldberg, 1985; Liebman, Honig, & Berger, 1976; Payne & Norfleet, 1986).

Pain patients are involved in many interpersonal systems, the most salient of which is usually the family (Kremer, Sieber, & Atkinson, 1985; Roy, 1984, 1985; Tarsh & Royston, 1985; Turk, Rudy, & Flor, 1985). Psychosomatic families have been described as characterized by enmeshment of members, rigidity, poor problem-solving capacity, and overprotectiveness (Liebman, Honig, & Berger, 1976; Minuchin, Rosman, & Baker, 1978). One member's role as the designated patient may serve to distract focus from other problems, avoid acknowledgment of conflict, and hold the family unit together. Bokan, Ries, and Katon (1981) use the term "tertiary gain" to emphasize that a central factor in many chronic pain problems may be the reluctance (conscious or otherwise) of other people to give up the advantages they gain from the patient's pain. Goldberg (1985) describes a few functions pain may serve in a family system: regulation of emotional closeness and distance, a means for negotiating power and control, and a "tacit collusion in which the patient's sick role and pain behavior is accepted and defended by the spouse (or significant other) in exchange for the patient's accepting and defending psychosocial inadequacies or pathology in the spouse" (p. 587).

Evidence that pain patients do tend to have more relatives with pain problems than controls is cited as support for continuity of family coping styles down the generations (Blumer & Heilbronn, 1982; Gentry, Shows, & Thomas, 1974; Mohamed, Weisz, & Waring, 1978; Payne & Norfleet, 1986). However, such data could also support genetic, learning, psychodynamic, or cognitive models of pain. There is also evidence that pain patients tend to mate with spouses who have somatic problems, or spouses whose pathology may be balanced by the patient's pain problem. Roberts and Reinhardt (1980) found that patients who failed to benefit from a pain treatment program were more likely to have spouses with high MMPI hypochondriasis and hysteria scores themselves. Ahern and Follick (1985) also found that the spouses' MMPI profiles were predictive of patients' treatment outcome. Mohamed et al. (1978) found consistency in the location of pain among patients, their spouses, and family members on both sides. These results were cited as supporting "significant other specificity" (Waring, 1977): the patient unconsciously selects the location of pain because of its meaningfulness to significant others. Haber and Roos (1985) noted that 38% of a sample of women presenting with chronic pain problems reported ongoing physical or sexual abuse in their marriages; somatization may have served both to deny marital problems and to modulate their husband's aggressiveness.

Other systems may also play a role in maintaining pain problems. A society's compensation system may tacitly require the patient to maintain a pain problem to ensure financial stability. The legal system may require the maintenance of disability to win a favorable settlement. The health-care system may promote continued somatization as a result of physicians' focus on traditional medical approaches to pain (Fordyce et al., 1986; Fordyce, 1988). Sternbach (1974a, 1974c) and Szasz (1968) described transactions between pain patients and health-care providers as "pain games" or "painsmanship," emphasizing the repetitiveness in these maneuvers as each tries to maintain the stability of role definition. Treatment of any of these factors, including the family's influence on pain problems, requires broad-range assessment tactics leading to interventions that change the rules of the entire system.

Cognitive and Information-Processing Approaches

Many researchers now suggest that the effects of childhood experiences, cultural learning, stressful life events, operant conditioning, and even sensory input may all be mediated through their influence on the individual's information-processing and perceptual style (Barsky, 1986; Chapman, 1978; Costa & McRae, 1985; Mechanic, 1972; Pennebaker, 1982; Pennebaker & Skelton, 1978; Weisenberg, 1984, 1987). The gate control theory of Melzack and Wall (1965, 1983) initiated the examination of the complex interactions of sensory, affective, evaluative and motivational influences on an organism's perception and interpretation of data. Psychological research on sensation, perception, information-processing, labeling, and attribution has also suggested some possible roles for cognitive factors in chronic illness.

Melzack and Wall stated that an individual's experience of pain is subject to modulation by a variety of physiologically mediated inhibitory and excitatory inputs. Psychological research indicates that an individual's prior experiences and present social context influence focus of attention as well as interpretation of stimuli. This appraisal in turn can influence the intensity of response and affective reaction to stimulation. Pennebaker (1982) notes that we have a limited attentional capacity; the attention we pay to internal (somatic) sensations will depend in part on the amount of external stimulation experienced. Thus, people become more aware of tickling in their throats during symphony intermissions, and the pain of tired muscles may not be noticed in the excitement of a first day of skiing but worsens in bed when outside stimulation is reduced. The client with sensory deficits, such as an older adult losing hearing, might be particularly prone to increasing somatic preoccupation as the external world loses its salience. Repetitive, boring jobs might also provide more opportunity for heightened attention to sensations such as back pain (Feuerstein, Sult, & Houle, 1985).

Appraisal and labeling of ambiguous sensations have been shown to be influenced by learning history and situational cues. The classic experiment by Schachter and Singer (1962) illustrated that an individual's labeling of autonomic arousal can be manipulated to reflect seemingly opposite states of "euphoria" or "anger" by the social cues modeled by a confederate. Anderson and Pennebaker (1980) showed that groups of students could be influenced to label an identical stimulus as "painful" or "pleasurable" simply through a slight change in the label provided by the experimenter. Each group later claimed there was no possible way the stimulus could have been experienced in the opposite category. Individuals constantly seek causal explanations for incoming data and constantly organize and reduce stimulation into meaningful categories.

Although this process must be physiologically based, an individual's internal organizational schemes are largely learned from experience. From a cognitive perspective, the preponderance of somatic illness and unresolved relationship conflict in pain patients' families supports the hypothesis that these clients learned early in life to selectively focus on somatic sensations and to interpret a wide variety of inputs in somatic terms. Pennebaker (1982) suggests precursors to the hypochondriacal personality style are family conflict, reinforcement of illness behavior, and insecurity about performance in other arenas (increasing self-consciousness, self-monitoring, and somatic input from autonomic correlates of anxiety) and a history of personal or modeled serious illness or physical trauma which provides a schema for organizing experience.

Once such schemas are organized, it is very difficult to change them owing to patients' tendency to selectively attend to data that confirm their preconceived hypotheses (Pennebaker, 1982) and to behave in ways that reduce the likelihood they will encounter contrary data, such as refusing to try increased exercise because they "know" it will only make them sicker. Several researchers have indicated that chronic pain patients tend to blur normal distinctions between painful and nonpainful situations, and may interpret a wide variety of experiences, particularly affective distress, in pain terms (Clark & Yang, 1983; Pennebaker, 1982; Pennebaker & Skelton, 1978; Yang, Wagner, & Clark, 1983). "The figure-ground organization of pain experiences tends toward stability when pain becomes familiar and is accepted as part of the normal perceptual routine. For chronic pain patients the tendency toward stability in experience is quite strong, and the pain tends to resist therapeutic interventions that would threaten the familiar, albeit unpleasant, perceptual experience" (Chapman, 1978, p. 199).

Recent research suggests that an individual's appraisal of his or her control over pain and associated disabilities may be an important predictor of chronicity vs. successful coping with the problem (Dolce, 1987; O'Leary, 1985). Such approaches are based on Bandura's (1977a) concept of self-efficacy: an individual's appraisal of personal resources and effectiveness will affect whether and how long he or she will actively attempt to cope with problems. Compared to normal individuals, less disabled pain patients, or medical patient controls, highly disabled chronic back pain patients have been described as less active, more prone to use medications, and more prone to use passively avoidant coping strategies associated with an attitude of generalized helplessness (Feifel, Strack, & Nagy, 1988; Keefe & Dolan, 1986; Rosenstiel & Keefe, 1983; Smith, Follick, Ahern, & Adams, 1986; Turner & Clancy, 1986).

Cognitive treatments aim to provide the patient with techniques to gain a sense of control over the pain experience as well as actually modifying the intensity, affective component, and behavioral sequelae of that experience. Social modeling is used to teach coping self-statements, problem-solving and goal-setting. Relaxation, imagery, biofeedback, and hypnosis have all been used to modify attentional focus as well as to provide the patient with an increased sense of mastery (Fernandez, 1986; Jessup, 1984; Orne, 1983; Orne & Dinges, 1984; Turner & Chapman, 1982a, 1982b; Zitman, 1983).

It could be predicted from the appraisal and labeling literature that the most difficult focus of treatment would be the patient's tendency to interpret a multitude of sensations and emotions as signs of illness. The cognitive-behavioral approach to pain management combines training in cognitive techniques with contingency management techniques, in the hope of improving the effectiveness of both approaches (Evans, 1985; Turk & Meichenbaum, 1984; Turk, Meichenbaum, & Genest, 1983). Behavioral experiences help to show patients they are capable of more than they assumed, increasing their sense of personal competence and combating their assumptions that limitations are due to illness. Cognitive techniques help to place affective, perceptual, and behavioral responses under the patient's control. The assumption is that long-term maintenance of behavioral changes will occur only if the patient has learned to attribute success to his or her own efforts (Dolce, 1987). Patients may be taught other skills such as assertive communication designed to support a view of themselves as competent and effective rather than as passive victims.

At this point little information is available on whether cognitive changes are necessary for behavioral gains to be experienced or maintained, although there are suggestions that cognitive treatment can result in changes of coping style and reduction of reported pain severity as well as behavioral changes (Dolce, Crocker, & Doleys, 1986; Turk & Rudy, 1986; Turner, 1982; Turner & Chapman, 1982b; Turner & Clancy, 1986, 1988). It is also unclear whether certain types of patients are more likely to benefit from cognitive approaches than others. There are some preliminary suggestions that individual variability in personality characteristics may affect degree of benefit from relaxation, self-hypnosis, and cognitive coping strategies; these self-help strategies are considered more likely to be useful for patients who have more self-esteem and already use more active coping measures (Ford, 1985; Harris & Rollman, 1985; Page & Schaub, 1978). It is not certain whether this pattern is specific to these treatments or reflects a general trend for such patients to do better in any treatment.

The Multidisciplinary Approach to Chronic Pain

Although the various approaches to chronic pain differ in the specifics of proposed etiologic and maintaining factors, all emphasize the need to understand an individual's suffering as a complex, multiply determined phenomenon that has an impact on all areas of the patient's life. They also share the assumption that this suffering can be modified or lessened. They tend to differ on whether this is best accomplished through addressing subjective, internal aspects of chronic pain, the objective behaviors associated with it that result in disability, or the social, cultural, and health-care systems that can serve to maintain it.

Despite disagreements on the active ingredients of treatment, pragmatic clinicians have increasingly advocated a multidisciplinary approach which more or less addresses all the different theories noted above. Such programs are usually inpatient packages lasting for several weeks which include various combinations of behavior modification, physical therapy, medication management, group or individual psychological counseling, education about modulating influences on pain, family therapy, vocational counseling, occupational/recreational therapy, relaxation training, biofeedback, hypnosis, guided imagery, etc. Disciplines represented by the treatment team may include nursing, physical therapy, occupational or recreational therapy, psychology, psychiatry, anesthesiology, vocational rehabilitation, social work, neurosurgery, and orthopedics (Aronoff, 1985; Aronoff & Evans, 1985; IOM, 1987; Keefe, Gil, & Rose, 1986; Swanson, Floreen, & Swenson, 1976; Swanson, Swenson, Maruta, & McPhee, 1976).

These programs combine techniques from many disciplines and theories in the interest of achieving a multidimensional goal: the relief of suffering in the most general sense of the word, not simply physical pain, and the reduction of costs to society engendered by these patients. Aronoff (1985, p. 509) provides a representative list of treatment goals as defined at the Boston Pain Center: 1) eliminating the source of pain when feasible, 2) teaching the patient to function within pain limitations, 3) improving pain control through conservative physical therapy and psychologic methods, 4) relieving drug dependence, 5) use of non-narcotic medications, if medication is necessary, 6) treating underlying depression, 7) addressing secondary gain issues, 8) improving family and community support systems, 9) providing access to vocational and occupational rehabilitation, 10) returning the patient to a functional and productive life-style, 11) decreasing the cost of medical care associated with chronic pain disorders, and 12) stopping patients from doctor-shopping in search of symptomatic relief.

Given the complex treatment goals of such programs, it is not too surprising that reports of treatment efficacy vary. The literature generally suggests that multidisciplinary programs result in improvements in a substantial proportion of patients at the end of treatment on at least some of these criteria, most notably improvement in physical functioning and activity, reduction of medication dependence, and subjective report of decreased pain (Cairns, Mooney, & Crane, 1984; Chapman, Brena, & Bradford, 1981; Guck, Skultety, Meilman, & Dowd, 1985; IOM, 1987; Keefe, Block, Williams, & Surwit, 1981; Keefe, 1982; Keefe, Gil, & Rose, 1986; Linton, 1982; Malec, Cayner, Harvey, & Timming, 1981; McArthur et al., 1987; Roberts & Reinhardt, 1980; Swanson, Floreen, & Swenson, 1976; Swanson, Swenson, Maruta, & McPhee, 1976).

It is difficult to draw more specific conclusions about treatment efficacy because of the lack of consistency in outcome criteria and measures used across studies, the lack of comparable nontreated control groups, lack of objective pre-post measures for comparison purposes, lack of long-term follow-up after treatment, differences in patient populations and selection criteria between programs with inadequate description of these factors, and difficulty comparing results based on patient self-report versus those based on more objective criteria (Aronoff, Evans, & Enders, 1983; Goldberg, 1982; Holzman et al., 1985; Keefe, Gil, & Rose, 1986; Linton, 1982; Turner & Chapman, 1982b; Turner & Romano, 1984a).

Just as important, multidisciplinary programs vary widely in the combination and method of application of different treatment components, making it difficult to compare program outcomes or identify the active components of treatment packages. Some apply the same package to all clients, whereas others tailor their programs to perceived needs of the particular individual. It is unclear whether treatment goals differ for individuals and, if so, how this is reflected in outcome statistics. Turk and Flor (1984) comment that it still "needs to be determined which patients profit from what treatment" (p. 225). Assessment approaches are vitally important in that effort.

Summary: The Need for Assessment

Current concepts of etiologic and maintaining factors in chronic pain have moved far beyond a model of pain as a sensory signal of tissue injury. Even a brief review of representative theories reveals the enormous complexity of chronic pain: it must be approached as a psychosocial as well as physiological phenomenon. The chronic pain patient can only be understood when the interaction of affective, cognitive, life history, learning and conditioning, social modeling, physiological, psychiatric, and systems influences, among others, is taken into account. Current pain treatment programs tend to take a pragmatic, eclectic view of the problem and attempt to attack as many facets and contributors to the chronic pain syndrome as possible.

Adequate assessment of chronic pain patients can help to address many of the problems inherent in the complex multidimensional models of chronic pain etiology and approaches to treatment described above. Two major goals of assessment strategies should be:

(1) To describe the characteristics of the typical pain patient, the average pain-patient personality. Such descriptions have relevance for discovering etiologic and maintaining factors in chronic pain states in general, for guiding clinicians in developing general treatment programs that address all these components of the chronic pain syndrome, and potentially for predicting the development of pain problems premorbidly from the match of a pain patient to this average description.

(2) To describe the differences among pain patients. Multidisciplinary treatment approaches require an enormous financial investment and the involvement of many professionals from diverse backgrounds. Adequate assessment of the constellation of factors contributing to a particular client's pain problem could potentially cut these costs by accurately predicting who might benefit from such a program, allowing selection of those patients most likely to show gains. Even more helpful, however, would be the ability to identify groups of patients with certain factors in common who will respond best to certain treatment components. Research on chronic pain patients has generally conformed to the same "uniformity myth" (Kiesler,

1966) that pervades psychotherapy outcome research in general. In searching for the overall characteristics of pain patients and the overall effects of various treatments, most researchers have overlooked the possibility of patient-by-treatment interactions (Bergin, 1971; Beutler, 1979). If subgroups of patients who have certain etiologic or maintaining factors in common could be identified, it is possible that matching them to an appropriate treatment could simultaneously cut costs and improve outcome statistics.

Both of these assessment goals have been most consistently addressed using the Minnesota Multiphasic Personality Inventory (MMPI). At this point other assessment instruments and approaches have not received enough attention in the literature to provide comparably extensive data. As will be shown in Chapter 2, however, there is still a need for research addressing clinical and demographic correlates of subgroups of patients obtaining different patterns on the MMPI. Description of profiles of pain patients is particularly important now that the test has been revised (see Chapter 3).

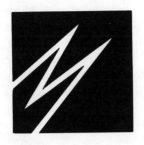

Chapter 2

The MMPI and Chronic Pain

Total Group Approaches: Describing the Chronic Pain Personality

The majority of researchers have treated chronic pain patients as a homogeneous group whose shared personality characteristics await discovery, description, and eventual modification. Many studies have tried to characterize the typical chronic pain patient. Such investigations provide important data needed to hypothesize and test theories of chronic pain etiology and maintenance such as those described earlier.

The available descriptive literature suggests that the mean chronic pain patient tends to be a high-school-educated Caucasian Protestant from a lower socioeconomic background; a blue-collar worker engaged in physically demanding, monotonous work. He or she is from 25 to 55 years old, was injured on the job, and has compensation available. If married, his or her marriage is likely to be marked by communication difficulties and unacknowledged conflict, and it is fairly likely that the spouse is having somatic problems as well. The patient is likely to be overweight and a smoker. He or she probably grew up in a large family with an atmosphere of conflict, possibly erupting in physical abuse but rarely acknowledged or discussed, and one or more family members probably suffered from depression or alcoholism. Family members may have served as models of physical or psychiatric disability, and the patient probably had bouts with illness and disability before the current problem, possibly including alcohol abuse (Andersson, 1981; Beals & Hickman, 1972; Craig, 1983; Edwards et al., 1985; Feuerstein, Papciak, & Hoon, 1987; Feuerstein, Sult, & Houle, 1985; Fishbain, Goldberg, Meagher, Steele, & Rosomoff, 1986; France, Krishnan, & Trainor, 1986; Gentry, Shows, & Thomas, 1974; Katon, Egan, & Miller, 1985; Klein, Jensen, & Sanderson, 1984; McArthur et al., 1987; Murray, 1982; Steinberg, 1982).

Psychologically, pain patients have been described as hypochondriacal (preoccupied with somatic symptoms and disease phobias, anxious and irritable, withdrawing from life problems), having hysterical personality styles (marked denial of psychological problems, inhibition of aggression, attention-seeking, dependent, suggestible, with somatic symptoms serving to resolve emotional conflict and express needs), and alexithymic (concrete, no language for feelings or abstract concepts; interpersonal and emotional expression is in "body language"). They may have assumed adult caretaking and work roles early in life, resulting in unmet dependency needs. They are often described as suffering from either obvious or masked depression, manipulative of social systems to meet their needs, and tending to see themselves as helpless and without resources or skills to take control of their lives (Aronoff & Rutrick, 1985; Blumer & Heilbronn, 1981, 1982; Catchlove et al., 1985; Crown, 1980; Engel, 1959; Evans, 1985; Feuerstein et al., 1987; Gentry et al., 1974; Murray, 1982; Sternbach, 1974a; Van Houdenhove, 1986).

Although a variety of measures and observational methods have been used in arriving at these descriptions, the most widely cited objective assessment device used with chronic pain patients is the Minnesota Multiphasic Personality Inventory (MMPI). This is a 566-item true-false self-report questionnaire. Items are grouped into scales which were originally developed in the 1940s to discriminate empirically between groups of patients with various psychiatric diagnoses and a group of "normal" adults. Raw scores on the scales are transformed into standardized "T scores," designed to have a mean of 50 and a standard deviation of 10 in the original normative sample. These scores are then plotted on a test profile. While diagnostic systems have changed and interpretive strategies are now based more on profile patterns of scores ("codetypes") and item content than on single scale scores, four validity scales and ten clinical scales have remained the standard set of MMPI scores reported across studies in a wide variety of patient populations (Dahlstrom, Welsh, & Dahlstrom, 1972, 1975; Graham, 1987; Keller, Butcher, & Slutske, 1990). These scales are briefly described in Table 2-1.

Mean MMPI Profile Configurations

Many of the personality characteristics listed above are based on correlates of MMPI mean profiles: the pattern of scale scores found when the MMPIs of a group of patients are averaged together. Studies presenting mean profiles of pain patients show great consistency in reporting one of two similar configural patterns. The first common profile is a "conversion V": highest elevations (T scores usually > 70) on scales Hs and Hy, with a relative absence of elevation on D (Adams, Heilbronn, Silk, Reider, & Blumer, 1981; Franz, Paul, Bautz, Choroba, & Hildebrandt, 1986; Gentry et al., 1974; Love & Peck, 1987; McGrath & O'Malley, 1986; Murray, 1982; Snyder, in press; Southwick & White, 1983). This configuration is interpreted as "denying any emotional problems; . . . a tendency to manifest marked somatic concern (complaints), to use denial and repression as major psychological defense mechanisms, to interpret problems in living in rational and socially acceptable terms, as well as a poor prognosis for remotivation and a contrasting appearance of being externally extroverted and sociable and internally self-centered, demanding, and dependent" (Gentry et al., 1974, p. 175).

The other common mean profile is characterized by elevations on Hs, Hy, and D: the "neurotic triad" (Adams et al., 1981; Beals & Hickman, 1972; Fordyce, Brena, Holcomb, DeLateur, & Loeser, 1978; Lair & Trapp, 1962; Murray, 1982; Snyder, in press; Sternbach, Wolf, Murphy, & Ake-

TABLE 2-1. Standard MMPI Scales

Validity Scales	Representative Descriptions of High Scores
?	Number of unanswered/doubly answered items.
L	Tendency to present overly favorable, virtuous self-image.
F	Tendency to endorse rare, unusual items reflecting disturbance, confusion, disorganization, or faking.
K	Subtle defensiveness, unwillingness to disclose personal information, positive self-image.
Clinical Scales	
1 (Hs)	"Hypochondriasis." Tendency to claim many vague somatic problems, unhappy, complaining, demanding, hostile.
2 (D)	"Depression." Pessimism, despondency, guilt, low self-esteem, and vegetative symptoms.
3 (Hy)	"Hysteria." Use of repression and denial to manage conflict. Experience stress somatically. Suggestible, outgoing, manipulative, uninsightful.
4 (Pd)	"Psychopathic Deviate." Impulsiveness, hostility, disregard for rules and authority, extraverted, manipulative, exhibitionistic, poor insight or empathy.
5 (Mf)	"Masculinity-femininity." Sex role attitudes and behavior. Range of interests, degree of passivity.
6 (Pa)	"Paranoia." Suspiciousness, guardedness, tendency to externalize blame, hostility, resentment.
7 (Pt)	"Psychasthenia." Anxiety, phobic preoccupations, tendency to intellectualize, obsessiveness, compulsiveness.
8 (Sc)	"Schizophrenia." Unconventionality, unusual ideas and experiences, social alienation, confusion, psychosis.
9 (Ma)	"Hypomania." Energy level, sociability, impulsiveness, optimism, impatience, grandiosity, irritability.
0 (Si)	"Social Introversion." Overcontrol, shyness, tension, guilt, withdrawal, social inadequacy.

Note: Consult MMPI sources for more thorough descriptions of scales and their empirical correlates; e.g., Dahlstrom, Welsh, & Dahlstrom, 1972; Duckworth & Anderson, 1986; Graham, 1987.

son, 1973). This profile is interpreted more in line with hypochondriasis and depression than with conversion hysteria, emphasizing passive-dependency, low self-esteem, anxiety, avoidance of performance demands, and masked hostility (Beals & Hickman, 1972; Snibbe, Peterson, & Sosner, 1980). The distinction between these two profiles is fuzzy at best (Cohen, 1987). The salient difference is purported to be the level of depression, with some researchers describing pain patients as quite depressed and hypochondriacal and others describing a relatively complacent, hysteroid denial of distress. However, definitions of the relative elevations of Hs, D, and Hy overlap a great deal, so that different authors may label the same profile configuration a conversion V in one case and a neurotic triad in the other.

Overall, the literature is remarkably consistent in finding that total-group average profiles of chronic pain patients have primary elevations on some pattern of the neurotic-triad scores. The "characteristic repression and denial and clinical depression which are implied in the neurotic triad" (Adams et al., 1981, p. 865) show up not only in chronic back pain samples, but also in chronic headache, arthritis, and pelvic pain groups (Dieter & Swerdlow, 1988; Domino & Haber, 1987; Ellertson & Klove, 1987; Kudrow & Sutkus, 1979; Rosenthal, Ling, Rosenthal, & McNeeley, 1984; Sternbach, Dalessio, Kunzel, & Bowman, 1980; Snyder, in press). Most studies do not report validity scale patterns or secondary scale elevations, but there is some evidence that relatively common peaks occur on K, Pd, Sc, and Pt (Cohen, 1987; Gentry et al., 1974; Heaton, Getto, Lehman, Fordyce, Brauer, & Groban, 1982; Jamison, Ferrer-Brechner, Brechner, & McCreary, 1976; McArthur et al., 1987; Swanson et al., 1976). These secondary elevations are quite consistent with pain patient personality descriptions reported in the literature, namely defensiveness and denial of psychological distress, proneness to manipulate others or obtain secondary gain through physical symptoms, and anxiety/muscle tension as associated symptoms. Some researchers have found that Sc elevations among pain patients tend to result from endorsement of unusual physical sensations rather than endorsement of items reflecting thought disturbance or social alienation (Moore, McFall, Kivlahan, & Capestany, 1988).

Problems with Total-Group Descriptions

While the consistency of characteristic MMPI patterns across many studies of pain patients is impressive, there is little evidence to suggest they are differentially representative of the chronic pain personality as opposed to other medical conditions. The conversion-V and neurotic-triad profiles are extremely common in medical populations in general, and particularly in populations of patients with chronic illnesses (Henrichs, 1981; Schwartz & Krupp, 1971; Swenson, Pearson, & Osborne, 1973). Although the mean chronic pain profile is generally more elevated on these neurotic scales than mean profiles of other medical conditions, several researchers suggest this is a function of degree of disability and life disruption rather than representing a distinct personality pattern characteristic of pain patients (Frymoyer, Rosen, Clements, & Pope, 1985; Naliboff, Cohen, & Yellen, 1982). Degree of elevation tends to rise with duration of pain, number of prior surgeries, and length of unemployment, and tends to decrease after successful treatment (Adams et al., 1981; Beals & Hickman, 1972; Gatchel, Mayer, Capra, Diamond, & Barnett, 1986; Sternbach et al., 1973).

Butcher and Tellegen (1978) cautioned that interpretation of MMPI mean profiles is complicated by the content heterogeneity of the standard

MMPI scales. They suggested analyzing individual item content and content homogeneous scales or subscales to provide a more accurate interpretation of the overall profile. Virtually no studies have examined pain patient performance on content scales other than the Harris-Lingoes subscales, which are subsets of items on each of the standard clinical scales (Harris & Lingoes, 1955). These studies, together with factor analyses and single-item examination of pain patient item responses, do not give a simple picture of the average chronic pain patient. While all studies find high endorsement of items directly reflecting somatic distress and pain-related disability, their findings differ on the more psychological components of the composite pain patient profile. Watson (1982) concluded that pain patients are hypochondriacal and depressed, but that item analysis shows little evidence of hysteroid denial, repression, and defensiveness. In contrast, Franz et al. (1986) reported that the average pain patient described himself as even more socially competent and self-confident than did normal controls, denied anger and aggressiveness, and did *not* possess hypochondriacal tendencies. Other researchers have shown that similar elevation levels on scales such as Hs and Sc may in fact reflect quite different combinations of item content, suggesting that scores on these scales may mean different things for different patients (McGrath & O'Malley, 1986; Moore et al., 1988; Prokop, 1986).

Inconsistent results such as these reflect the heterogeneity of chronic pain patients. The greatest problem with research addressing the chronic pain personality is that mean profiles and group averages obscure individual differences and possible pain patient subgroups. Few studies report the variability surrounding the mean MMPI profile, giving the erroneous impression that the profile is characteristic of all patients in the sample. Several studies have found that demographic, pain, and treatment history average descriptions differ markedly among treatment settings (Deyo, Bass, Walsh, Schoenfeld, & Ramamurthy, 1988; Holzman, Rudy, Gerber, Turk, Sanders, Zimmerman, & Kerns, 1985). Fordyce (1976) warns of the "illusion of homogeneity" in both patients and treatments: researchers and clinicians too often assume that labeling a person as a "chronic pain patient" or a treatment as "cognitive" means that the patient and treatment conform to the typical characteristics of each.

Correlates and patient descriptions based on group averages cannot be assumed to apply to all or even a majority of patients in the sample. It is possible to produce a conversion-V mean profile in a sample of patients even though that particular codetype is not the most frequent pattern in the sample (Naliboff, Cohen, & Yellen, 1983). This certainly could affect the overall efficacy of treatments or accuracy of theoretical formulations based on characteristics of the typical pain patient. As a result, the MMPI literature on chronic pain reflects a growing tendency to look beyond group averages and concentrate on pattern analysis and subgrouping of pain patient profiles.

Subgrouping Approaches

Prediction of Treatment Outcome

One purpose of treatment outcome research is to identify subgroups of patients that differ in response to treatment. However, most studies have concentrated on developing predictors from total sample characteristics. The accuracy of these predictors is necessarily affected by the heterogeneity of the sample. It is difficult to draw general conclusions about outcome prediction because of the variety of treatment methods and outcome criteria used, lack of adequate control groups, lack of long-term follow-up, as well as the heterogeneity of patient populations studied. Numerous researchers have criticized the current pain patient treatment outcome literature for these deficiencies (Aronoff, Evans, & Enders, 1983; Kleinke & Spangler, 1988; Linton, 1982; Turner & Chapman, 1982a, b; Turner & Romano, 1984a).

The majority of outcome studies attempt to predict which patients presenting for traditional medical treatment will show sustained benefit from invasive procedures such as surgery, chemonucleolysis, or epidural stimulation. Psychological tests such as the MMPI are typically added to the standard medical evaluation in the hope that personality dispositions will be relevant to the individual's rehabilitation prospects. Many such studies have shown that greater elevations on scales Hs and Hy are related to poorer outcome (Blumetti & Modesti, 1976; Chapman & Brena, 1982; Herron, Turner, & Weiner, 1986; Oostdam, Duivenvoorden, & Pondaag, 1981; Turner, Herron, & Weiner, 1986; Wiltse & Rocchio, 1975), which has been interpreted as evidence of rigid defenses and use of somatization to avoid psychological and life problems (Blumetti & Modesti, 1976). Other researchers have not found that elevated Hs and Hy predict medical treatment failure (Brandwin & Kewman, 1982; Hagedorn, Maruta, Swanson, & Colligan, 1982; Hubbard, 1983; Waring, Weisz, & Bailey, 1976; Watkins, O'Brien, Draugelis, & Jones, 1986). Some have found D alone (Brandwin & Kewman, 1982) or in combination with elevations on Hs and Hy (Wilfling, Klonoff, & Kokan, 1973) to be better predictors of failure. Overall, however, the literature tends to support the view that high elevations on the neurotic-triad scales, particularly on Hs, are associated with poor response to invasive treatments (Love & Peck, 1987; Snyder, in press). The implication is that multiple factors contribute to the client's problem syndrome and a single-mode treatment such as surgery is not enough to cure these other life difficulties.

The usefulness of these associations for classification and prediction at the individual level is questionable, however. There is often a large overlap between successful and failed groups when sorted by elevated Hs and Hy scores, and the elevation and pattern of neurotic-triad scores tend to change with chronicity of the problem rather than being stable premorbid predictors of vulnerability to chronic pain (Beals & Hickman, 1972; Fordyce, 1979; Garron & Leavitt, 1983a; Swanson, Maruta, & Wolff, 1986). Thus, the assumption that a chronic pain personality can be identified premorbidly is probably not valid. The MMPI can better indicate the degree of functional impairment already present, and it is likely to be this impairment that predicts poor outcome from a single-modality treatment such as surgery.

Indeed, studies predicting outcome of more complicated multidimensional pain treatment programs have not uniformly found a strong connection between neurotic-triad scores and treatment success. Almost everyone entering such programs has high elevations on these scales; therefore, prediction within such populations may need to rely on alternative MMPI interpretive strategies (Love & Peck, 1987; Rylee & Wu, 1984). Although some studies have found that degree of somatic preoccupation and denial of other life problems (conversion-V profile) tend to be predictive of poor outcome in general chronic pain populations (McCreary, Turner, & Dawson, 1980; Strassberg et al., 1981), again there is considerable overlap between successful and unsuccessful patient groups, with many studies finding no differences or even positive effects of certain scale elevations such as D or Hy (Beals & Hickman, 1972; Jamison et al., 1976; Kleinke & Spangler, 1988; Roberts & Reinhardt, 1980; Rylee & Wu, 1984; Trief & Yuan, 1983). Brennan et al. (1986-87) suggest "the predictive value of these psychological tests stems less from their reflection of a psychological state or attitude with respect to pain, and more from their tendency to reflect ongoing level of pain, disability, and other pain sequelae" (p. 373).

A major flaw in any attempt to lump outcome studies together is that treatment methods and outcome measures vary considerably, as do patient characteristics. Several studies have suggested that different predictors may be more accurate in predicting certain aspects of outcome than others, and that the performance of predictors may vary with characteristics of the patient population as well as the treatment applied to the patients (e.g., Strassberg et al., 1981; Trief & Yuan, 1983). Love and Peck (1987) conclude from their review that outcome prediction within multimodal pain clinics must go beyond looking for elevated neurotic-triad profiles, which are very common in this population and are not necessarily predictive of outcome. Instead, they suggest taking other scale elevations into account, such as elevated Pa and Sc scores which could indicate long-standing psychological difficulties. "Subgroup analysis may therefore have implications for multimodal treatment programs . . . and further work in this area is strongly recommended" (p. 8).

Other Attempts at Patient Classification

Despite the complexity of factors entering into chronic pain problems, there have been relatively few attempts to define subgrouping dimensions that could improve description of pain syndromes and improve treatment planning and outcome prediction. Most classification attempts have been based on single dimensions, a few of which will be reviewed below.

Demographic variables. Relatively little work has been published that subgroups patients by demographic variables. Sternbach et al. (1973) provided evidence that composite measures, such as average MMPI profiles, can obscure the heterogeneity in pain populations. They noted differences in the mean profiles for male and female subsamples: men were reported to appear more depressed, angry, and passive for their sex than women, whose profiles were closer to the norm. In contrast, Strassberg et al. (1981) found that female chronic pain patients scored higher on the MMPI than do male pain patients. Despite these suggestions that the experience and correlates of chronic pain might be different for men and women, most studies have utilized all-male populations or combine males and females in their statistics, so no conclusions can be made at this time. Conclusions for such variables as age and education are similarly limited (Guck et al., 1986; Murray, 1982), although increasing chronicity and unemployment are generally associated with more evidence of psychopathology on the MMPI and less likelihood of successful outcome.

Functional vs. organic pain. The major dichotomy into which numerous researchers have tried to classify patients is "functional" vs. "organic" pain. The former implies that the pain problem is caused or maintained by psychosocial factors, whereas the latter assumes a physiologic basis. This distinction is difficult to justify even on a purely medical basis: the gate control theory now demonstrates how extraordinarily complex the neurophysiologic bases of pain experiences may be, making it virtually impossible to rule out some organic contribution to any particular individual's pain problem. Conceptualization of chronic pain problems has moved away from this arbitrary distinction to more emphasis on assessing the degree of "functional overlay" or "excess disability" (Fordyce, 1976) involved in a patient's pain problem.

Assessment approaches have mirrored this changing view of pain problems, although the attempt to classify patients into functional or organic groups dies hard. Hanvik (1949, 1951) first described a method of discriminating functional and organic pain patients on the basis of MMPI profiles. He found that patients classified as functional tended to score higher on scales Hs, Hy, Pt, Sc, and Pd, with the overall profile characterized by a conversion-V pattern of hypochondriasis and hysteria with relatively little depression. Several other researchers have reported that functional patients are characterized by elevated profiles, evidence of greater psychopathology, and a conversion-V or neurotic-triad pattern (e.g., Freeman, Calsyn, & Louks, 1976; Gilberstadt & Jancis, 1967; Lair & Trapp, 1962; McCreary, Turner, & Dawson, 1977). However, these researchers and others have cautioned that conversion-V profiles occur in the organic population as well, and the degree of overlap between groups makes it impossible to use such profiles for individual diagnosis (Adams et al., 1981; Osborne, 1985; Rook, Pesch, & Keeler, 1981). Other researchers, in contrast to Hanvik, have failed to find differences between organic and functional groups even when using mean profiles (Cox, Chapman, & Black, 1978; Hendler et al., 1988; Leavitt, 1985; Schwartz & Krupp, 1971; Sternbach et al., 1973; Stone & Pepitone-Arreola-Rockwell, 1983).

Attempts to develop MMPI scales that discriminate between organic and functional groups have fared poorly as well. Neither the Low Back Scale (Lb) (Hanvik, 1949) nor the Dorsal Scale (DOR) (Pichot, Perse, LeBeaux, Dureau, Perez, & Rychawaert, 1972) has demonstrated any consistent ability to distinguish organically maintained pain from purely psychological pain or to distinguish low back patients from psychiatric or psychosomatic, nonpain patients (Calsyn, Louks, & Freeman, 1976; Elkins & Barrett, 1984; Freeman, Calsyn, & Louks, 1976; Haven & Cole, 1972; Rosen, Frymoyer, & Clements, 1980; Sternbach et al., 1973; Towne & Tsushima, 1978; Tsushima & Towne, 1979). In general, classification of patients into organic and functional categories has not proven particularly replicable or useful in treatment planning. A review by Snyder (in press) concludes "findings from these studies suggest that high scores on the MMPI, and particularly on those scales comprising the neurotic triad, confirm a significant psychological component to the patient's pain complaints and functional limitations, but do not rule out underlying physical pathology." More complex classification schemes based on characteristics occurring across these groups, such as particular patterns of psychological disturbance or maintaining factors, may prove more useful (Elkins & Barrett, 1984; Rosen et al., 1980; Trief, Elliott, Stein, & Frederickson, 1987).

Medication usage. A few studies have classified patients by medication usage and examined the associated characteristics of these groups. Turner, Calsyn, Fordyce, & Ready (1982) assigned 131 multidisciplinary pain clinic patients to groups according to their drug use: 30% used no addictive medications, 33% used narcotics but not sedatives, and 37% used both narcotics and sedatives. Patients in the latter two groups had histories of more hospitalizations and surgeries than the nondrug group, and the narcotic/sedative users reported more impairment and had higher Hs and Hy scores than the other groups. McCreary and Colman (1984) reported similar results when they grouped patients by no drug use, aspirin-type use, narcotics alone, or narcotics combined with other medications. The last group was the only group to show the "typical pain patient" pattern of high bodily concern and denial of psychological difficulties, characterized by higher Hs and Hy scores and more intense, affectively toned pain reports. The no-drug-use group reported the least activity limitation, even though they reported as much pain as the aspirin or narcotic group. The narcotic users were characterized as more personality disordered, with low frustration tolerance: their primary MMPI elevation was on Pd.

Although cause and effect cannot be determined from these studies, the authors present some speculations on different personality patterns and pain maintenance factors operating in these groups. Turner et al. speculated that the combined narcotic/sedative users might be the group with the largest psychosocial component to their pain problem, in that the dependent sick-role lifestyle helps them avoid demands and responsibilities associated with being well. McCreary and Colman agreed that the combined drug user group contained the most disturbed individuals, but noted this might be a result of their drug use. They described the narcotics alone group as more sociopathic, using pain symptoms in a manipulative fashion primarily as a means to obtain drugs. Clearly, classifying patients into these categories could have implications for treatment choice and differential outcome prediction, although these studies did not address either issue. Unfortunately, the generalizability of these drug-use-related MMPI patterns is questionable, since other researchers have failed to find the same distinctions between drug abuse and nonabuse groups (Maruta, Swanson, & Finlayson, 1979; McNairy, Maruta, Ivnik, Swanson, & Ilstrup, 1984). Henrichs (1987) suggests the MacAndrew Addiction scale might be a useful addition to classification strategies based on configural patterns of MMPI scores.

Depression. Depression is another variable that has been suggested as a basis for classifying patients. Dworkin, Richlin, Handlin, and Brand (1986) found that treatment response in depressed vs. non-depressed chronic pain patients was predicted by different patterns of variables. For non-depressed patients, predictors of success included number of treatment visits, lack of financial compensation, fewer previous types of treatments, and locus of pain in the back. Depressed patients, on the other hand, were more likely to improve if they had ongoing employment and a shorter duration of pain. The authors interpreted this as indicating the greater need for activity and personal involvement in treatment for patients who are depressed, making this an important classification variable to be used in treatment choice.

Krishnan, France, Pelton, McCann, Davidson, and Urban (1985) also suggested that depression status could have important implications for differential treatment. They noted that symptoms of anxiety were more common in patients with depression, particularly those diagnosed as major depressive. They suggested that treatments such as biofeedback, relaxation training, and antidepressant medications would be particularly useful with this subclass of patients to reduce their anxious over-reactivity to pain and the resulting disability. As noted earlier, many researchers suggest that antidepressant medications and activity can simultaneously improve mood and lower pain perception for a subgroup of depressed pain patients.

MMPI research on the role of depression in chronic pain has been inconclusive, largely owing to definitional problems. While investigators seem to agree that interpretation of D should be modified by elevations on at least the Hs and Hy scales, there has been little consistency in defining their relative patterns (Snyder, in press). In fact, studies frequently label a profile as conversion V, which is typically interpreted as a non-depressive pattern, even when the D scale is equal to or higher than Hs and Hy (Cohen, 1987).

Compensation status. Classification of patients based on evidence of secondary gain is exemplified by studies of compensation status. This literature is generally as inconclusive as the other single-dimension classification schemes. Elevated pain reports and elevated Hs, D, Hy, and Pd scales on the MMPI have been associated with ongoing compensation or litigation (Beals & Hickman, 1972; Pollack & Grainey, 1984; Shaffer, Nussbaum, & Little, 1972; Sternbach et al., 1973). This has been interpreted as reflecting positive reinforcement of pain behaviors, conscious malingering to manipulate the system for financial gain, the effects of litigation and compensation in focusing the patient's attention on somatic symptoms, and/or actual increased disability of this group in relation to employed groups unrelated to the compensation issue (Carron et al., 1985; Fordyce, 1976, 1984; Painter, Seres, & Newman, 1980). However, other investigators have found no differences between compensation claimants and nonclaimants on various measures including reports of pain severity, MMPI patterns, level of psychological disturbance, or treatment outcome (Chapman, Brena, & Bradford, 1981; Leavitt, Garron, McNeill, & Whisler, 1982; Mendelson, 1984; Trabin, Rader, & Cummings, 1987; Trief & Stein, 1985).

Just as with the other classification schemes discussed, grouping patients by compensation status alone is probably too simplistic to result in reliable, meaningful patient correlates and treatment predictions. Other moderating variables must be added to the picture. For example, Dworkin, Handlin, Richlin, Brand, and Vannucci (1985) examined the relationships between compensation, litigation, employment status, and treatment response in 454 chronic pain patients. They found that both compensation and lack of employment predicted poorer short-term outcome when univariate analyses were used. However, only employment predicted long-term outcome, and prediction of short-term outcome using multiple regression analysis resulted in compensation dropping out as a significant predictor. Thus, they suggested that activity and employment may be the most important determinants of the effects of compensation. Similarly, Patrick (1988) suggested that workers' compensation recipients should not be assumed to comprise a homogeneous group. She found that patients judged as "work-ready" by their compensation counsellors obtained a normal-limits MMPI profile on the average, despite the fact that most of this group had been receiving compensation benefits for more than six months. Kleinke and Spangler (1988) found that although patients receiving workers' compensation did more poorly than noncompensated patients on both admission and discharge treatment measures, there was no difference in the groups' amount of improvement during a multidisciplinary pain program. Trabin et al. (1987) found that compensated versus noncompensated pain patients did not differ on a variety of behavioral outcome measures in a multidisciplinary program even though the compensated patients continued to be more likely to complain of greater subjective pain. Thus, research suggests this subgrouping variable should not be used unilaterally to draw negative conclusions about a patient's level of motivation or likelihood of benefit from treatment.

In fact, across several studies the most consistent finding is that being employed at the beginning of treatment predicts better outcome. Overall, "despite the common belief that compensation and litigation are disincentives to the successful rehabilitation of chronic pain patients, the literature increasingly reveals that there is no direct effect" (IOM, 1987, p. 245). These studies illustrate the importance of using multivariate rather than univariate methods in discovering the most important predictive factors in chronic pain conditions.

The need for more complex strategies. Given the multiply determined nature of chronic pain problems, it seems unlikely that subgrouping patients along single dimensions will lead to more than minimal improvements in the accuracy with which treatment efficacy can be predicted. Like the artificial organic/functional dichotomy, such attempts "serve only to oversimplify the complex psychological processes involved in the pain experience" (Bradley, Van der Heide, Byrne, Troy, Prieto, & Marchisello, 1981, p. 95).

Multivariate methods such as discriminant analysis and regression can aid in combining many scores in an optimally predictive fashion and may provide leads to the most important dimensions within a complex set of predictors. However, these methods still assume homogeneity in the patient group studied and their treatment needs. Predictive equations based on weighted sums across scales have usually not generalized well to new populations and outcome criteria (Aronoff & Evans, 1982; Guck et al., 1987; Reich, Steward, Tupin, & Rosenblatt, 1985). One way to address this complexity would be to abandon the search for the chronic pain personality and instead look for subgroups of patients who are similar to each other in their pattern of scores across a number of measures tapping a number of areas. Just as one cannot predict job performance from interests without taking abilities into account, it seems reasonable to expect that prediction of pain-treatment outcome (in itself a complex phenomenon) would be improved by using profiles of scores that modify each other's meaning.

In actual practice, this is the approach implicitly or explicitly used by clinicians in arriving at treatment decisions. Several assessment devices as well as a clinical interview may be used, and the clinician weighs individual responses in light of the overall pattern of information. However, each clinician's scheme is likely to differ substantially from others, and for research purposes it is difficult to quantify and replicate these pattern-recognition approaches.

Multidimensional personality tests such as the MMPI do not, of course, summarize all the factors that might be relevant in subgrouping patients. However, personality measures do seem to be a good starting point, since theoretically many life-history and demographic factors gain predictive importance only through their effect on the individual's coping style, affective status, self-appraisal, and view of the environment (Harris, 1982). Thus, while use of the MMPI alone is probably too limited an approach, personality measures have been shown to have validity in predicting general patterns of behavior and may represent a way of measuring final common pathways, in terms of cognitive, affective, and behavioral dispositions, of a variety of life experiences. Research utilizing the MMPI can also offer an assessment model that may be expanded to include other types of measurement data in the future.

Configural Subgrouping of MMPI Profiles

Codetype grouping. Several researchers have attempted to define homogeneous patient subgroups by sorting MMPI profiles into similar types. The criterion of similarity has usually been the particular investigator's clinical judgment of relevant groups.

Sternbach (1974a, 1974b) described four profile types he commonly encountered in his clinical practice and his impressions of their correlates and outcome implications. Figure 2-1 illustrates the profiles for reference, since these four groups have been cited for comparison in numerous subsequent studies. He labeled the first profile type "Hypochondriasis," defined by a primary elevation on Hs and secondary elevations on Hy and D, forming a neurotic triad. These patients were described as very preoccupied with a variety of somatic symptoms, many of them unrelated to pain. He felt that this profile was most common in patients with a clear organic basis for their pain, and inability to ignore their continuing sensory input was a major reason for their likely treatment failure.

The second profile group was labeled "Reactive Depression," defined by an elevation on D. These patients were described as depressed in response to the effects of pain in their lives and as having good premorbid adjustment. They tended to respond well to antidepressant medication, and the profile was considered to predict successful outcome.

The third profile was the familiar conversion V, which he labeled "Somatization Reaction." Correlates included somatic preoccupation along with denial of psychological or interpersonal problems, with the implication that the somatic focus represents repression of psychological conflict. Sternbach felt this profile indicated potential for moderate treatment success because the patient had already made some adjustment to his or her condition.

The last profile was labeled "Manipulative Reaction," defined by an elevation on Pd in addition to the neurotic scales (Hs, D, Hy). These patients were described as con artists who used their symptoms to manipulate the staff, their families, and social systems for their own ends. Alcoholism, drug abuse, and litigious behavior were considered common correlates.

Unfortunately, Sternbach's classification rules and patient population are not clearly described, nor does he present any empirical support for the correlates he ascribes to these profile types. Other codetyping studies provide little assistance in validating his subgrouping scheme, because each tends to use its own unique classification rules also based on clinical experience.

Louks, Freeman, and Calsyn (1978) classified a sample of 74 VA back pain patients' MMPIs into six configural groups. Their first category, "Denial," was defined primarily by an elevation on K and accounted for only 4% of their patients. "Conversion V with Defensiveness," defined as $K < 60$ and (Hs$> = $D and Hy$> = $D) or (Hs$>D>Hy>70$) or (Hy$>D>Hs>70$), accounted for 27% of the patients. Twelve percent of the patients were classified as "Conversion V without Defensiveness," defined as both Hs and Hy$>$D, and $K> = 60$ but $<$ either Hy or Hs. The fourth group, "Depressed/Anxious," was defined as either D or

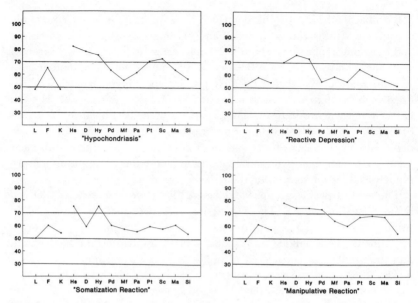

FIGURE 2-1. MMPI Profile Subgroups Described by Sternbach (1974a)

Pt> = 70 and the highest of the clinical scales; 14% of the sample fell into this category. The "Psychotic" category required that at least two of scales Pt, Pa, Sc, and Ma had to be elevated, and at least one of them had to be 5 points above the "nonpsychotic" scales. Thirteen percent of the sample fit this category. The remaining patients either were classified as "Normal" (13%) or were unclassified because their profiles did not fit a category or fit more than one (15%).

It is difficult to make any comparisons between Sternbach and Louks, Freeman, and Calsyn because there is little similarity in their classification schemes and the rationale for the typology used in the Louks study seems questionable at best (Bradley, Prieto, Hopson, & Prokop, 1978). Louks's definitions of "Conversion V" could include profiles other researchers would classify as hypochondriacal or even depressed; their definition of "Conversion V without defensiveness" could include profiles with very high K scores and conversely the "with defensiveness" profiles actually have low K scores; and the definition of a "normal" profile is unclear. Overall, since they also failed to present any data addressing differential correlates of these classifications, the Louks et al. study provides little information other than further evidence that a variety of personality profile patterns exist in a pain patient population.

McCreary, Turner, and Dawson (1979) grouped 76 chronic back pain patients into five codetypes which they felt had been indicative of psycho-pathology in previous studies of somatizing patients without chronic pain.

They predicted that patients classified into one of these profiles would have significantly poorer outcome from conservative medical treatment than patients not so classified. Their final sample consisted of 66 patients who returned outcome measures. Groupings used for prediction were based on the pattern of highest scales, regardless of elevation, although they included a frequency table breaking down codetypes into "severe" (T scores above 70) and "mild" (T scores greater than 55) categories. Their five "poor risk" profiles included:

(1) Primary elevations on Hs and D. Eight percent of their final sample fell into this codetype, with 5% qualifying as severe. The authors expected that this profile reflects "numerous physical complaints with relatively less demonstrable physical pathology, and they seem to have learned to use their complaints to help them deal with emotional conflicts" (p. 279).

(2) Primary elevations on Hs and Hy, which characterized 29% of their sample with 12% classified as severe. These clients were predicted to "show somatic preoccupation, but typically deny depression and emotional conflicts and strongly resist the implication that they may need psychiatric care" (p. 279).

(3) Primary elevations on D and Hy, predicted to characterize patients "with complaints of chronic tension along with feelings of inadequacy, and . . . repression of unacceptable feelings" (p. 279). Twelve percent of the sample had this codetype, with 6% classified severe.

(4) Primary elevations on Hs, D, and Hy, which was described as "similar to the above neurotic codetypes" (p. 279) and accounted for 24% of the sample, 17% severe.

(5) Combinations of Hs and/or Hy with Sc, thought to characterize patients who "often show unusual physical complaints associated with symptoms of severe psychopathology" (p. 279). Eight percent of the sample fell into this category, which required an elevation of Sc above 70 but did not specify necessary elevations for Hs and Hy.

Patients with one of these five profiles did have poorer outcomes than other patients, the authors concluding that subgrouping patients by codetype substantially improves prediction of outcome. However, the use of these particular codetypes as poor risk groups resulted in an unacceptably high false positive rate: 61% of patients with good outcomes were erroneously classified as poor risks. This may have resulted from the use of codetype rules that did not take elevation into account; the profiles of many of their patients would probably have been classified as within normal limits by other investigators. Their procedure might have been improved by using only elevated profiles and by adding a category for elevated Pd scores. Like the studies cited above, they failed to provide data validating their descriptions of differential correlates of their codetype groups. In fact, they effectively obscured any subgroup effects by lumping all identified pathological profiles into one poor-risk group.

Long (1981) gave the MMPI to 44 patients who were to receive surgery for low back pain, and grouped them six to eighteen months later as surgery successes (N = 22) or failures (N = 22) based on self-reported pain relief and resumption of normal activities. The success and failure groups did not differ on age or number of prior surgeries. The failure group reported less education than the successful group, consistent with previous research suggesting better educational background and job skills increase the probability of successful rehabilitation. Total group mean scale scores and profile patterns did not seem to offer much outcome-relevant information. The mean profile in both groups showed characteristic elevations of Hs and Hy, and the only single-scale difference was a greater mean elevation on Hs in the failure group.

In contrast, "configurational grouping of the MMPI profiles yielded eight subgroups that bore a striking relationship to surgical outcome" (Long, 1981, p. 747). Profiles were sorted according to clinical judgment; although Long states he used scales Hs, D, Hy, and Pd as the primary classification determinants to be consistent with previous research, the subjective nature of his sorting scheme makes it impossible to directly compare his study to others. His results are suggestive nevertheless. All patients who had normal-limits profiles (no elevations) before surgery fell into the successful group at outcome. The patients with an elevation only on Hy were also successes, as were those who had elevations on Hs, D, and Hy without the conversion-V pattern. In contrast, all the patients who had elevations on Hs and Hy without an elevation on D fell into the poor-outcome group. An elevation on Pd was also predictive of treatment failure. Five of the six patients with an elevation only on Hs were failures, as was one person with a "clearly abnormal profile" (undefined).

These results provide some support for Sternbach's prediction of differential outcome associated with his four profile types. Long's "Hs alone" category roughly corresponds to Sternbach's "Hypochondriasis" group, and, as predicted, these individuals did not show much benefit from treatment. As Sternbach predicted with his "Reactive Depression" group, an elevation on D greatly improved the likelihood of a successful outcome. Long's "conversion-V" group did not do as well as Sternbach suggested "somatization reactions" might. However, there was some evidence that elevations on Hy might be associated with more success than elevations on Hs alone, which would be consistent with Sternbach's description of these clients as having found some degree of adjustment to their pain problem. Long's data also support Sternbach's prediction that elevations on Pd either alone or in association with other scales predict poorer outcome.

Generalizations based on these comparisons must be made cautiously because both the sample populations and the treatment methods differ markedly (Sternbach's was a mixed pain-clinic sample of acute and chronic cases, varying on extent of known organic involvement, and Long's was a neurosurgery clinic sample who were all considered to have sufficient organic findings to warrant surgery). Neither study described the classification rules in detail, and neither broke down their samples by potentially important variables such as sex.

In contrast, Heaton, Getto, Lehman, Fordyce, Brauer, and Groban (1982) described their sample characteristics and objective profile classification rules in detail. Again, the configural rules were based on the senior author's personal judgment. Their sample, 169 consecutive admissions to a multidisciplinary pain clinic, was more typical of chronic pain patients than that of Long (1981): the majority (93.5%) were considered to have a static pain syndrome with no physical reason to expect further deterioration, and only half the sample were considered to have any objective evidence of an organic basis for pain. The sample was mixed in sex and in location of pain.

Heaton et al.'s total sample mean profile was typical of that found in many other studies, with primary elevations on Hs and Hy and a secondary elevation on D. However, they noted that "considering only population mean scores on the MMPI obscures individual profile differences that may predict important behavioral syndromes in chronic pain" (p. 167). MMPI profiles were sorted into seven categories, four described as corresponding to Sternbach's (1974a, 1974b) categorization. These seven categories, shown in Figure 2-2, were:

(1) Hypochondriasis (6% of sample), characterized by a primary elevation on Hs and corresponding to Sternbach's category of the same name.

(2) Reactive depression (17% of sample), characterized by peak elevation on D well above Hy and Hs, corresponding to Sternbach's similar category.

(3) Normal group (10% of sample) with no clinical elevations.

(4) Somatization reaction (18% of sample), the conversion-V pattern corresponding to Sternbach's category of the same name.

(5) Somatization reaction with depression (18% of sample), also known as the neurotic triad.

(6) Psychotic/borderline group (9% of sample), characterized by a generally elevated profile including prominent elevations on Pa, Pt, and Sc.

(7) Manipulative reaction group (5% of sample), characterized by a prominent elevation on Pd, as described in Sternbach's group of the same name. The neurotic-triad scales were also clinically elevated.

Heaton's categories make rational sense as a refinement and extension of the clinically relevant groups suggested by Sternbach, providing a breakdown that intuitively matches some of the factors reviewed earlier as potential contributors to chronic pain problems. However, the true clinical relevance of codetype categories is dependent on empirical support for their discriminative and predictive utility. Heaton does not provide a great deal

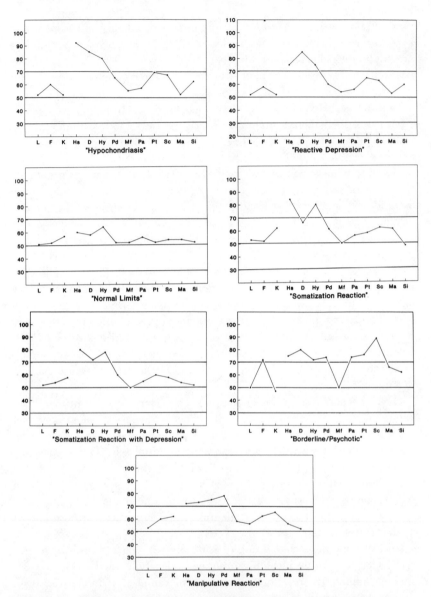

FIGURE 2-2. MMPI Profile Subgroups Described by Heaton et al. (1982)

of clarification of this issue, despite his more objectively defined classification scheme.

Naliboff, Cohen, and Yellen (1983) provided some data on extra-test correlates of MMPI profile types among a chronic low-back-pain population (N = 72). Profile sorting rules were primarily based on the first four MMPI clinical scales and were designed to match those of Sternbach (1974a) and standard MMPI interpretive manuals. Two profiles were broken down into elevated and nonelevated forms, similar to McCreary et al.'s (1979) presentation of mild and severe codetype forms. The six resulting profile types were:

(1) Unelevated depression (8% of sample): D greater than Hy and greater than Hs but less than a T score of 70.

(2) Unelevated somatization (12% of sample): Hs and Hy both at least 7 T score points greater than D, but both less than 70.

(3) Elevated depression (18% of sample): same as #1 but with D greater than or equal to a T score of 70.

(4) Elevated somatization (15% of sample): same as #2 but Hs and Hy both elevated at or above a T score of 70.

(5) Manipulative reaction (22% of sample): Scales Hy and Pd greater than a T score of 70.

(6) Hypochondriasis (16% of sample): Hs at least 7 T score points higher than D and Hy, and greater than or equal to a T score of 70.

As in most of the other configural studies, these rules did not take elevations on other clinical scales into account in modifying group membership. Naliboff et al. went back over the sample and counted the number of profiles containing primary elevations on the major psychotic scales, Pa or Sc. A surprisingly large number of patients, 18% of the sample, had one of these scales clinically elevated and higher than Hs and Hy. If, as might be expected, these patients present a different array of treatment needs than those without clinical elevations on the psychotic end of the MMPI profile, the configural sorting schemes based only on Hs, D, Hy, and Pd have serious shortcomings.

Naliboff et al. improved on other studies by examining age, sex, self-reported limitation owing to pain, and chronicity of illness in relation to MMPI codetype. The only difference between profile groups was that higher elevations were more likely to be associated with greater self-reported limitation. As the authors noted, the lack of differences "again demonstrates the heterogeneity of these populations even when divided according to age, gender, and chronicity of illness" (p. 846). It is interesting that the total group profile for this study was the familiar conversion-V configuration, even though this pattern was not the most frequent profile in the sample— further corroboration that this pattern "in fact is an artifact of averaging several clinically distinct profiles" (p. 846). Naliboff et al. did not expand on the clinical correlates of the distinct profiles beyond the data noted above and did not present outcome data.

A study that did provide empirical evidence of treatment-relevant correlates of MMPI profile types was reported by Atkinson, Ingram, Kremer, and Saccuzzo (1986). Fifty-two male consecutive admissions to an inpatient pain-treatment program were assigned psychiatric diagnoses on the basis of scores on the Hamilton Rating Scale for Depression (Hamilton, 1960), the Beck Depression Inventory (Beck, Ward, Mendelson, Mock, & Erbaugh, 1961), and structured diagnostic interviews. The investigators then looked at the relationship of psychiatric symptomatology to MMPI profile type. They limited their codetypes to three combinations of scales Hs, D, and Hy, identified as a hypochondriasis group (major elevation on Hs, secondary elevations on D and Hy), a depression group (major elevation on D, secondary on Hs and Hy), and a somatization group (the conversion-V pattern). Rules for classifying profiles were clearly described and resulted in classification of 83% of the sample (33% somatization, 27% depression, 23% hypochondriasis).

The three MMPI profile types differed significantly on presence or absence of psychiatric diagnosis. This was largely due to the concentration of psychiatric diagnoses, particularly major depression, in the depression profile category and the lack of psychiatric diagnoses in the somatization (conversion-V) pattern. The frequency of psychiatric diagnoses in the hypochondriasis category fell between these two. These differences were obtained in spite of the fact that, as usual, there was no difference between profile groups in evidence of organic involvement.

Although the data do not address whether psychiatric problems are a cause or a result of chronic pain problems, the authors speculate that the high D group might reflect affective disturbance in reaction to the stress and loss associated with chronic pain, while the depressed patients scoring in the hypochondriasis category might be those with personal and family histories of preexisting psychiatric problems who are expressing affective distress and justifying their maladjustment through somatic preoccupation. Longitudinal data would be needed to explore this hypothesis and the differential treatment implications of these two depression etiologies. However, their results do clearly indicate that MMPI profile subtypes may have treatment implications in terms of identifying patients for whom "treatments aimed at major depression, in addition to pain itself, should be included in interventions" (p. 412).

A recent study by Adams, Heilbronn, and Blumer (1987) confirmed the clinical salience of four principal profile types in a chronic pain population. They provided an expert MMPI interpreter with individual profiles of 72 chronic pain patients and asked him to blindly sort them into natural groupings that would have different interpretive significance. Without being told that these profiles came from pain patients, the interpreter classified the profiles into four major groups very similar to the groupings suggested by other research: normal limits (30% of sample), conversion V (34%), depressive reaction (14%), and general elevation—neurotic triad plus elevations on Sc and Pt—(22%). The authors stated this procedure provided greater support for the significance of these profiles than some other studies because their clinician was using the entire profile of scores, instead of just the neurotic triad, in making his decisions. A nice addition to this study was their provision of frequencies of all possible two-point code combinations in the sample. Although predictably they found that combinations of scales Hs, D, and Hy accounted for the majority of the profile high points, it is interesting to note that even in this small sample, 14 patients (19%) had two-point codes that did not include *any* of the neurotic-triad scales. The most common unique code had high points on Pa and Pt, occurring primarily among the generally elevated group Adams et al. called "mixed neurosis." Again, this study provides ample support for the heterogeneity of patients within pain samples.

Cluster analysis. Although the classification approaches cited above show promise in defining subgroups of patients with shared treatment-relevant characteristics, they were based on researchers' preconceived classification schemes with little empirical validation that these characteristics actually form reliable and meaningful patient groups. Many of the strategies used only the first four clinical scales of the MMPI, ignoring moderating effects of other scales in the profile. Recently, several investigators have employed cluster analysis to explore the complex relationships inherent in an entire profile of assessment data, with the hope of discovering empirically which patient characteristics are reliably associated with each other and can be used to discriminate treatment-relevant subgroups of patients.

Cluster analysis in its broadest definition is "the general logic, formulated as a procedure, by which we objectively group together entities on the basis of their similarities and differences" (Tryon & Bailey, 1970, p. 1). When the entities to be grouped are variables such as test scores measured across several individuals, the clustering procedure is known as factor analysis. Cluster analysis in its narrower definition is the opposite procedure: it is a method for grouping objects on the basis of the similarity of their patterns of scores across multiple variables. A common example would be the attempt in medicine to group patients by syndromes, different patterns of intercorrelated individual signs and symptoms (Green, 1978; Tryon & Bailey, 1970). Theoretically, cluster analysis differs from discriminant analysis (also a multivariate method for classifying subjects) because it is not necessary to know the group membership of a few individuals ahead of time, or even how many meaningful subgroups exist. It provides a method for identifying subgroups of patients whose patterns of scores are maximally similar to each other and maximally different from the patterns of subjects in other groups (Norusis, 1985).

There are several methods of performing a cluster analysis. Most studies of chronic pain patients have used a hierarchical clustering procedure; the program starts by treating each individual as a separate cluster and then progressively combines similar individuals into larger and larger clusters, ending with the total sample (Green, 1978; Norusis, 1985; SPSS, 1986;

Tryon & Bailey, 1970). Since cluster solutions may vary with the computer program used, similarity measure chosen, and the procedure used to determine the optimal number of clusters, it is important for researchers to describe their procedure and assumptions carefully (Blashfield, 1980). There is no single correct number of clusters existing in a data set; the researcher must determine the optimal combination of between group difference, within group similarity, and meaningfulness of profile patterns for his or her particular application.

Cluster analysis is certainly not a magical procedure providing totally objective, maximally predictive patient groups. As with factor analysis, the adage "garbage-in, garbage-out" applies: although cluster analysis may improve predictive power by exploiting the complicated relationships between variables, its usefulness will be limited by the relevance and comprehensiveness of the variables used to define subgroups. Clusters can be generated even from random data sets (Blashfield, 1980). Thus, it is vital to validate solutions both in terms of their replicability in other samples and their interpretability through correlations with other demographic, behavioral, and outcome data.

The studies reviewed below use MMPI scales as their variables, and thus can be criticized on the grounds that other important variables are excluded from the clustering algorithm. However, just as with the configural subgrouping studies, their methods can be justified as exploratory pilot approaches to a complicated problem, and multidimensional measures of current personality dispositions may potentially reflect the influence of many other life-history factors.

Several researchers using the MMPI have at least partially replicated each other's cluster solutions, and a few have begun to test correlates of the obtained groups. The majority of these studies have been the work of Bradley and colleagues (Bradley, 1983; Bradley, Prokop, Gentry, Van der Heide, & Prieto, 1981; Bradley, Prokop, Margolis, & Gentry, 1978; Bradley & Van der Heide, 1984; Prokop, Bradley, Margolis, & Gentry, 1980; Bradley, Van der Heide, Byrne, Troy, Prieto, & Marchisello, 1981). In 1978 Bradley et al. reported applying hierarchical cluster analysis to the MMPI profiles of three independent samples of chronic low-back-pain patients, performing analyses separately for males and females because of previous suggestions of sex differences on mean MMPI profiles (e.g., Sternbach et al., 1973). The authors stated that establishing replicability of clusters was of fundamental importance "since it would be essential to use replicable profile groups in future studies of treatment outcome as a function of specific therapeutic operations and homogeneous LBP patient groups" (p. 255).

Over a three-year period, the researchers obtained MMPIs from 233 male and 315 female low-back-pain patients admitted for evaluation to a university medical center "because of a lack of response to traditional medical-surgical treatments and/or a questionable physiological basis for their pain" (p. 255). The male and female samples were each divided into three cohorts, consisting of all patients evaluated in any particular year. A cluster analysis was performed separately for each cohort using the three validity scales and ten clinical scales of the MMPI. The researchers decided to examine only those solutions consisting of five or fewer subgroups, because of the suggestion by Sternbach that chronic pain patients could be characterized by four principal profiles. Cluster solutions for the cohorts were then compared to determine the division that best replicated across the subsamples.

Four general profile types were found to replicate across the female samples. The first subgroup (23% of sample) was characterized by elevations on the neurotic-triad scales. The second group (39% of sample) was a normal-limits profile with relative high points on scales K, Hs, and Hy. The third group (13% of sample) might be described as a "general-elevation" group, with Hs, D, Hy, Pt, and Sc all clinically elevated. The final group (24% of sample) was characterized by the conversion-V pattern. Thus, groups 1, 2, and 4 differed primarily in the elevation and relative pattern of the neurotic-triad scales, while group 3 had a markedly different profile including more indicators of affective distress, anxiety and obsessionality, and paranoid or psychotic thinking.

A similar procedure applied to the male cohorts resulted in three replicated groups. The first two groups were very similar to the women's samples: a neurotic-triad profile (44% of sample) and a normal-limits profile with relative elevations on K, Hs, and Hy (46% of sample). The third cluster was characterized by elevations on F, Hs, D, Hy, and Sc (10% of sample). Interestingly, there was no male cluster comparable to the female conversion-V group. However, the same pattern was maintained of one set of groups differing primarily on relative elevations on the neurotic triad, versus another group marked by more severe neurotic and even psychotic symptoms and depression. Figures 2-3 and 2-4 illustrate the mean MMPI profiles derived for the four female clusters and the three male clusters; these have been the basis of comparison in all subsequent clustering studies.

There were no systematic differences in age or educational level among subgroups for either the male or female sample. The authors did not provide other data on correlates of the subgroups, but speculated about the characteristics of the three groups found to be common to the male and female populations. They compared the elevated neurotic-triad group to Sternbach's (1974a) "hypochondriasis" group, noting that it might be indicative of a somatogenic component to pain and of respondent rather than operant pain problems. Such patients might be expected to be poor treatment risks because of difficulty shifting their focus away from their multiple physical symptoms.

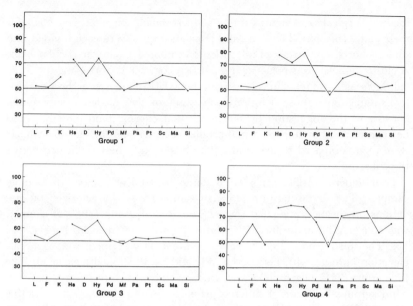

Figure 2-3. Mean MMPI Profiles for Female Clusters (Bradley et al., 1978)

The normal-limits group was compared to the clinical correlates reported by Marks, Seeman, and Haller (1974) for the "K + " profile identified in an inpatient psychiatric population. Marks et al. described these individuals as having severe dependency conflicts but reluctant to admit psychological conflict. The authors speculated that this might be an appropriate description of a subgroup of the chronic pain population, which would be consistent with theories suggesting pain patients tend to have histories of unmet dependency needs until the pain problem provides an acceptable reason for depending on others' financial and emotional support. Speculations regarding characteristics of the third group, possessing elevations on Hs, D, Hy, and Sc, were again based on Marks et al.'s list of codetype correlates in a psychiatric population. Such individuals would be described as somatically preoccupied, depressed, emotionally isolated, and conflicted over emotional dependency. Thus, the authors suggested this group might use the sick role to meet their dependency needs and avoid emotional threat in a socially acceptable manner.

The conversion-V group, found only in the female population in this study, was compared to Sternbach's similar group and the inference made that these individuals had learned to derive satisfaction from the sick role. They tended to be focused on one symptom rather than on multiple complaints, and the prognosis for successful treatment was considered better than in the hypochondriacal group.

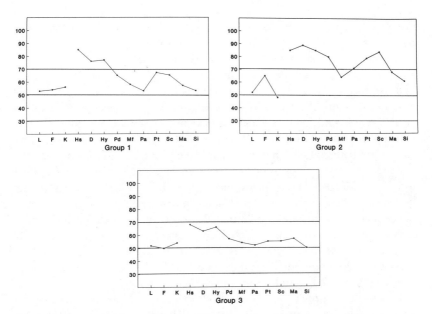

Figure 2-4. Mean MMPI Profiles for Male Clusters (Bradley et al., 1978)

This original study established the possibility of deriving replicable clusters of pain patients with similar personality profile patterns and provided some beginning speculations on the different characteristics of these patient groups. The authors called for further studies to replicate these groups in other populations and to examine behavioral correlates: "It would then be possible to conduct controlled investigation of the question 'What specific treatments may be applied to what LBP patient groups to best modify what specific, pain-related behaviors?'" (p. 272).

Several studies have addressed the replicability and correlates of these patient clusters in other samples of chronic pain patients. Prokop et al. (1980) studied a sample of patients with multiple pain complaints, ranging from headache to extremity pain to total-body pain but excluding patients with low back pain alone. The authors replicated the procedure used by Bradley et al., dividing the male and female samples into three cohorts corresponding to year of admission, performing separate cluster analyses on each of these cohorts, and then looking for clusters that replicated across the groups.

For the female samples (N = 221), no subgroups replicated across all three cohorts. However, three clusters did replicate across two of the cohorts: a neurotic-triad profile, a normal-limits profile, and a conversion-V profile. For the male sample, again replicable clusters were found across only two of the three cohorts. Of the four clusters identified, the first and second groups were similar to the female sample's neurotic-triad and normal-limits profiles; the third group was marked by a peak on D; and the fourth was characterized by elevations on most of the clinical scales.

Two of the groups identified in this study, the neurotic-triad pattern and the normal-limits pattern, were common to both men and women not only in this sample but also in the back pain sample presented by Bradley et al. (1978). Both studies provided evidence of sex-related differences in patterns of personality traits; the conversion-V pattern was an identifiable cluster in both studies in the female group but not among the males. Among the males, Prokop et al. found an elevated profile group similar to one identified for both males and females by Bradley et al.; they suggested appropriate treatment for this group might involve psychiatric components. It is interesting to note that Prokop et al.'s elevated profile group included elevations on Pd, possibly incorporating the manipulative reaction clients identified by Sternbach. In addition, their profile cluster with elevations on D might correspond to Sternbach's reactive depression group, which he predicted would be an indicator of good prognosis.

Prokop et al. provided personality descriptions of each of these cluster groups which were very similar to those of Bradley and colleagues. However, all of these personality descriptions were speculative, based on published codetype correlates for psychiatric samples or the investigators' personal experiences with pain patient profiles. No empirical data addressing profile correlates were presented. In addition, the differences in the cluster solutions found by these studies are difficult to interpret without further cross-validation to sort out the effects of type of pain vs. selection characteristics of patients in the particular setting studied.

Several other studies have addressed the replicability of MMPI profile clusters and have begun to provide validity data by examining their external correlates. Armentrout, Moore, Parker, Hewett, and Feltz (1982) gave the MMPI and a pain-history questionnaire to 240 male chronic pain patients evaluated over a three-year period at a VA hospital. The sample was quite heterogeneous in age, education, chronicity of problem, site of pain, and compensation status. Their cluster analysis results replicated the three male groups described by Bradley and colleagues: 25% had normal-limits profiles, 58% had neurotic-triad patterns, and 16% had "psychopathologic" profiles with multiple elevations on F, Hs, D, Hy, Pd, Pa, Pt, and Sc.

The authors compared these groups on a number of extra-test variables. There were no significant group differences on education, income, age, IQ, assertiveness scores, surgical history, duration of pain problem, or compensation status. The psychopathology group members were more likely to be divorced, more likely to have multiple symptoms, and reported greater severity of pain and negative impact of pain in their lives than the other groups. The normal-limits individuals were most likely to be employed. On the pain-severity and life-impact variables, the neurotic-triad group tended to fall between the other groups on almost every aspect of functional limitation, affective disturbance, interpersonal problems, etc.

The authors comment that this study adds to literature indicating "a remarkable consistency to the psychological dimensions of pain, in spite of the high variability in the organic substrates of pain problems" (p. 209). The data suggest that the degree of psychopathology reflected in the MMPI subgroups is related to the severity of pain and degree of life disruption experienced. The results fit with a model utilizing suffering as the salient focus of treatment rather than pain in a narrow sensory definition, and suggest that treatment approaches aimed at reducing emotional problems and maladaptive cognitive styles may in addition reduce the patient's experience of pain and related disability.

Leavitt and Garron (1982) provided a similar description of differences in pain experience associated with these three groups. Rather than statistically deriving clusters in their sample of 150 patients hospitalized for treatment of low back pain, they hand-sorted MMPIs into configural groups to match those identified in Bradley et al.'s male sample, namely the normal-limits, conversion-V, and general-elevation patterns. No differences were found on age, education, marital status, sex or race distribution, surgery history, or duration of pain. Groups did differ on self-report of their pain experience, as broken down into sensory and affective components. The normal-limits group reported less severe pain on all dimensions studied. The conversion-V and general-elevation groups reported similar aspects of sensory pain, but the general-elevation group reported more intense suffering associated with their pain experience. The authors speculate that "more openly admitted psychiatric disturbances are associated with magnification of mood-related attributes of pain" (p. 305).

Bernstein and Garbin (1983) did not address correlates of clusters, but did add to the literature finding consistency in cluster solutions. They derived five clusters from the MMPI profiles of 77 female pain-clinic patients. Their first three clusters were very similar to the neurotic-triad, normal-limits, and conversion-V profiles found by Bradley et al. (1978) and by Prokop et al. (1980) in their female samples. The first and last of these are similar in configuration to Sternbach's hypochondriasis and somatization profiles. A fourth cluster seemed to correspond to the general-elevation profile found by Bradley et al. for both men and women, and by Prokop et al. and Armentrout et al. (1982) for men only. A fifth cluster, not identified in other studies, was characterized by elevations on Hs, D, Hy, and Pd, and was described as similar to Sternbach's hypochondriacal and manipulative profiles combined.

McGill, Lawlis, Selby, Mooney, and McCoy (1983) designed a study to replicate former cluster solutions and to explore the relationship between group membership, self-reported pain history, and treatment response. Forty-six women and 46 men were selected at random from patients admitted to a multimodal low-back-pain treatment program during a one-year period. A hierarchical cluster analysis was performed on the total sample, with four profiles designed to match those found by Bradley et al. (1978) added to seed the clustering process. This procedure resulted in the identification of four clusters corresponding to the three profiles found by Bradley et al. (1978) to replicate across male and female cohorts, plus the conversion-V profile they had found only in the female sample. This fourth group also had a clinical elevation on Pd, similar to the somatization/manipulative reaction group noted by Bernstein and Garbin (1983). McGill et al. repeated their analysis separately for males and females, and found the same four profile groups in these two subsamples.

McGill et al. used discriminant analysis and univariate analyses of variance to identify several pain-history variables that differed across the groups. Their data supported Sternbach (1974a) and Bradley et al. (1978) in describing the neurotic-triad group as influenced by respondent conditioning and as being most likely to maintain focused attention on physical stimuli. These patients had histories of more surgeries and hospitalizations than the other groups, and on the average had been vocationally disabled longer than they had had a pain problem. The latter suggested they may have had other physical complaints predating pain and tended to "respond to any external stimulus in a psychophysiological way" (p. 90). The authors suggested they might respond best to treatments focusing on respondent conditioning and treatment of depression.

The second group, characterized by normal-limits profiles, reported the least pain, the least hospitalizations and surgeries, the shortest duration of pain, and the shortest vocational disability. The authors suggested these might be "pain copers" who would be most likely to respond to traditional medical management or a program focused on positive coping techniques; if they could be treated at this point they might not develop the more entrenched coping styles of the conversion-V group. This description contrasts with the suggestion of Bradley et al. that these individuals were denying dependency problems and therefore would not be expected to respond well to traditional treatment.

The third group, with generally elevated profiles, tended to report the most subjective pain both at admission and discharge, consistent with other reports (Armentrout et al., 1982; Leavitt & Garron, 1982; Rosen et al., 1987). There was also a nonsignificant trend for this group to be least likely to have reported benefit from previous treatment. The authors labeled these individuals "pain decompensators," suggesting that an initial approach using antipsychotic medication and individualized reinforcement might be more beneficial than treating pain symptoms directly.

Their fourth group was associated with self-report of longer pain duration and was less likely to be associated with a clear pain precipitant. The authors suggested this profile might represent a coping reaction to the experience of pain, as patients adopt defenses against any psychological or physiological experiences that might exacerbate pain. The data do not directly address this issue, and their explanation of this profile in terms of previous descriptions of the conversion V appears to ignore the elevation on Pd which is also indicated in their tables, and the associated possibility of secondary gain maintaining part of the patient's illness behavior.

Identification of distinct correlates of these cluster groups is primarily useful if these different patterns have implications for treatment outcome. In spite of clear differences in pain histories, McGill et al. found no differences among groups in outcome variables measured at discharge, including change in drug use, hours out of bed, range of motion, rating of goal attainment, and rating of physical improvement. They noted that these negative results could be interpreted three ways: "First, the four groups may not respond differently to treatment in spite of the distinctive histories. Second, because the program was multimodal, elements may have been included that were specifically helpful to each group, thus concealing any differential response to treatment. Third, since data were obtained only at immediate follow-up, it is not known if there may be differences in the long-term treatment response" (pp. 91-92).

Bradley et al. (1981) studied 96 men and 218 women from a university back-pain clinic in a large northeastern city. The authors replicated two female subgroups and two male subgroups previously identified in other studies (Armentrout et al., 1982; Bradley et al., 1978; McGill et al., 1983), namely the elevations on Hs, D, Hy, and Sc found in males by Bradley et al., the subclinical neurotic-triad profile for men, the elevated neurotic triad with a secondary elevation on Pd for women, and an elevated profile with peaks on Hs, D, Hy, Pd, and Sc for women. They also found a novel male cluster marked by elevations on D, Pd, Pt, and Sc, a normal-limits cluster for men and for women, and a subclinical depression profile for women. They did not report frequencies for these groups, so it is difficult to gauge the significance of the novel clusters in this sample. The authors note that it is impossible to determine whether their unique profile patterns reflect differences in urban vs. rural settings, ethnic composition of samples, differences between public, private, VA, inpatient, and outpatient programs, or the use of volunteer subjects rather than consecutive admissions: "It is necessary, then, for future investigators to consistently report important demographic characteristics of their subject samples if meaningful comparisons may be made across studies" (pp. 171–172).

Despite the differences in some of their clusters from previous studies, Bradley and colleagues (Bradley, Prokop, Gentry, Van der Heide, & Prieto, 1981; Bradley, 1983; Bradley & Van der Heide, 1984) replicated some of the general correlate patterns reported elsewhere. They found a positive relationship between elevation of profile and self-report of pain intensity and disruption of daily activities. This relationship was complicated by the fact that elevations on the neurotic-triad scales alone were associated with more self-reported affective disturbance and disruption of activities *as a function of pain* than were profiles characterized by elevations on this triad along with Pd and Sc. The implication might be that more of the latter group's suffering and disability could be attributed to premorbid characterological and psychiatric disturbance rather than a direct function of the pain problem per se. Alternatively, the former group's tendency to deny psychological problems might be reflected in greater attribution of affective problems to their pain alone.

Atkinson et al. (1986) addressed the association of psychiatric disorders, particularly depression, with distinct clusters of MMPI profile types. They did not perform a new cluster analysis on their sample of 51 consecutive admissions to a VA inpatient pain-treatment program, but instead used a least-squared differences procedure to assign patients' MMPI profiles to the closest of the three male clusters described by Bradley et al. (1978). This resulted in a hypochondriasis neurotic-triad profile (39% of sample), a general-elevation profile (43% of sample), and a subclinical profile with relative elevations on Hs and Hy (18% of sample). Both the elevated profiles were significantly more likely than was the normal-limits profile to be associated with an RDC psychiatric diagnosis. The frequency of depression was highest in the general-elevation profile as measured by RDC diagnosis and by scores on the Beck and the Hamilton depression inventories. The groups did not differ in age, in chronicity, or in judged presence of organic basis for the pain.

Hart (1984) cluster analyzed the MMPIs of 70 male patients referred to a university medical center for treatment of chronic pain. He used a hierarchical clustering procedure with initial seeding by four marker profiles designed to match Bradley et al.'s solution (1978). The neurotic-triad group accounted for 33% of the men, 21% had profiles characterized by a subclinical elevation on Hs and Hy, 24% had generally elevated profiles, and 21% had conversion-V profiles. The results replicated previous studies in finding these to be distinct profile configurations identifiable within a heterogeneous pain-patient population, and confirmed several previous studies finding that the conversion-V pattern can be reliably identified in men as well as in women.

A recent study by Rosen, Grubman, Bevins, and Frymoyer (1987) provided a strong replication of previous cluster solutions plus a broad range of correlate data. The authors' sample differed from others in including acute pain patients as well as others differing in pain chronicity and organic status. They replicated two normal-limits and three clinically elevated clusters across sexes and across two different clustering methods. Patients in the two nonelevated groups tended to be younger, with a shorter duration of pain, the fewest previous treatments for pain or mental distress, the least activity limitation, and were most likely to be working. Group

3, the most common elevated profile, was a conversion-V pattern. These patients had the longest current pain episodes, the most frequent reports of pain and activity limitation, and had the poorest physical capacity of any group. Compared to normals, they were judged as exhibiting disability in excess of physical findings and were more likely to have had mental-health treatment. Their adoption of the sick role was not as entrenched as that of Group 4, whose mean profile fit the hypochondriasis pattern found elsewhere. Compared to other groups, Group 4 patients were the oldest, with the longest history of back pain, usually of unknown etiology. They had the most previous surgeries, blamed problems on their work environment, had severe vocational disabilities, and were likely to be receiving compensation. They were the group judged most often to have disability in excess of physical findings.

The fifth group found by Rosen et al. corresponded to other investigators' general-elevation profile. These patients did not have as severe physical disabilities as the other elevated groups, but were marked instead by severe psychological impairment. They had average physical and functional capacity, yet a high rate of financial compensation, perhaps related to having the highest rate of previous mental-health intervention.

Rosen et al. did not present outcome data on their groups, but did speculate about some potential treatment-by-personality interactions that could be predicted from their findings. They suggest that the patients with normal-limits profiles "should respond satisfactorily to ordinary education and reassurance," those with conversion-V patterns "may be appropriate for psychological intervention that focuses on facilitating coping with the stresses of illness and disability and controlling subjective pain and pain behavior," and the hypochondriasis group "should receive psychological intervention geared toward reducing their illness behavior *and* reducing depression and interpersonal skill deficits that may be promoting the sick role." Finally, patients with the most pathological profiles should receive psychotherapy or medications aimed at their psychological disorders rather than behavioral interventions for pain (p. 597).

Although Rosen et al. did not test their differential treatment predictions, three recent studies have joined McGill et al. (1983) in examining the relationship of MMPI profile clusters to treatment outcome. McCreary (1985) submitted the profiles of 401 low-back-pain patients to a cluster analysis, dividing the male and female subsamples each into two cohorts for cross-validation purposes. The author also utilized a different cluster-analytic procedure than previous studies to provide a stricter test of cluster replicability. At admission, patients filled out questionnaires rating their intensity of pain during the previous week in relation to various activities. They then received conservative medical treatment consisting of exercises, instructions on body mechanics, and analgesic medication. Six months after finishing treatment, they were sent outcome evaluation forms repeating the questions they had answered at admission. Fifty-four percent of the patients returned the outcome questionnaire.

Five clusters were obtained and were replicated on the cross-validation samples. Four of these clusters were common to both sexes: a general-elevation profile, a neurotic-triad profile, an unelevated profile with highest scores on Hs, Hy, Pd, and Ma, and an unelevated neurotic-triad pattern. An elevated conversion-V pattern was found only for women. Larger percentages of men than women fell into the general-elevation group (27% vs. 4%), and there were more women than men in the unelevated neurotic-triad profile. There were no ethnic differences between groups. Patients in the third profile group were more often single, were younger, and along with the other nonelevated profile group were more likely to be working full-time, as opposed to groups 1 and 5 which were most likely to be unemployed. The patients with subclinical profiles also reported significantly lower pretreatment pain intensity and activity limitation, consistent with other studies.

The general-elevation group and the elevated conversion-V group showed the highest pain intensity at six-month follow-up and had the least change in scores from pretreatment to follow-up. The two subclinical profile groups had the lowest follow-up pain scores and the greatest decrease in pain scores from pretreatment to follow-up. None of the demographic variables related to successful outcome except being employed. These findings did not hold as consistently when the male and female samples were analyzed separately; subgroup membership was generally a better predictor of outcome in men than in women. The elevated neurotic triad was a predictor of poor outcome in males but good outcome in females. The authors note that the suggestion of sex differences in outcome prediction needs replication studies.

Moore, Armentrout, Parker, and Kivlahan (1986) also examined outcome correlates of MMPI clusters, using an all-male sample of 57 patients admitted to a six-week inpatient VA multimodal pain-treatment program. Patients were assessed on several self-report measures two to five months before treatment, upon admission to treatment, and immediately following treatment. The authors speculated that the lack of association between cluster membership and outcome reported by McGill et al. (1983) might have been an artifact of lack of overall treatment efficacy. Accordingly, they first established the efficacy of their treatment program as defined by improvements in scores on the dependent self-report measures. All dependent measures except sleep and time sitting improved significantly from admission to end of treatment.

A least-squares difference procedure was employed to assign patients to the closest of three MMPI clusters reported by Armentrout et al. (1982) and Bradley et al. (1978), consisting of a subclinical profile, a general-elevation profile, and a neurotic-triad profile. The authors did not report pretreatment correlates of subgroup membership. Despite the range of outcome variables used, there was no evidence for differential outcome by cluster membership.

Guck, Meilman, Skultety, and Poloni (1988) also examined treatment-outcome differences among MMPI cluster groups. Their large sample consisted of 635 chronic pain patients (305 men and 330 women) admitted to an inpatient university medical-center multidisciplinary pain program from 1973 to 1985. They used Bradley's procedure of cross-validating clusters within each sex and chose final clusters based on similarity to previous studies. Their three male clusters generally matched prior descriptions of a subclinical profile, a neurotic-triad profile, and a general-elevation profile. Among the women, four replicated clusters were found corresponding to the subclinical, general-elevation, neurotic-triad, and conversion-V patterns found by other researchers.

Comparison of cluster groups on pretreatment variables revealed that the general-elevation group among the men was associated with more pretreatment pain hospitalizations and surgeries, and a higher probability of being divorced. The cluster groups among the women were not differentially associated with any of the pretreatment measures. When the cluster groups were compared on self-report questionnaire items measuring outcome an average of two years after treatment, few or no consistent cluster correlates were found. The authors conclude that this study extends the previous research finding no differential effects across cluster groups from short-term to long-term outcome.

There could be several explanations for the lack of group differences, beyond the obvious possibility that cluster membership has no predictive utility. McGill et al., Moore et al., and Guck et al. reported outcome of comprehensive, multidisciplinary inpatient treatment programs which might obscure interactions between individual personality types and individual treatment components. Moore et al.'s results suggest that patients showed improvement over a wide variety of measures, including reductions in all MMPI scales, which "may reflect a generalized improvement in psychological functioning following treatment and may be related to the comprehensive nature of this treatment program. Less comprehensive treatment might produce more focal changes on the MMPI as well as differential treatment outcome for MMPI subgroups" (p. 62). It is interesting to note in this regard that McCreary's study found subgroup membership was predictive of outcome of a specific type of treatment program, in this case conservative medical management.

Obviously, this is a very new research area and more studies are needed to explore the predictive utility of personality cluster methodology. Guck et al. note that current state-of-the-art outcome measures may be inadequate to accurately test treatment outcome differences—most studies still use self-report measures without augmenting them with more objective data. Overall, the cluster literature to date has shown remarkable consistency in finding a few common replicable profiles across studies, while also continuing to illustrate pain patient heterogeneity by the differences in less common profiles and in correlate patterns. Costello, Hulsey, Schoenfeld, and Ramamurthy (1987) summarized the literature on the four most common patterns (normal limits, conversion V, hypochondriasis, and general elevation), concluding that these types are now quite well established. They propose a set of classification rules to allow patient-typing even without a computer, so that hypotheses based on cluster studies can begin to be tested in general clinical practice.

The use of these rules in the general clinical setting seems premature, since even Costello et al. note that no data are available on the expected base rates of each type using such a classification scheme. Cluster procedures by definition classify the total sample, whereas typing rules such as theirs can be expected to result in "a shrinkage or loss of subjects as great as 20-40%" (p. 208). Their rules are designed to match individual profiles to the mean profile of each cluster type; in actuality, there has been little research into the amount of variability within cluster analytically derived groups. Henrichs (1987) illustrates that forcing all profiles within a sample into one of a few cluster groups can result in a wide variety of profile types within each group—the same criticism leveled at total-group approaches to chronic pain patient assessment. He suggests purifying cluster groups by retaining only those patients who most closely match the mean profile shape for that cluster, predicting that this will improve correlate descriptions and the predictive power of such typologies.

Although little work has been done in this area, a report by Snyder and Power (1981) illustrates that treatment-relevant subgroups may exist even within the larger groups identified by many cluster studies. They broke down one commonly occurring MMPI profile type by cluster analyzing a sample of normal-limits pain-patient profiles. They obtained five distinct clusters, with the least elevated profile corresponding to patients with the least diffuse pain complaints, the most likelihood of being treated on an outpatient basis, the least history of previous surgery or psychiatric treatment, the least family history of pain complaints, and the least change in work status. Given that this group of patients also tended to be younger, it is unclear without longitudinal research whether unelevated profiles change with time to reflect chronicity of the problem and changes in the individual's mode of coping with pain. At this point there has been no replication or expansion of Snyder and Power's work with normal-limits profiles.

Summary and Conclusions

Objective, replicable assessment strategies are an essential tool in the search for characteristics of pain patients that have implications for preventive and treatment strategies. Self-report personality tests should be only one part of a comprehensive assessment approach, supplemented by medical, behavioral, and demographic data. The use of personality measures can be justified because of their potential to capture patient dispositions that may be common pathways of many life experiences. "If two persons produce similar profiles by the method of verbal response to a structured objective inventory, they do so because they have experienced their psychological, familial, and biological environments in roughly similar ways, and such experiences serve as partial determinants of their current perceptions of their psychological environments [and physical health]" (Harris, 1982, p. 33). Studies utilizing group averages on the MMPI are remarkably consistent in finding elevations on the neurotic-triad scales, interpreted as indicating somatic preoccupation along with denial and repression of psychological conflict. Studies differ somewhat on the relative elevation of the depression scale, with some researchers emphasizing the conversion hysteria aspect of pain patients' symptomatology and others describing pain patients as quite depressed and hypochondriacal. In both cases, greater elevations on the neurotic-triad scales have been associated with greater functional disability, chronicity, reliance on medications, complaints of more severe pain intensity, and poor response to traditional medical or psychological treatment (Snyder, in press). High Hs and Hy scores do not, however, rule out the possibility of an organic component to a client's problems even when they do suggest a strong functional component.

Given the enormous complexity of influences on the experience of pain and the degree of disability associated with it, it is not too surprising to find a variety of interpretations of the pain-patient personality or even that individual patients tend to differ in important respects from either of the typical profiles found in research using group averages. The "illusion of homogeneity" (Fordyce, 1976) has prevailed for too long. Instead, "the goal of research concerning the assessment of chronic pain should be to contribute to the understanding of what specific treatments may be applied to what pain patient subgroups to best alter what pain-related experiences, behaviors, and attributes" (Bradley et al., 1981, pp. 111–112).

Classification of patients into dichotomous groups based on functional vs. organic status, presence or absence of depression, medication use, presence or absence of pain-related compensation, etc., are first steps in this direction but may not, as yet, substantially improve treatment choice or outcome prediction. The implications of each of these single-dimension classifications may be greatly modified by other variables.

Recent subgrouping studies using MMPI patterns are a prototype of multidimensional schemes that may potentially capture important interactions between variables distinguishing different groups of patients. Research using configural sorting and statistical clustering of MMPI profiles has demonstrated that several distinct subgroups of patients can be identified. Several of these distinctive profile patterns have now been replicated across pain patient populations and by different investigators, even across diverse pain groups such as headache patients (Rappaport, McAnulty, Waggoner, & Brantley, 1987). The most robust configurations seem to be the conversion-V pattern, the neurotic-triad pattern, the normal-limits profile, and the general-elevation profile. Other patterns have emerged in some studies and not others, such as a reactive depression pattern and a manipulative reaction pattern.

The reasons for differences in subgroups across studies remain unclear. The first step in finding treatment-relevant groups of patients must be establishing the reliability of obtained subgroups, so it will be important for future research to clarify this issue. Researchers must clearly delineate the characteristics of their patient samples to allow better determination of the factors that may contribute to different solutions. It would make sense, for instance, to discover more groups in a highly heterogeneous sample of pain patients than in one that had already been carefully selected for homogeneity.

In this same regard, the tendency for researchers to use small samples in their cluster and configural studies may result in unique clusters as statistical artifacts, or conversely may obscure the effects of rare but important personality patterns. Bradley (1983) suggests a subject-to-variable ratio of at least 5:1, which would require a population size of at least 65 for a cluster analysis using 13 MMPI scales. In fact, a good replication study would require a much larger sample to provide separate analyses for men and women: the effect of sex on profile subgroup solutions remains unclear, but enough studies have found differences that it seems important to assess sex effects. Cross-validation of cluster solutions by dividing the sample into cohorts is also highly recommended to improve reliability; this again requires larger samples than reported in many studies. With larger, well-defined samples and cross-validation procedures, it would be possible to evaluate whether studies finding more than four important clusters were merely flukes or indeed identified important but infrequent replicable patterns specific to certain pain-patient populations.

Once replicability of various MMPI patterns has been established, their validity must be tested by demonstrating that group membership has differential implications for behavioral, cognitive, and/or affective correlates of the pain problem and for treatment choice and outcome. The major deficiency in many studies is the lack of empirical data supporting speculations about the correlates of these proposed clinically relevant profile types. Many expert clinicians have described interpretive schemes based on the supposed significance of various scale configurations (e.g., Fordyce, 1979; Lawlis & McCoy, 1983; Sternbach, 1974a, 1974b), but there is still little data available to support these assumptions. Naliboff et al. (1983) provide a good summary of the state of the art: there is "only minimal evidence for specificity in terms of MMPI profiles associated with a particular disease or symptomatology (e.g., pain). The MMPI codetypes describe, instead, a variety of ways in which patients can react psychologically to a disorder. In order to confirm the utility of this sort of classification scheme (which is already in wide clinical use), research must continue to focus on both refinement and cross-validation of sorting rules as well as the validity of profile typologies with respect to specific behaviors, psychosocial problem areas, and treatment potential" (p. 847).

This monograph is designed to provide a foundation for applying the rich tradition of chronic pain research and clinical applications of the MMPI to its revision, the MMPI-2 (Butcher, Dahlstrom, Graham, Tellegen, & Kaemmer, 1989). The revision differs from the MMPI in several important ways, differences that may have an impact on the applicability of previous research to the revised form and may offer interpretive advantages. The research study described in this monograph was designed to evaluate the MMPI-2 total group, codetype, cluster group, and correlate data for a large sample of chronic pain patients. Goals were to establish the degree of generalizability of MMPI research to the MMPI-2 and to expand the research base on chronic pain patients by providing new correlate data for MMPI-2 subgroups, using extra-test information as well as the new MMPI-2 content scales.

Chapter 3

The MMPI Restandardization Project: MMPI-2

The need for a revision of the MMPI has been discussed for a number of years (Butcher, 1972; Butcher & Owen, 1978), and several studies examining the relevance of the original MMPI norms for contemporary use have been reported (Colligan, Osborne, Swenson, & Offord, 1984; Parkison & Fishburne, 1984). However, the official test norms have remained the same as when the MMPI was first published in 1942 (Hathaway & McKinley, 1940; Hathaway & McKinley, 1943). In 1982 the University of Minnesota Press, which holds the copyright to the MMPI, initiated a project to revise the MMPI and establish new nationally representative norms for the instrument. A revision team was appointed consisting of Professors James N. Butcher and Auke Tellegen of the University of Minnesota, W. Grant Dahlstrom of the University of North Carolina, and John R. Graham of Kent State University in Ohio. The revision team was charged with the task of modifying the existing item pool, adding new items, and collecting new normative data on the instrument.

Development of the MMPI-2

Changes in the MMPI Item Pool

The revision of the MMPI sponsored by the University of Minnesota Press was designed to simultaneously "preserve as many of the well substantiated original MMPI clinical correlates as possible, while expanding the item pool to cover some additional problem areas" (Butcher, 1989). To meet this goal, a special form of the MMPI booklet, the AX (adult experimental) version, was developed specifically for use in the restandardization research. The booklet included all 550 original MMPI items, but 82 of these were rewritten slightly to eliminate sexist wording, modernize idioms, or clarify syntax. (Ben-Porath and Butcher [1988] demonstrated that changes in item wording did not substantially affect endorsement frequency or item-scale correlations in a college sample.) The 16 repeated items in the original MMPI were deleted. Finally, 154 provisional new items dealing with such content domains as treatment compliance, suicidal thoughts or behavior, family conflict, drug abuse, etc., were added to cover content areas previously underrepresented in the item pool. These additional items brought the length of the MMPI AX form to 704 items.

Collection of New Normative Data

National standardization sample. A major change in the MMPI-2 is the inclusion of a new national normative reference group upon which all T scores are based. The contemporary normative sample, described in Butcher, Dahlstrom, Graham, Tellegen, and Kaemmer (1989), is composed of adults from communities in seven states chosen to provide geographic diversity: California, Minnesota, North Carolina, Ohio, Pennsylvania, Virginia, and Washington. A variety of methods was used to recruit subjects, but most were contacted through invitation letters sent to household addresses randomly generated by a direct-mail marketing firm. Subjects were paid a nominal amount to come to a group testing location in their area and complete the MMPI-2 along with associated research forms described below. In an effort to match the demographic characteristics of the 1980 census, subjects were added to the normative sample from a Washington state Indian reservation and from several military bases. The final community sample used in developing norms for the MMPI-2 consisted of 1138 men and 1462 women, after excluding protocols that did not meet specified validity criteria. As noted in the manual, the sampling methods were relatively successful in obtaining proportional representation of black and American Indian minority groups, but Hispanic and Asian subpopulations are underrepresented. The normative sample also tends to be somewhat biased toward higher socioeconomic levels and educational status compared to the general U.S. population, although it is heterogeneous on these variables.

Psychiatric sample comparison group. The MMPI was originally developed for use with psychiatric patients, and it is with this population that the majority of clinical and research applications of the MMPI are still undertaken. As part of the revision of the MMPI, a large sample of inpatient psychiatric patients was tested with the research forms used in the national restandardization. This sample included 137 inpatients from Fallsview Psychiatric Hospital in Ohio (Graham & Butcher, 1988) plus 286 psychiatric inpatients tested at Hennepin County Medical Center and Anoka State Hospital in Minnesota (Roberts, 1987). Fallsview Hospital is a state-supported hospital providing short-term care, primarily psychotropic medication, for patients of lower socioeconomic status. Hennepin County Medical Center is a large county hospital with two adult psychiatric units; it serves primarily economically disadvantaged patients from the Twin Cities area in Minnesota. Anoka State Hospital is a long-term treatment facility; the majority of its patients are court committed. The psychiatric sample included all testable subjects admitted to Hennepin or Fallsview or resident at Anoka during the study period. Primary diagnoses for the sample were: 20% schizophrenia, 26% depressive disorders, 16% other psychotic disorders, 10% adjustment disorders, 9% bipolar disorders, 8% substance-abuse disorders, and 11% other disorders (J. Graham, personal communication, 10/1/88). This sample was used in refining the new content scales described below, as well as providing data about the performance of the MMPI-2 in clinical samples, and will be used as a comparison group later in this monograph.

Development of New Norms

At the scale level, the largest differences between the MMPI and the MMPI-2 are likely to result from differences in the norming procedures. The normative sample for the MMPI was collected in the 1940s; several previous studies (Colligan et al., 1984; Diehl, 1977) have questioned the applicability of these norms to modern populations. Norms for the MMPI-2 are based on the large national sample described above, chosen to match general demographic characteristics of the 1980 U.S. census. Scores from this sample provided the raw-score distributions used to develop T-score transformation tables for each scale.

Traditionally, raw scores on MMPI scales were converted to standardized T scores with a mean of 50 and standard deviation of 10 in the original Minnesota normative sample. These T scores were linear transformations of the raw-score distributions, retaining the positive skew shown by all the clinical scales in the original norms and also retaining the wide variation in range shown across the scales. Colligan et al. (1984) pointed out that these differences in raw-score distributions can make interpretation and comparison of linear T scores misleading, since percentile equivalence cannot be assumed: a T score of 70 may cut off quite different proportions of the population on different scales. The T-score transformation they suggested and employed in their Mayo Clinic regional normative study converted each scale's distribution to a standard normal distribution. However, this procedure results in greatly lowering scores that would be highly elevated on the original T scores, can change codetype configurations substantially, and reduces the interpretive range on each scale.

The MMPI-2 committee used a new approach developed by Auke Tellegen and designed to reduce the discrepancies between scale distributions while retaining the greatest discrimination at the high end of each scale. It was considered desirable to retain the positively skewed shape of each scale's score distribution as an accurate reflection of the distribution of psychopathological characteristics in the population rather than artificially forcing these to fit the normal curve. Tellegen developed "uniform" T scores by combining the raw scores of the eight clinical scales (Hs, D, Hy, Pd, Pa, Pt, Sc, and Ma) into a composite distribution, then regressing the component scales against the composite to obtain T-score conversion formulas (Tellegen, 1988a; Butcher, Dahlstrom, Graham, Tellegen, & Kaemmer, 1989). This procedure was expected to result in some changes in scale elevations and codetype patterns compared to the original norms, but not to change the distribution of any particular scale as much as a normalizing procedure would.

The new uniform T scores result in somewhat lower profile elevations than the linear transformations, which could affect interpretive strategies based on strict score levels or codetype patterns. Ahles, Yunus, Gaulier, Riey, and Masi (1986) have noted that scoring pain patients' MMPIs with the "normalized" T scores of Colligan et al. (1984) results in substantially fewer patients being classified as psychologically disturbed. Although uniform T scores are not expected to lower profiles as much as normalized T scores, there is still a potential for interpretive confusion unless the pattern of changes introduced by these new T scores is clearly specified. When using the MMPI-2 scales for clinical assessment, the MMPI-2 Restandardization Committee suggested a shift in level of interpretive significance (Butcher, Dahlstrom, et al., 1989). The "critical" level of elevation has been changed to a T score of 65, appearing to be the optimal point for separating the normative sample from various clinical groups. The degree of change from linear T scores to uniform T scores remains an empirical question within particular clinical samples and is one of the issues to be addressed in this study with chronic pain patients.

Biographical Information and Life Events Forms

Two forms were developed to provide extra-test information about the restandardization sample and were also administered to a subset of the psychiatric sample as well as other clinical comparison groups of interest. The Biographical Information Form was designed to provide general demographic and life-history information about tested subjects, including information on educational background, occupation, income, race, and marital status. Questions also included information on alcohol and drug use, psychiatric and medical treatment history, and family history of psychiatric or substance-abuse problems.

The Life Events Form was adapted by the MMPI-2 Restandardization Committee from Holmes and Rahe (1967). It was included as a measure of degree of life stress in the six months before taking the MMPI-2. Because this was an adaptation and not a standardized instrument, the committee examined only single item responses and a total endorsement score rather than differentially weighting the items. In addition, recent research has generally failed to support the incremental validity of using weighted scores as opposed to unit weights for life events items (see review by Williams & Uchiyama, in press).

MMPI-2 Content Scales

An additional innovation in the MMPI-2 that may prove of value in assessing chronic pain patients is the development of new content scales incorporating some of the new items as well as original MMPI items. Throughout the history of MMPI applications, users have attempted to augment interpretation of the content-heterogeneous standard validity and clinical scales with content-homogeneous scales. Inclusion of new items in the MMPI-2 provided the opportunity of developing a new set of scales (Butcher, Graham, Williams, & Ben-Porath, 1989). These scales were developed through a multi-step strategy. First, a rational subgrouping was performed by the first three authors assigning items to content-homogeneous groups. Next, psychometric criteria were applied, requiring item groupings to be internally consistent across several samples. Items that correlated more highly with another scale than with their own were eliminated, as were a few items that appeared on many scales, thus providing little discriminative validity. The authors examined item content to maintain the face validity of each scale, and developed external correlates based on clinical samples, including the psychiatric population described above, and on behavior ratings from the normative study. (See Table 3-1 for scale descriptions.)

Final Form of the MMPI-2

Following the extensive standardization data collection, the development of new norms, and the development of a number of additional scales, the 704 item Form AX item pool was reduced to a total of 567 items to comprise the final MMPI-2 booklet. In this phase of the project the MMPI Restandardization Committee maintained as a goal the preservation of the original validity and clinical scales. Primary goals in the item deletion stage were to eliminate many items that people have found particularly objectionable (Butcher & Tellegen, 1966) and to remove nonworking items that did not appear on the clinical scales, widely used supplementary scales, or the new content and supplementary scales. The item membership of the basic validity and clinical scales is largely equivalent to the original version, though a few items on each scale were reworded and five scales (F, Hs, D, Mf, and Si) are slightly shorter. Thus, at the raw-score level there is the potential for slight shifts in score patterns from the MMPI to the MMPI-2.

The MMPI-2 and Chronic Pain Patients

At this time, the only study to examine the significance for chronic pain patients of some of the changes incorporated in the MMPI-2 was reported

TABLE 3-1. MMPI-2 Content Scales
(Adapted from Butcher, Graham, Williams, & Ben-Porath, 1989)

Scale	Description of Content and Correlates
ANX (Anxiety)	General symptoms of anxiety and tension, sleep and concentration problems, somatic correlates of anxiety, excessive worrying, difficulty making decisions, willingness to admit to these problems.
FRS (Fears)	Many specific fears and phobias including animals, high places, insects, blood, fire, storms, water, the dark, being indoors, dirt, etc.
OBS (Obsessiveness)	Excessive rumination, difficulty making decisions, compulsive behaviors, rigidity, feelings of being overwhelmed.
DEP (Depression)	Depressive thoughts, anhedonia, feelings of hopelessness and uncertainty, possible suicidal thoughts.
HEA (Health Concerns)	Many physical symptoms across several body systems: gastrointestinal, neurological, sensory, cardiovascular, dermatological, and respiratory. Reports of pain and of general worries about health.
BIZ (Bizarre Mentation)	Psychotic thought processes, auditory, visual, or olfactory hallucinations, paranoid ideation, delusions.
ANG (Anger)	Anger control problems, irritability, impatience, loss of control, past or potential abusiveness.
CYN (Cynicism)	Misanthropic beliefs, negative expectations about the motives of others, generalized distrust.
ASP (Antisocial Practices)	Cynical attitudes, problem behaviors, trouble with the law, stealing, belief in getting around rules and laws for personal gain.
TPA (Type A)	Hard-driving, work-oriented behavior, impatience, irritability, annoyance, feelings of time pressure, interpersonally overbearing.
LSE (Low Self-Esteem)	Low self-worth, overwhelming feelings of being unlikable, unimportant, unattractive, useless, etc.
SOD (Social Discomfort)	Uneasiness around others, shyness, preference for being alone.
FAM (Family Problems)	Family discord, possible abuse in childhood, lack of love and affection in the family or marriage, feelings of hate for family members.
WRK (Work Interference)	Behaviors or attitudes likely to interfere with work performance, such as low self-esteem, obsessiveness, tension, poor decision making, lack of family support, negative attitudes toward career or coworkers.
TRT (Negative Treatment Indicators)	Negative attitudes toward doctors and mental-health treatment. Preference for giving up rather than attempting change. Discomfort discussing any personal concerns.

by Cohen (1987). Cohen administered the experimental form (Form AX) of the MMPI to 80 chronic pain patients from three pain-treatment programs in Minneapolis; 40 of his patients are incorporated in the study described later in this monograph. Cohen showed that the item changes from the MMPI to the MMPI AX form did not substantially affect the expectable mean profile when the original MMPI norms and scoring were used: he obtained a neurotic-triad average profile just as has been reported so frequently in other studies. Cohen went on to sort the profiles into groups according to Sternbach's (1974a) criteria. He found 23% could be classified as a conversion-V pattern, 20% fit a neurotic-triad profile, 14% were within normal limits, 14% had a high point on the depression scale, and 13% fit a 1-3-4 pattern, termed "manipulative reaction" by Sternbach. Cohen noted that these figures were comparable to those found in previous studies and supported the continuity of previous MMPI research to the revised items of the MMPI-2.

Cohen (1987) also compared chronic pain clusters found with the MMPI to those found when MMPI-2 item changes are incorporated. He replicated Bradley's cluster analysis procedure separately for men and women, although his sample size (31 men and 49 women) was somewhat small for this procedure and did not allow for replication cohorts within each sex. Cohen, like other researchers, identified four clusters corresponding to the normal-limits, neurotic-triad, general-elevation, and conversion-V profile types, although elevations and proportions of these varied somewhat between men and women and in comparison to previous studies. He concluded that the same general patterns occur with MMPI-2 items as with original MMPI items, supporting continuity of research across this aspect.

Cohen's study did not address the other major changes incorporated in the new form, such as the use of MMPI-2 norms or the use of the new MMPI-2 scales, since the normative data and additional scales were not available at the time his study was completed. This makes it difficult to generalize from his data to performance on the completed MMPI-2. In addition, no data were presented on the behavioral correlates or treatment outcome of Cohen's subgroups, and he did not present information on the new content scales in the pain patient population. The study reported in the next two chapters is the first to examine performance of the final version of the MMPI-2 in a large population of chronic-pain-syndrome patients.

Chapter 4
The Chronic Pain
Research Project

Setting

Data for this study were collected at the Sister Kenny Institute Chronic Pain Rehabilitation Program in Minneapolis, Minnesota. Sister Kenny Institute, a division of Abbott Northwestern Hospital, is a rehabilitation facility founded in 1942 to help patients suffering from polio. Today, a full range of inpatient and outpatient rehabilitation and follow-up programs is offered to a wide variety of individuals, including those with spinal cord or brain injury, stroke, amputations, birth defects, speech disorders, arthritis, chemical dependency combined with physical disability, and chronic pain (Sister Kenny Institute, 1984).

The chronic pain program at Sister Kenny is a three-week intensive multidisciplinary rehabilitation package whose "primary goal is to return the injured worker to the workplace" (Sister Kenny Institute, undated program pamphlet). Clients are evaluated only by referral from a physician; the majority have been through extensive workups and treatments before coming to the institute. Many of the patients treated in the program are in the Workers' Compensation system, but this is not a criterion for admission. Referrals first receive a total medical evaluation; approximately 30-40% of those screened are admitted to the program. Primary reasons for refusing admission are severe chemical dependency or psychiatric problems, clear psychopathy/malingering, lack of insurance coverage, or discovery of a medical condition that would require a different treatment approach. Psychological tests, including the MMPI, are *not* part of the initial screening for acceptance into the program (D. Jones, program director, personal communication, 7/24/86).

Clients are accepted into the program on either an inpatient or outpatient basis, depending largely on whether they live in the area and whether medication management/weaning is to be a part of their treatment. Approximately 15-20 patients participate in each three-week program; they enter together and most of their treatment is in a group. The program itself is organized around physical therapy and active exercise rehabilitation, but it also includes great emphasis on stress management, relaxation training and biofeedback, acupressure, therapeutic recreation, educational seminars, vocational planning, and individual counseling. The clients' families are involved during the second week of the program for one and a half days, in an effort to educate them about chronic pain rehabilitation and enlist their support in helping the client return to normal functioning (D. Jones, personal communication, 7/24/86; Sister Kenny Institute, undated program pamphlet).

Upon completion of the three-week intensive program, clients are expected to participate in the Program of Aftercare (PACE). They return to Sister Kenny once a month for six months along with the rest of their group, participating in a full day of follow-up evaluation, vocational planning, pain management seminars, refresher sessions of relaxation, exercise, acupressure, etc., and individual and family counseling as needed. "The primary goal of the PACE program is a return to full and productive living, both at home and at work. Patients are encouraged to become self-reliant in the management of their pain problem. Increased activity and productivity are the criteria of success" (Abbott Northwestern Hospital, 1984). According to recent Sister Kenny statistics, over half of the program's participants are back at work by the end of the PACE follow-up program, and after a year 96% of those workers are still employed (Sister Kenny Institute, undated program pamphlet).

Subjects

Chronic Pain Sample

The subjects recruited for this study included all consecutive admissions to the Sister Kenny Chronic Pain Rehabilitation program over a two-and-one-half-year period (March 1985 to August 1987). As described below, research materials were substituted for the psychological testing package routinely administered to patients upon their arrival at the institute. The only exceptions to this policy were individuals who had already taken the MMPI in the past year or so, and a two-month period (October 1986 to December 1986) during which the program directors experimented with making psychological testing voluntary. Those subjects who volunteered for testing during that period were not included in the final subject pool because they could not be assumed to be representative of their patient groups. In addition, a small group of patients either refused the testing outright or failed to complete their forms during the program.

Excluding the two months of incomplete testing, a total of 38 groups of patients entered Sister Kenny during the research period. Of the 590 patients entering these groups, complete and usable MMPI-2 data were obtained on 502 (85%). Although data are not available on the untested subjects, it is possible that there may be a slight bias in the tested sample toward more successful or cooperative patients. However, given the large total sample size, the somewhat unusual fact that the MMPI was not used at Sister Kenny to screen out any potential patients, and the fact that 85% of all admissions to the Sister Kenny program were tested, it seems reasonable to assume that the tested sample is largely representative of this chronic pain population and is likely to provide MMPI-2 data covering a variety of chronic pain syndrome symptom constellations.

Normative and Psychiatric Sample Comparison Groups

One of the major changes from the original MMPI to the MMPI-2 was the new national normative reference group upon which all T scores are based. Any description of pain patient performance on the MMPI-2 must include comparisons with this normative group (described in Chapter 3). Although the Sister Kenny Institute chronic pain sample is largely drawn from Minnesota and other Midwestern states, regional comparisons reported in the MMPI-2 manual do not suggest significant regional differences in average MMPI-2 profiles, making it unnecessary to use a regional normative group instead of the national normative sample. In addition, data from the psychiatric sample collected as part of the MMPI Restandardization Project were used to augment the normative data at times as a comparison and contrast with the chronic pain patients' MMPI-2 performance. It is hoped that such comparisons help characterize what is unique to pain patients in contrast to what is typical of the normal population or of patients suffering from psychiatric disorders. Although the most meaningful control group for diagnostic uses of the MMPI-2 with pain patients would be a medical population, MMPI-2 data on such a group were not available at the time of this study.

Measures

MMPI Restandardization Project Forms

The AX form, consisting of a printed item booklet and machine-scorable answer sheet, is the form of the MMPI that was administered to patients in this study as well as to the national normative sample and the psychiatric sample discussed earlier. Thus, data were collected on all 704 old, revised, and new items, making it possible to score patients' MMPIs according to the original scoring rules and norms as well as to the new scale memberships and norms developed for the MMPI-2, which consists of 567 of the items comprising the AX form.

The biographical information and life events machine-scorable forms were also administered to the chronic pain sample and a subset of the psychiatric sample. It should be noted that these two forms, along with the AX form, are entirely self-report in nature. Although the normative sample subjects were assured of complete confidentiality, and the pain and psychiatric samples were told their answers on the life events and biographical information forms would be confidential, there was no external measure against which to evaluate the accuracy of the self-descriptions reported on these instruments.

Chart Review Form

To augment the information provided by the biographical information and life events forms, a form was designed for abstracting demographic, medical and psychiatric history, and treatment information from the Sister Kenny pain patients' hospital charts. This form was designed to cover a wide variety of information that might differentiate groups of pain patients. Raters were to complete the information based on the patients' intake, discharge, and PACE summaries, progress notes during the program and PACE, and any medical records included in the chart that had been sent from the patients' home physicians. Certain data were fairly standard in the charts, including reports of Beck Depression Inventory (Beck et al., 1961) scores at intake, and less commonly at discharge. Not surprisingly, data relating to description of the pain problem itself were more frequently available in the charts than was information about the patients' pre-pain life-style, psychiatric history, and family history. The chart review form was found to be overly inclusive because much of the desired information could not be accurately or reliably obtained from clinical charts which had not been written with research in mind. Chart information can be expected to reflect more sources of information about the patient than self-report measures alone, yet charts varied in the variety, availability, internal consistency, and sources of these data. In many cases it was not possible to tell whether the source of information had been the patient's report or an outside evaluation.

Because abstracting the chart information often required some summary ratings or clinical judgment on the part of the abstracter, a subset of charts (N = 63) were reviewed independently by various combinations of two of the six individuals who participated in this task. Reliabilities were then computed for the variables abstracted from the charts. Kendall's tau was used to evaluate interrater agreement for ordinal variables such as rating scales. Fleiss's (1971) generalization of coefficient kappa to the case of differing combinations of raters was used to test the interrater agreement for nominal variables such as marital status or site of pain. Variables for which interrater agreement was not significant at .05 or less were not included in further analyses. Variables eliminated owing to poor interrater agreement included most family history information other than that relating to parents, and most personal history variables including history of eating disorder, anxiety disorder, or unspecified psychiatric disorder. Many of the problems with rating seemed to result from the chart form asking for more detail than was available in charts, such as a detailed family history or psychiatric history. In addition, several outcome ratings were dropped owing to lack of information for the majority of patients: the only outcome ratings that could be retained were those for physical exercise, medication reduction, vocational goals, weight reduction, and depression reduction.

Unfortunately, two of the ratings of contributors to the patients' overall impairment also had to be dropped owing to poor reliability. These were anxiety/stress problems and illness conviction/phobic overguarding, which might have been expected to correlate with elevated Pt scores. Finally, the ratings of intensity of pain behaviors exhibited by the patient were dropped owing to lack of agreement. This is probably not too surprising given that the raters had no chance to actually observe the patients themselves, and there was a great deal of inconsistency in descriptions of patients' behavior in the charts.

Procedures

Data Collection

Before this research project was begun, patients entering the Sister Kenny program were routinely given the MMPI and the Beck Depression Inventory their first day in the group. During the research testing period, all patients were asked to complete the AX version of the MMPI and the biographical information and life events forms. Although patients could choose whether or not to participate, the original MMPI was a required part of their program and for most of them the additional forms and extra items did not seem to deter participation. They were informed that their MMPI results would be used as part of their treatment planning in the program, but the other forms and any information abstracted from their charts would be kept completely confidential.

Patients were expected to complete the forms independently and return them within the first few days of the program. Although most patients completed all three forms, a minority turned in only one or two of the forms (Table 4-1). A total of 507 patients participated in the research project. Upon examination of the data, one person was eliminated because he was only thirteen years old and another four subjects were deleted because of invalidating scores on the Cannot Say scale. Other than requiring a Cannot Say score of 35 or less, no other validity criteria were used to screen out patient profiles because this study was designed to illustrate the variety of profile patterns to be found among a large chronic pain population.

The next phase, chart reviews, was conducted from September 1987 through May 1988. Charts were reviewed by a team of six judges consisting of the first author, two third-year medical students, and three undergraduate assistants who had taken courses in abnormal psychology. All had been given reading materials describing the chronic pain syndrome and assessment of chronic pain, and all had participated in rating several

TABLE 4-1. Sample Ns for Each Data Form

Sample	Bio. Info.	Life Events	Chart Review
Normative (N = 2600)	2600 (100%)	2600 (100%)	0
Chronic Pain (N = 502)	480 (96%)	479 (95%)	463 (92%)
Psychiatric (N = 423)	286 (68%)	286 (68%)	0

practice charts and discussing questions and disagreements that arose from them. Even after this training considerable interrater disagreement remained on several measures, which seemed largely a function of incomplete or inconsistent chart information. However, in some instances, the raters' lack of clinical expertise probably resulted in less accurate or useful data than might have been obtained with professional clinicians as judges, particularly in the case of psychiatric history and current psychiatric status. Raters were specifically instructed not to look at the MMPI profiles of patients if they were included in the charts, so that ratings would be made independently of MMPI results.

Chart information was sought for all patients who had completed MMPIs during their stay in the program. Of the 502 patients with usable MMPI data, charts were located for 463. The remaining 39 charts had been misfiled or misplaced and could not be located for the purposes of this research project. Data that had been collected in the early 1980s for the normative and psychiatric samples were available on the same AX form, biographical information form, and life events form used in this study. The chart data were specific to the chronic pain population, so no comparisons are possible on those variables. The life events and biographical information form data were available only for a subset of the psychiatric sample (the Hennepin County and Anoka Hospital patients), so all comparisons using those data employed only those patients. Table 4-1 summarizes the number of individuals completing each form for each sample. All subjects included in this table had complete AX form MMPI data.

Sample Comparisons on Non-MMPI Measures

Table 4-2 illustrates and contrasts the general demographic characteristics of the three patient samples used in this study, derived from the biographical information form. Compared to the normative sample, both the pain sample and the psychiatric sample are on average less educated, less likely to report managerial or professional careers, and more likely to be divorced. The pain sample tends to be more homogeneously Caucasian than the other samples, possibly an artifact of being primarily a Minnesota sample as compared to the other two. The psychiatric sample on average is somewhat younger than the normative or pain samples and is more likely to

TABLE 4-2. Demographic Characteristics of Pain, Normative, and Psychiatric Samples

Variable	Pain (N = 502)		Normative (N = 2600)		Psychiatric (N = 423)	
Sex						
% Men (n)	53	(268)	44	(1138)	55	(232)
% Women (n)	47	(234)	56	(1462)	45	(191)
	Men	Women	Men	Women	Men	Women
Age						
Mean	39.8	40.3	41.7	40.5	31.0	33.6
S.D.	10.3	11.6	15.3	15.2	9.8	11.7
Range	18-74	19-76	18-84	17-85	16-75	18-85
Race						
% Asian	0.4	0.4	0.5	0.9	0.9	0.5
% Black	6.2	4.5	11.1	12.8	10.4	8.4
% Hispanic	1.9	0.9	3.1	2.5	0.0	0.5
% White	87.9	90.6	82.0	80.8	83.5	84.2
% Other	3.6	3.6	3.3	3.0	5.2	6.4
Education (yrs)						
Mean	11.7	12.3	15.0	14.4	12.5	12.2
S.D.	2.2	2.1	2.8	2.4	2.5	2.1
Range	3-18	3-18	3-20	2-20	2-20	6-19
Marital Status						
% Married	70.4	58.8	72.3	61.1	7.9	18.3
% Widowed	0.4	3.0	1.1	5.3	3.5	2.6
% Divorced	11.6	21.9	5.2	11.0	18.4	30.9
% Separated	4.1	3.0	2.0	2.3	5.7	8.9
% Never married	13.5	13.3	19.4	20.3	63.6	38.7
Usual Occupation						
Laborer	34.0	23.7	11.6	5.0	35.1	15.1
Clerical	2.1	16.6	3.3	22.6	5.3	20.0
Skilled craftsperson	27.0	1.4	14.5	3.5	14.2	4.9
Manager	3.3	4.3	14.8	7.5	4.9	1.1
Professional	14.1	23.2	42.2	40.0	11.6	5.9
None of above	19.5	30.8	13.6	21.3	18.2	29.7

Note: Except for age and sex, which were known for all subjects, biographical data are reported as percentages of those responding to each item. The numbers of subjects completing each form in each sample are noted in Table 4-1.

report having never been married. However, all three samples are quite heterogeneous on all variables except race, and there is considerable overlap between them on these basic demographic characteristics.

Data from the chart review form, biographical information form, and life events form were examined to provide a description of this pain clinic sample and to choose variables to be included in MMPI scale, codetype, and cluster correlate analyses described later. Appendix A illustrates the characteristics of the total group of pain patients for which information was abstracted on the chart review form (N = 463). The categories on several variables do not completely match those on the original chart form (available from the authors) because some items were recoded based on information written in by raters. Other items were excluded if raters marked them as missing or uncodable for more than half the sample. Appendix B contains the pain sample's self-description on the biographical information form.

Chart review and biographical information variables entered into the correlate analyses described later included almost all the data presented in the appendixes. However, in some cases data were combined into smaller or potentially more meaningful categories, such as coding "completion status" and "aftercare status" according to evidence of noncompliance. Extremely infrequent variables, such as whether a patient was receiving Veteran's Disability Compensation, were dropped from analyses in favor of using combined measures, such as whether the patient was receiving *any* pain-related compensation. Similarly, family-history variables were combined into larger categories such as "any first degree relative with a pain problem" rather than looking at individual family members. However, the more detailed breakdowns provided in Appendixes A and B give a good overall description of this sample's characteristics.

Further information about the characteristics of the pain sample was obtained by contrasting their performance on the biographical information form and life events form with that of the normative and psychiatric samples. No comparisons could be made on the chart review data because this information was unique to the pain sample. Tables 4-3 and 4-4 illustrate the biographical information items that were significantly different between the pain and psychiatric and the pain and normative samples, respectively. Statistics used to contrast the groups were chi-squares for nominal data, Mann-Whitney U tests for ordinal data, and t-tests for the difference between means of continuous variables. In total, the samples were compared on 39 biographical information variables, separately for each sex. Because of the large number of comparisons, the alpha level used to indicate a significant difference was set at $p < = .0012$, equivalent to an overall alpha of $< = .05$ for 39 comparisons (Bonferroni criterion, Grove & Andreasen, 1982). This procedure, followed throughout most of the analyses reported here, was designed to provide some correction for the possibility of chance relationships occurring among so many contrasts.

Appendix C includes the item-endorsement percentages on the life events items for each of the three samples, separately for each sex. Again, the Bonferroni criterion (divide desired overall alpha by number of comparisons) was used to decide which differences would be considered significant.

TABLE 4-3. Differences between Pain and Psychiatric Samples on Biographical Information Form Data

<u>Different for Both Men and Women</u>
Age (pain group older)
Education (pain group less educated)
Household income (pain group higher)
Describe self as disabled (more likely for pain group)
Receiving disability compensation income (more likely for pain group)
Currently looking for work (less likely for pain group)
Currently live in own home (more likely for pain group)
Lived most of life in city (less likely for pain group)
Have ever been given a ticket for speeding (more likely for pain group)
Have ever been arrested for other than a motor vehicle violation (less likely for pain group)
Have ever been treated for an emotional problem (less likely for pain group)
Have ever been hospitalized for emotional problems (less likely for pain group)
Currently in psychological or psychiatric treatment (less likely for pain group)
Have ever been in treatment for drug or alcohol problems (less likely for pain group)
Have had an operation or major physical illness in the last year (more likely for pain group)
Have a physical handicap (more likely for pain group)
Have used and/or had a problem with drugs (less likely for pain group)

<u>Different for Men Only</u>
Father's education (lower for pain patients)
First degree relative with history of treatment for emotional problems (pain group less likely)
Second degree relative with history of treatment for emotional problems (pain group less likely)

<u>Different for Women Only</u>
Describe self as on leave from job (pain group more likely)
Have had problems with alcohol use (pain group less likely)

Tables 4-5 and 4-6 list the text of those items that discriminated between the pain and psychiatric and the pain and normative samples. An overall measure of stressful life events during the six months before testing was computed by adding together all the separate life events items endorsed. As in many of the other variables reported in these tables, the pain sample fell between the normative and psychiatric samples on this measure. For men, the mean number of life events items was 4.1 for the normative sample, 7.8 for the pain sample, and 9.0 for the psychiatric sample. For women, the normative sample mean was 4.7, the pain group mean was 8.1, and the psychiatric sample mean was 9.7. T-tests showed the pain sample mean to differ from both other sample means at $p < = .05$.

The distributions of biographical information, chart review, and life events items suggest both the similarity of this chronic pain population to others reported in the literature and the heterogeneity apparent in such

TABLE 4-4. Differences between Pain and Normative Samples on Biographical Information Form Data

Different for Both Men and Women

Education (pain group less educated)
Total household income (pain group lower)
Currently employed (less likely for pain group)
Currently a student (less likely for pain group)
Currently on leave from job (more likely for pain group)
Describe self as disabled (more likely for pain group)
Occupation (pain group less likely to be professionals)
Receiving disability compensation income (pain group more likely)
Receiving welfare income (pain group more likely)
Father's and mother's education (pain group lower)
Father's occupation (pain group lower SES: labor rather than professional)
Lived most of life in city (pain group less likely)
Currently taking any medications prescribed by a doctor (pain group more likely)
Ever been treated for an emotional problem (pain group more likely)
Currently in psychological or psychiatric treatment (pain group more likely)
Ever been hospitalized for emotional problems (pain group more likely)
Ever been in treatment for drug or alcohol problems (pain group more likely)
Had an operation or major physical illness in the last year (pain group more likely)
Have a physical handicap (pain group more likely)
Last time visited a physician (pain group more recent)
Drug use: pain group more likely to deny history of recreational use, but also more
    likely to admit history of problems with drug use
Alcohol use: pain group more likely to deny social use, but more likely to have had
    problems with alcohol
First degree family member treated for chemical dependency problems (pain group
    more likely)

Different for Men Only

Currently retired (less likely for pain group)
Receiving pension income (pain group less likely)
Ever been given a ticket for speeding (more likely for pain group)
Ever been arrested for anything other than a motor vehicle violation (pain group more
    likely)

populations. The characteristics of the Sister Kenny average patient closely matched those summarized in the literature review: most of these patients were white, lower SES, high-school educated or less, married with families, and were in their prime working years. They tended to come from fairly large families, had working-class parents, and rather large minorities had parents, siblings, or spouses with chronic illness, pain, or chemical dependency problems. The average Sister Kenny patient was injured on the job, quit or changed jobs as a result of pain, was receiving disability compensation for his or her pain problem, had pain lasting several years and had been unemployed for over a year, had a primary complaint of back pain, but also complained of several other pain sites. He or she had

TABLE 4-5. Life Events Items Discriminating Pain from Normative Sample

Different for Both Men and Women
Personal injury or illness
Sexual difficulties
Change in financial status
Change in number of arguments with family members
Unable to pay mortgage or loan
Change in living conditions
Change of personal habits
Change in recreation
Change in social activities
Change in sleeping habits
Change in number of family outings or holidays
Change in eating habits

Different for Men Only
Marital separation
Trouble with in-laws

Different for Women Only
Change in health of family member
Business difficulties or loss
Son or daughter leaving home

Note: All differences were in the direction of greater life stress for the pain sample.

TABLE 4-6. Life Events Items Discriminating Pain from Psychiatric Sample

Different for Both Men and Women
Fired from job
Change in living conditions
Change in residence
Minor violations of the law

Different for Men Only
Jail term
Business difficulties or loss
Begin or end school

Different for Women Only
Pregnancy
Change in schools

Note: All differences were in the direction of greater life stress for the psychiatric sample.

received numerous forms of treatment before entering the pain program, and was suffering from depression along with the physical complaints.

The variety of responses to some of the items supports the hypothesis that treatment-relevant subgroups exist within this patient population. For example, about 20% of the patients still had litigation pending at the time of their admission to the program, which could potentially affect their motivation for improvement. About half the sample was considered depressed enough to warrant treatment with antidepressant medications, and sizable groups had histories of treatment and even hospitalization for emotional problems. Alcohol abuse and narcotic dependency were salient issues for large subsets of the sample, and others had histories of behavior suggesting antisocial tendencies.

Comparisons of the pain sample with the normative and psychiatric groups suggested that the pain sample falls between these two on a continuum of distress and life disruption. It should be noted that although pain patients are often described as denying emotional and psychological distress, this group as a whole admitted to significantly greater histories of emotional problems, mental-health treatment, chemical dependency problems, and even family histories of psychiatric and chemical dependency problems than the normative sample. In terms of stressful life events, the pain sample actually scored as more similar to the psychiatric patients than to the normative sample, suggesting that they view their lives as full of changes and upheaval. None of these factors was as extreme as in the psychiatric sample, with the predictable exception of complaints about physical illness and disability.

In general, these forms and comparisons provided data that support the similarity of this chronic pain sample to those from other inpatient multidisciplinary programs reported in the literature. However, it should be noted that generalizability of research results found in this study will be affected by the degree of similarity of new samples to this research population. Thus, the extensive sample description included in this chapter and the appendixes was designed to facilitate comparisons and allow the reader to assess the applicability of these MMPI-2 findings to his/her own patient population.

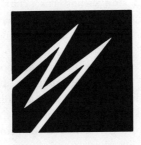

Chapter 5

Chronic Pain and the MMPI-2: Empirical Analyses

In this chapter, we report a number of empirical analyses designed to delineate the self-report personality characteristics of chronic pain patients as assessed by the MMPI-2. First, descriptive aspects of the pain patients' responses on the MMPI-2 norms were contrasted with the original MMPI norms to determine if similar patterns occur on both forms of the test. The MMPI-2 clinical, validity, and supplementary scales were contrasted for various pain patient subgroups to determine if such variables influence MMPI-2 patterns.

Next, the analyses addressed differences between chronic pain patients, psychiatric inpatients, and the normative sample to determine how well the MMPI-2 can differentiate between populations with different characteristics and degrees of psychopathology.

Finally, analyses were performed to determine how the MMPI-2 can be employed to separate chronic pain patients into more homogeneous subgroups, and to determine whether these groups correlate with other treatment-relevant information.

Characteristics of Chronic Pain MMPI-2 Mean Profiles

Mean Profiles Using MMPI-2 and Original MMPI T Scores

Mean profiles for men and women were computed using MMPI-2 scoring and T-score conversions, and were compared to the profiles obtained using the original MMPI norms and T scores (Hathaway & Briggs, 1957). The differences between these two methods include slightly longer versions of several scales in the original scoring, a different set of norms against which profiles are compared, and a different method of converting raw scores to T scores. The total group mean profiles for each method, separately for each sex, are presented in Figures 5-1 and 5-2. Both systems use K-corrected scores because all previous studies have used K-corrections and there are no data available suggesting that omission of the K-correction would improve predictive accuracy of profiles within the chronic pain population.

Although the mean profiles shown in Figures 5-1 and 5-2 illustrate that the new norms and T-score conversions result in a generally lower profile, the overall shape of the profiles was maintained from the MMPI to the MMPI-2. The mean distributions for men and women as scored by old norms correspond to the neurotic-triad or hypochondriasis profile often found in studies of average chronic pain profiles. The profile is marked by secondary elevations on Pd, Pt, and Sc, again matching the configurations found in previous studies. This provides further support for the

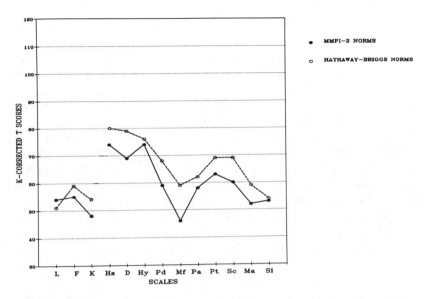

FIGURE 5-1. Mean MMPI Profile for Chronic Pain Men, Hathaway-Briggs Norms vs. MMPI-2 Norms

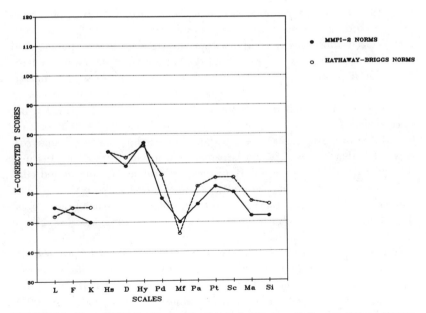

FIGURE 5-2. Mean MMPI Profile for Chronic Pain Women, Hathaway-Briggs Norms vs. MMPI-2 Norms

comparability of the Sister Kenny population to other chronic pain program samples previously reported in the literature.

At first glance, the change from old to new norms seems to reduce the clinically elevated scales from Hs, D, and Hy to only Hs and Hy, which could result in underinterpreting the degree of depression and distress associated with a client's somatic preoccupation. However, the MMPI-2 Restandardization Committee (Butcher, Dahlstrom, Graham, Tellegen, & Kaemmer, 1989) has suggested that a T score of 65 be used as the clinically elevated cutoff point for the new norms, as opposed to a T score of 70 on the old Hathaway-Briggs norms. If this criterion is used, the MMPI-2 mean chronic pain profile matches the original mean MMPI profile in having a neurotic-triad pattern of scores for both sexes, even though their relative elevation has shifted slightly. Indeed, if the interpretive range is lowered by 5 T-score points, for interpretive purposes the two versions of the mean profiles are virtually identical. With the exception of that shift in elevation, there seems to be good continuity between the old and new versions of the MMPI in summarizing the average of a large group of chronic pain patients. The data in this study support the $T> = 65$ interpretation cutoff.

Effect of Subgrouping Variables on Mean Profiles

Because researchers have suggested that mean chronic pain profiles may differ according to some basic subgrouping variables, profiles were contrasted according to sex, compensation status, whether the patient had litigation in process, site of pain, and the chronicity of the pain problem. Entire profiles of scores were contrasted by using a multivariate analysis of variance (MANOVA) with the scale scores as dependent variables and the subgrouping variables as factors. All analyses were performed using K-corrected T scores. Although Butcher and Tellegen (1978) have suggested that in most cases raw scores should be used for statistical analyses, it was felt that T scores would be more appropriate in this case because they provide direct comparability to the way profiles are interpreted clinically. In addition, the new uniform T scores provide more similarity of scale distributions across scales within the profile than is true of raw scores, thus reducing the possibility of one long scale carrying more weight in analyses than shorter scales.

In comparing male (N = 268) and female (N = 234) mean profiles, the Mf scale was left out of the analysis because it would by definition separate the groups. Even so, the MANOVA results indicated that the male and female profiles differed significantly (p value for Hotelling's $T^2 = .003$). However, examination of the univariate F-tests for individual scales revealed that only two (scales K and Hs) differed significantly at $p< = .05$.

As can be seen by comparing Figures 5-1 and 5-2, these differences were actually quite small: 2 points apart on K and 3 points on Hs.

Despite the lack of large differences between the mean profiles of men and women, all subsequent analyses in this and remaining sections were run separately by gender. Because chronic pain has been considered to be largely influenced and maintained by psychosocial factors, which are likely to differ for men and women in this society, it seems most reasonable to examine the sexes separately.

Other subgrouping variables examined were: 1) whether or not the patient was receiving any disability compensation related to the pain problem; 2) whether or not the patient still had litigation pending when he or she entered the program; 3) primary site of pain (back vs. neck/shoulder vs. headache vs. extremity vs. abdominal/pelvic); 4) whether the patient had ever had surgery for the pain problem; and 5) length of the pain problem (less than 2 years vs. 2 to 5 years vs. 6 to 10 years vs. 11 years or more). Because none of these comparisons of overall profiles was significant at $p < = .05$ for either sex, no further exploration of individual scale differences was considered justified.

Although some of the previous research in this area has suggested that mean pain profiles may differ according to some relatively simple subgrouping variables, results from this sample did not support this prediction. The one significant difference was found between sexes, and this seemed mostly to be an artifact of large sample size rather than a finding that would result in clinically meaningful interpretive differences.

The similarity of mean profiles across primary site of pain does fit with previous studies that find the same elevation of neurotic-triad scores across chronic pain subpopulations. Indeed, it would be surprising to find too many differences considering that the majority of patients complained of several other pain sites in addition to their primary complaint. However, it does seem somewhat surprising that chronicity or severity of the pain problem, as measured both by history of surgery and by length of the patient's difficulties, was not associated with more elevated profiles as had been found in previous studies. A possible explanation is that *all* of these patients had pain of sufficient duration to have achieved "chronic" profiles; certainly the majority of the sample had experienced major life disruptions for at least several months before entering the program. This is not the type of sample that might be seen at an outpatient clinic; they had already been through the gamut of conservative treatments for pain.

The lack of differences between mean profiles on the compensation and litigation variables accords with more recent literature on these patient subgroups. This is an important finding, supporting the contention that, at least among patients in a chronic pain program, no "litigation profile" can be clearly distinguished from the majority of patients complaining of chronic pain. This is not to say that the MMPI-2 is of no use in suggesting the influence of secondary gain issues. Secondary gain is probably a more complicated concept among these patients than simply whether or not financial reinforcement is available. In addition, it must be kept in mind that obviously malingering or psychopathic individuals had been selected out of this population during the admission process. If the MMPI had been given to all applicants, more differences might have emerged.

Content and Supplementary Scale Scores

Summary statistics were computed in the male and female total samples for all of the newly developed content scales as well as for four commonly used supplementary scales (A, R, Es, and MAC). Scales A and R were developed by Welsh (1956) and correspond to the first two factors in the MMPI, commonly referred to as Anxiety and Repression. Scale Es was developed by Barron (1953) to discriminate between neurotic patients who responded to psychotherapy versus those who did not; it is referred to as Ego Strength. MAC, the MacAndrew alcoholism scale, was developed to discriminate between alcoholic and nonalcoholic psychiatric outpatients; it has since proven useful as a broader measure of addiction potential (MacAndrew, 1965; see also Graham, 1987 for further discussion of all these scales). Table 5-1 summarizes by sex the distributions of the standard validity and clinical scales, new content scales, and four supplementary scales. Although these are the only scales to be considered further here, Appendix D presents distribution information on some other MMPI supplementary scales and subscales for comparison with other studies or for use in future research.

Figures 5-3 and 5-4 present the mean profiles of content-scale scores for male and female patients, respectively. As was done with the standard validity and clinical-scale profiles, content-scale profiles were compared across subgroups broken out by sex, compensation status, litigation status, length of pain problem, whether the patient had received surgery for his or her problem, and site of primary pain complaint. Again, only the comparison across genders resulted in a significant overall MANOVA (p-value for Hotelling's $T^2 < .001$). Examination of univariate F-tests for each scale showed three to be significantly different for men and women at $p < = .05$: Anger (ANG, $p = .002$), Antisocial Practices (ASP, $p < .001$), and Cynicism (CYN, $p < .001$). Comparison of the mean profiles in Figures 5-3 and 5-4 reveals that all of these differences were in the direction of the men having more elevated scores compared to the norms for their sex. However, none of the differences exceeded 5 T-score points.

Examination of the scale distributions in Table 5-1 and the mean content-scale profiles in Figures 5-3 and 5-4 gives much the same picture of the average chronic pain profile as was found with validity and clinical scales

TABLE 5-1. Chronic Pain Sample Scale Statistics (T Scores)

Scale	Men (N = 268)					Women (N = 234)				
	Mean	SD	Median	Min	Max	Mean	SD	Median	Min	Max
Validity Scales										
CS	49.4	7.9	47	47	118	51.4	11.7	47	47	120
L	53.6	10.0	52	35	96	55.1	9.6	57	33	86
F	55.2	13.2	51	36	120	53.3	11.0	51	37	96
K	48.0	10.6	47	30	77	49.9	10.4	50	30	78
Clinical Scales										
Hs	74.5	10.8	75	35	110	74.3	11.0	74	46	101
D	68.5	12.3	68	38	102	69.4	14.1	68	40	105
Hy	74.0	13.6	74	45	119	77.1	12.9	77	43	113
Pd	59.2	12.0	59	34	90	58.4	11.8	58	32	94
Mf	46.2	9.0	46	30	79	50.3	9.1	50	30	84
Pa	58.0	13.8	57	32	112	56.5	12.0	56	31	96
Pt	62.5	14.1	62	34	113	62.4	12.0	62	34	92
Sc	60.3	14.2	58	31	120	60.4	11.6	60	33	96
Ma	51.9	10.9	51	31	94	51.5	11.2	49	31	82
Si	53.1	11.6	52	31	90	52.1	11.3	51	30	79
New Content Scales										
ANX	60.6	12.2	60	35	92	60.2	12.1	59	34	86
FRS	52.2	10.4	51	35	97	51.8	10.9	51	31	91
OBS	53.4	11.5	50	33	84	51.7	10.3	50	32	83
DEP	61.5	12.2	59	36	99	60.5	11.0	59	39	88
HEA	70.3	11.6	70	37	103	68.5	11.4	68	36	100
BIZ	52.4	11.1	51	39	94	51.8	9.5	52	39	84
ANG	55.6	11.9	53	32	86	52.4	10.7	52	31	84
CYN	52.4	10.7	51	32	83	49.0	9.5	48	32	77
ASP	52.5	11.2	51	30	94	48.0	8.8	47	33	75
TPA	50.9	10.5	50	30	89	49.9	10.1	48	33	86
LSE	55.5	12.3	53	35	101	55.8	11.6	54	35	92
SOD	51.7	11.4	49	32	89	50.7	10.0	49	32	77
FAM	52.8	11.5	50	33	88	51.5	10.5	50	32	89
WRK	58.8	11.9	57	36	92	57.8	12.0	57	34	88
TRT	56.7	12.1	54	35	94	55.0	11.1	53	35	97
Supplementary Scales										
A	56.7	12.7	54	36	89	55.5	11.4	55	35	80
R	53.5	10.2	52	32	83	55.5	10.1	54	31	83
Es	38.9	9.0	36	30	65	39.3	8.8	39	30	68
MAC	55.0	10.3	53	30	83	52.1	10.3	53	30	86

Note: Scales Hs, D, Hy, Pd, Pa, Pt, Sc, Ma, and new content scales ANX to TRT are all reported as uniform T scores. All other scales are linear T scores. Clinical scales are K-corrected.

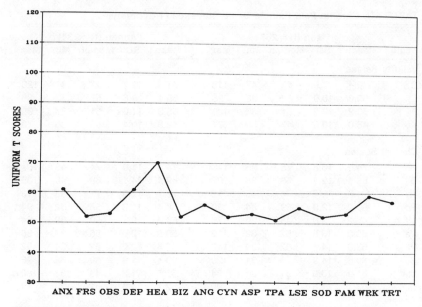

FIGURE 5-3. Content-Scale Mean Profile for Chronic Pain Men (N = 268)

alone. Among the content scales, the only scale elevated above a T score of 65 for either sex is HEA, Health Concerns. The item content in this scale shows up in the clinical scales as contributing to elevations on Hs and Hy. As would be predicted from the clinical scale profile, secondary peaks on the content scale profile appear for scales containing anxious (ANX) and depressive (DEP) item content. This corresponds closely to the Hs, D, Hy configuration with a subclinical elevation on Pt shown in the clinical profiles and confirms that those elevations indeed reflect content appropriate to the scale names. The slight elevation on Work Interference (WRK), a scale designed to measure a variety of item content relevant to poor work adjustment, certainly seems expectable and accurate in this population, as well as the lesser peaks on LSE (Low Self-Esteem) and TRT (Negative Treatment Indicators). On the supplementary scales, both men and women scored more than one standard deviation below the normative sample mean on the Ego Strength scale, which could fit the image of these patients as non-psychologically minded and rather passive/dependent in their approach to life. Overall, however, it is interesting that this sample deviated very little from the national normative group except on measures of preoccupation with health. Indeed, the women as a group actually scored slightly *lower* than the normative female sample on measures of cynicism and antisocial attitudes (CYN and ASP), perhaps reflecting some of the naïveté and conformity often associated with elevations on Hy.

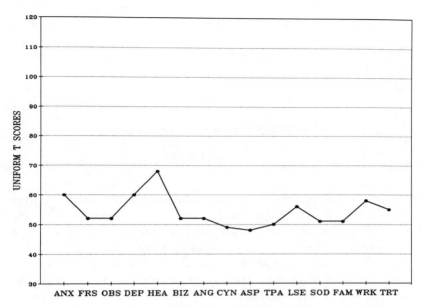

FIGURE 5-4. Content-Scale Mean Profile for Chronic Pain Women (N = 234)

The lack of content-scale-profile differences across subgrouping variables such as litigation status and pain chronicity parallels the results found with the clinical scales. These breakdowns seem to be either too simplistic or unrelated to personality patterns as measured by the MMPI-2 in this population. The differences across sex are small, but correspond to the first author's subjective impression when reading charts that the men in the sample tended to be more embroiled in conflictual relationships with employers or the compensation system than the average woman in the sample. It is impossible to know from these data whether the men had histories of more antisocial behavior or anger problems than the normative sample before their pain onset, or whether their elevations on Anger, Antisocial Practices, and Cynicism scales reflect their experience combating the medical, compensation, and/or employment systems.

Examination of mean profiles on the content scales supports their usefulness as a supplement to the clinical scales, serving to confirm the type of content reflected in elevations on the content-heterogeneous clinical scales. It also provides further confirmation that this sample as a whole is quite similar to others summarized in the literature via average profiles. However, Table 5-1 illustrates how inappropriate it would be to assume that all chronic pain patients conform to this averaged personality description. Scores on individual scales ranged from as low as 30 to as high as 120, the full range of T scores possible on the MMPI-2. The standard deviations for most of the scales were higher than those in the entire normative sample, suggesting that this sample is even more heterogeneous than a large group of people randomly solicited from around the country. These results strongly suggest the need to explore possible subgroups among the pain patient population, as will be discussed later.

Comparison of MMPI-2 Results across Samples

Profiles and Scale Distributions

Description of the average chronic pain patient MMPI-2 profile was further refined by comparing profiles and individual scale distributions to the psychiatric sample and the normative sample. Tables 5-2 and 5-3 present the mean T scores by sex and sample for clinical and content scales, respectively. Comparisons of the mean clinical and content-scale profiles of the pain and psychiatric samples can be found in Appendix E. The pain patients' mean clinical-scale profile and mean content-scale profile were each compared, using multivariate analyses of variance, to those of the normative sample and those of the psychiatric sample, separately for each sex. All comparisons were based on T-score distributions, K-corrected in the case of the relevant clinical scales. All eight overall profile comparisons (pain vs. psychiatric on clinical scales by sex, pain vs. psychiatric on content scales by sex, pain vs. normative on clinical scales by sex, and pain vs. normative on content scales by sex) were highly significant (p-value for Hotelling's $T^2 < .001$).

The particular scales contributing to these differences varied somewhat, although with such large samples even small mean differences were statistically significant. For example, in comparing the male pain sample with the male normative sample, all clinical scales were significantly different at $p < .05$ even though the means might differ by as little as 3 T-score points. On the content-scale profile, the male pain and normative samples differed significantly on all scales except Type A (TPA). Differences on both profiles were in the direction of greater elevations for the pain sample, with the exception of scales K and Mf. For the women, the pain and normative samples differed on all mean clinical-scale scores except K and Mf, and on all content scales except Social Discomfort (SOD), Type A (TPA), and Cynicism (CYN). Again, differences were almost entirely in the direction of the pain sample having higher elevations than the normative sample.

Differences on individual validity, clinical, and content scales between the pain and psychiatric samples were significant for all scales except L, D, and ANG (Anger) for the men and L and D for the women. For the content scales all of these differences were in the direction of higher scores

TABLE 5-2. Clinical Scale T-Score Distributions (K-Corrected), Pain Sample vs. Normative and Psychiatric Samples

Scale		Men (N = 268)			Women (N = 234)		
		Pain	Norms	Psych	Pain	Norms	Psych
L	Mean	53.6	50.0	52.2	55.1	50.0	53.1
	S.D.	10.0	9.9	11.1	9.6	9.9	12.9
F	Mean	55.2	49.9	78.7	53.3	50.0	81.0
	S.D.	13.2	10.1	25.6	11.0	10.0	24.3
K	Mean	48.0	50.0	46.1	49.9	50.0	44.9
	S.D.	10.6	9.9	11.1	10.4	9.8	10.4
Hs	Mean	74.5	50.0	61.4	74.3	50.0	60.2
	S.D.	10.8	10.0	13.6	11.0	9.9	13.9
D	Mean	68.5	50.0	67.9	69.4	49.9	67.6
	S.D.	12.3	9.9	15.9	14.1	9.9	16.3
Hy	Mean	74.0	50.2	62.1	77.1	50.0	61.1
	S.D.	13.6	10.1	15.7	12.9	10.0	15.3
Pd	Mean	59.2	50.0	70.0	58.4	50.0	69.7
	S.D.	12.0	10.0	15.2	11.8	9.9	14.3
Mf	Mean	46.2	50.1	54.5	50.3	50.1	53.6
	S.D.	9.0	10.0	10.6	9.1	9.9	11.1
Pa	Mean	58.0	50.1	73.7	56.5	50.0	73.2
	S.D.	13.8	10.1	20.5	12.0	10.0	21.3
Pt	Mean	62.5	50.1	72.1	62.4	50.1	67.3
	S.D.	14.1	10.0	18.5	12.0	9.9	16.0
Sc	Mean	60.3	50.1	77.6	60.4	49.9	73.9
	S.D.	14.2	10.0	21.3	11.6	9.9	18.7
Ma	Mean	51.9	50.0	59.2	51.5	50.1	57.4
	S.D.	10.9	10.0	13.7	11.2	10.0	14.1
Si	Mean	53.1	49.9	59.6	52.1	50.0	59.3
	S.D.	11.6	10.0	13.3	11.3	9.9	11.0

for the psychiatric sample, with the exception of the pain sample's peak on HEA (Health Concerns). The psychiatric patients also scored higher than the pain patients on all validity and clinical scales except L, K, Hs, D, and Hy.

Comparison of the three samples' average profiles continued to support the view of pain patients as more distressed and dysfunctional than the normative sample, but reporting fewer psychiatric problems than an inpatient psychiatric sample. While it is not surprising to find that in general the pain sample reported greater physical distress and less emotional distress than the psychiatric sample, it *is* somewhat surprising to

TABLE 5-3. Content Scale T-Score Distributions, Pain Sample vs. Normative and Psychiatric Samples

Scale		Men			Women		
		Pain	Norms	Psych	Pain	Norms	Psych
ANX	Mean	60.6	50.0	65.1	60.2	49.9	64.5
	S.D.	12.2	9.8	14.5	12.1	10.0	14.0
FRS	Mean	52.2	50.0	58.1	51.8	50.0	59.0
	S.D.	10.4	10.0	15.3	10.9	9.9	13.2
OBS	Mean	53.4	49.8	59.6	51.7	50.0	61.9
	S.D.	11.5	9.8	13.8	10.3	9.8	13.5
DEP	Mean	61.5	50.2	70.3	60.5	49.9	68.4
	S.D.	12.2	10.0	16.0	11.0	10.0	14.8
HEA	Mean	70.3	50.0	61.7	68.5	50.0	61.8
	S.D.	11.6	10.0	15.1	11.4	9.9	14.9
BIZ	Mean	52.4	50.0	66.4	51.8	50.3	67.7
	S.D.	11.1	9.7	19.9	9.5	9.7	17.8
ANG	Mean	55.6	50.0	56.9	52.4	49.9	57.9
	S.D.	11.9	9.9	12.2	10.7	9.8	13.9
CYN	Mean	52.4	50.0	56.6	49.0	50.0	57.9
	S.D.	10.7	10.0	12.8	9.5	9.8	12.1
ASP	Mean	52.5	50.0	58.6	48.0	49.9	59.4
	S.D.	11.2	9.9	12.7	8.8	9.9	13.0
TPA	Mean	50.9	49.9	53.7	49.9	49.8	57.2
	S.D.	10.5	9.9	12.8	10.1	9.9	13.6
LSE	Mean	55.5	50.0	64.5	55.8	50.0	63.7
	S.D.	12.3	10.0	14.8	11.6	9.9	14.7
SOD	Mean	51.7	49.9	57.9	50.7	50.0	57.1
	S.D.	11.4	10.0	13.1	10.0	9.9	10.8
FAM	Mean	52.8	50.1	65.0	51.5	49.9	64.3
	S.D.	11.5	9.9	15.8	10.5	9.8	13.8
WRK	Mean	58.8	50.0	65.1	57.8	50.0	65.3
	S.D.	11.9	9.9	14.8	12.0	9.9	15.0
TRT	Mean	56.7	50.0	65.3	55.0	50.0	65.9
	S.D.	12.1	10.0	16.2	11.1	9.9	15.2

find that the Depression (D) scale distributions were largely the same in these two samples. Rather than denying depression or expressing it solely through somatic preoccupation, this large group of pain patients reported the same degree of affective distress as a group of patients who had been hospitalized specifically for psychiatric problems. Examination of the Har-

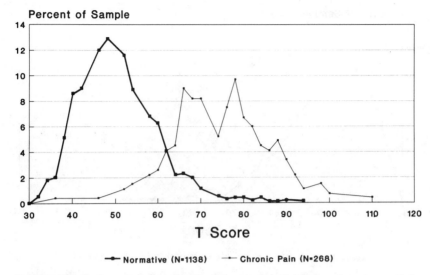

FIGURE 5-5. Uniform T-Score Distributions for Hs, Normative Sample vs. Pain Sample (Men)

ris-Lingoes subscales shown in Appendix D confirms that the D scale elevation for pain patients is not merely an artifact of their multiple physical complaints; the average pain patient scored high on subscales of subjective depression and mental dullness as well. Examination of the subscales of the Hysteria (Hy) scale also tends to refute the image of the average pain patient as denying all emotional distress; while the Hy elevation is largely composed of somatic items and "lassitude-malaise" items, the sample as a whole did not obtain high scores on the "inhibition of aggression," "denial of social anxiety," or "need for affection" subscales.

For most of the scales compared across samples, significant differences were obtained even though average scale means differed very little. The clinical significance of these differences was examined by superimposing plots of the different samples' distribution of scores on each of the scales. For example, Figure 5-5 contrasts the normative and pain sample men's score distributions on their most discrepant clinical scale, Hs. Figure 5-6 shows the women's distribution of the content scale showing the most discrepancy, HEA (Health Concerns), with the addition of the psychiatric sample's distribution. In contrast, Figure 5-7 shows the pain vs. normative and psychiatric distributions of Pa for men, a scale for which the distributions largely overlap. Because in all these comparisons, the relative scale distributions looked very similar for men and for women, only one gender will be illustrated. For the majority of clinical and content scales, distributional comparisons approximated the shapes shown for Pa in Figure

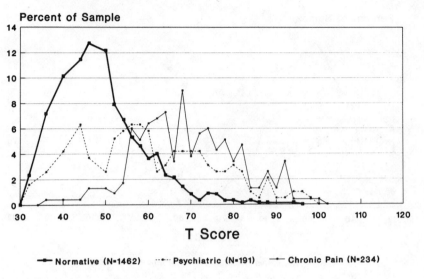

FIGURE 5-6. Uniform T-Score Distributions for HEA, Normative Sample vs. Psychiatric and Pain Samples (Women)

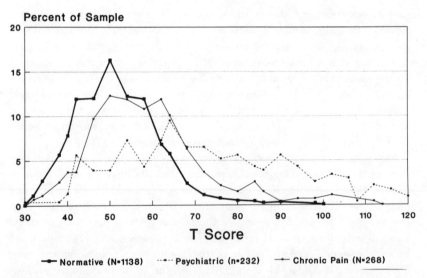

FIGURE 5-7. Uniform T-Score Distributions for Pa, Normative Sample vs. Psychiatric and Pain Samples (Men)

5-7: the pain sample scored slightly higher than the normative sample, the psychiatric sample higher than either other sample, and a large degree of overlap occurred between the pain sample and the other two. The only

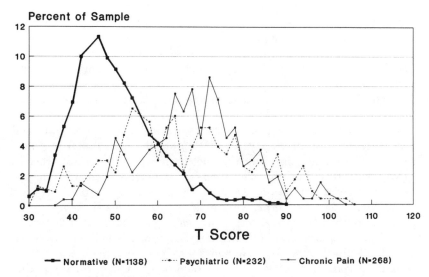

FIGURE 5-8. Uniform T-Score Distributions for D, Normative Sample vs. Psychiatric and Pain Samples (Men)

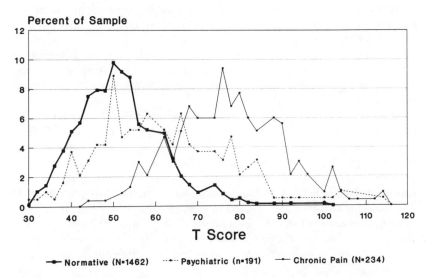

FIGURE 5-9. Uniform T-Score Distributions for Hy, Normative Sample vs. Psychiatric and Pain Samples (Women)

exceptions to this pattern were on the neurotic-triad scales of Hs (Figure 5-5), D (Figure 5-8), and Hy (Figure 5-9), and on the content scale HEA (Figure 5-6). For scales Hs, Hy, and HEA, the distribution of scores for pain patients was shifted well to the right of either the normative or psychiatric distributions. For scale D, the pain sample's distribution closely approximated both the range and shape of the psychiatric sample distribution, compared with the normative sample's lower scores on this scale. Because of the similarity of many of the distributions, only these comparisons will be illustrated here. The mean scores in Tables 5-2 and 5-3 illustrate the general characteristics of the other scale distributions across samples.

These results clearly show that scales measuring somatic complaints and health preoccupation (Hs, Hy, and HEA) are the most useful in differentiating the chronic pain group as a whole from other populations, whereas MMPI scales that were originally designed to differentiate other psychiatric disorders from a normative population do not clearly separate the pain group from either the normative sample or the psychiatric sample. The pain group provides a good test of the validity of the MMPI-2 somatic preoccupation scales, and in this case clearly supports their effectiveness. Examination of Figures 5-5, 5-6, and 5-9 suggests that the best cutoff for clinical interpretation of these scales should be lower than 70, supporting the MMPI Restandardization Committee's recommendation (Butcher, Dahlstrom et al. 1989) that a T score of 65 be used as the cutoff for interpreting elevations on the MMPI-2 as clinically deviant. However, It must be noted that without a medical population for comparison, elevations on these scales can be interpreted only in terms of preoccupation with somatic problems and a tendency to complain of physical distress compared to the normative population. This is not the comparison that is needed to differentiate potential chronic pain patients from other medical patients. A study using a medical patient control group will be needed to address this issue.

Although other scales are not particularly useful in differentiating the pain population from the comparison groups used here, they may be useful in subdividing the pain patients themselves. The preceding results suggest the MMPI-2 may prove useful in differentiating potential chronic pain patients from other patients, but further research with more appropriate control groups is needed. Another important issue is whether a group of pain patients can be differentiated into subgroups within the larger population. The range of scores shown across all the clinical and content scales suggests this may be the case; some patients score very much like the normative sample while others score close to the extremes of the psychiatric sample, depending on the scale. This supports the need to examine heterogeneity within scales and configural patterns, which will be reported below in the analyses of pain subgroups.

Item-Level Comparisons

The content of MMPI-2 items distinguishing the three samples was examined further by comparing the individual item-endorsement frequencies across the normative, pain, and psychiatric groups. Appendixes F and G list the item-endorsement percentages for all 567 items in all three samples for men and women, respectively. The pain sample endorsement percentages were compared with the psychiatric and normative samples separately. Appendixes H through K illustrate which items differed the most between samples.

Examination of the content of items differing in endorsement between the samples suggests that compared to the normative sample, pain patients seemed to be reporting a combination of somatic complaints, depressive and anxious content, and difficulty finding the energy or concentration to perform usual tasks. As a group, they were notably *not* reporting a high degree of family conflict, antisocial behavior or attitudes, or paranoid/psychotic symptoms. These areas of content served to differentiate them from the psychiatric sample, who tended to endorse such items more frequently. In contrast, items dealing with depressive content did not show up in the list of content differentiating psychiatric and pain groups, except for the extremes of suicidal ideation and intent. Thus, information derived from item-level comparisons was consistent with results of scale and profile comparisons.

The analyses presented examined the average characteristics of the total group of chronic pain patients in comparison to nonpain samples. Further research will be necessary to establish when the MMPI-2 is useful in screening a heterogeneous population for potential chronic pain problems. The preceding results support the continuity of research using the MMPI to the MMPI-2 and suggest some general characteristics of pain patients' responses on this test. However, this study does not directly address the issue of screening for functional contributions to pain problems owing to the lack of a medical patient control group and the relative homogeneity of the Sister Kenny population: all patients were selected because they had chronic multifactorial problems judged to be suitable for a multidisciplinary reactivation program.

Analyses of Chronic Pain Subgroups

Another possible use of the MMPI-2 is to help in subgrouping patients within an already selected chronic pain population, in order to most appropriately match treatment components to particular patients. The point in the assessment process at which this is done varies by program. Many use the MMPI to screen all referrals, whereas others, such as Sister Kenny Institute, use it *after* admission to add or confirm information about the patient's needs within their treatment and aftercare programs. Since the population has already been screened and selected as appropriate for the

Sister Kenny program, it is obvious that these patients will be more homogeneous in many ways than a population being screened at a general
medical clinic. Nevertheless, the hope of researchers using MMPI scale,
codetype, and cluster analyses has been that these patients can be differentiated along treatment-relevant dimensions. The subgrouping analyses
presented here represent attempts to replicate and expand that literature
using the MMPI-2.

Subgrouping by Single Scale Elevations

Probably the simplest way to break down the total pain sample into
subgroups is by contrasting those who score high on a particular scale
with those in the rest of the sample who do not. This can also provide
information about the unique correlates of elevations on particular scales
within the sample, regardless of the scores on other scales in the profile.
Correlates of each validity, clinical, and content scale were sought by
contrasting patients scoring in the top quartile of the frequency distribution
(75th percentile or above) for that scale against all patients scoring at the
74th percentile or below. Variables contrasted between groups included the
41 life events items and the total life events score, 39 biographical information items, and 108 chart-review items. A modified Bonferroni criterion
was used to choose the alpha level to be considered significant for these
comparisons (Green, 1982). It was decided that the strict criterion of
dividing an alpha of .05 by *all* possible comparisons would result in an
overly conservative test for this exploratory study. Instead, the Bonferroni
criterion was applied separately for each scale and each source of correlate
data for that scale. Thus, for each scale the life events items were considered
significantly associated with elevations on that scale if they were significant
at $p < = .0012$, equivalent to an overall alpha of .05 divided by 41, the
total number of life events items. An alpha of .05 was considered significant
for the total life events score, since this was a summary score which should
be more reliable than single items. For the biographical information form,
variables were considered significantly associated if p was $< = .0013$, equivalent to an overall alpha of .05 divided by 39 comparisons. Associations
with the chart review form variables were considered significant if p
was $< = .0005$, equivalent to an overall alpha of .05 divided by 108
comparisons.

The statistical tests used to measure association between the various
correlate variables and group membership (high quartile vs. bottom three
quartiles) were chi-square tests for nominal variables such as history of
psychiatric hospitalization, Mann-Whitney U tests for ordinal data such
as the chart-review rating scales, and t-tests for ratio data such as age,
education, or Beck Depression Inventory scores. Appendixes L and M

summarize the items found to correlate significantly with scores in the upper quartile of each of the validity, clinical, content, and supplementary scales.

The correlates presented in Appendixes L and M provide some evidence that the MMPI-2 can identify psychopathology even within this highly homogeneous sample. However, they also demonstrate a lack of specificity for most of the MMPI-2 scales when studied in this manner. Various indicators of depression tended to correlate with almost all MMPI-2 measures of psychopathology, suggesting that variability on many of the MMPI-2 scales reflects differences in general level of distress and dysphoria rather than the symptoms found to be specific to each scale in more heterogeneous populations. The MMPI-2 scales designed to measure depression, anxiety, and low self-esteem (D, Pt, ANX, DEP, LSE, A) seem useful in identifying patients who have or have had difficulty with depressive symptoms, and in general this seems to be the major dimension along which patients varied in this sample. For example, elevations on the new content scales Work Interference (WRK) and Negative Treatment Indicators (TRT), designed to identify patients likely to have problems with work or treatment, correlated positively with non-MMPI-2 measures of depression, and Es (Ego strength) correlated negatively with indicators of psychopathology. Unfortunately, treatment outcome data in this sample were quite limited, so it is not possible to judge whether these correlations accurately predict a negative effect of depression on subsequent treatment outcome and work adjustment. Another smaller group of correlate data to emerge was the association of history of various characterologic problems (alcohol and drug use, arrest history, violence) with scales Pd, Ma (men only), Antisocial Practices (ASP), Anger (ANG), and MacAndrew (MAC). This suggests that the MMPI-2 can identify these potential problems even within a patient population that had been screened to exclude individuals with blatantly psychopathic characteristics. However, it was not possible to determine whether for specific patients these elevations reflected current difficulties or past history information.

These results are likely to underestimate the amount of patient information associated with MMPI-2 scale elevations, because of the self-report nature of much of the potential correlate data and the possible unreliability or inaccuracy of ratings and outcome data culled from charts, along with the strict significance criteria used in analyses. While this allows great confidence in the significant correlates that *did* emerge, it does not allow for conclusions in the opposite direction—that particular patient characteristics are *not* associated with MMPI-2 performance. Some items were simply too infrequent in this population to result in strong associations. Others were probably not routinely noted in charts. For example, the lack of a note indicating a history of psychotic symptoms may not necessarily mean the patient did not have such a history. This could make for rather muddy comparison groups, attenuating associations with the MMPI-2 scales. On the other hand, measures that did show strong associations such as the Beck Depression Inventory were routinely given to almost all patients and the results were clearly noted in the charts.

Subgrouping patients by single scale elevations is also likely to result in a lack of differential correlates across scales because the scales themselves are intercorrelated. For example, patients scoring in the top quartile of Pt are likely to also have high scores on D and even Sc. Thus, by contrasting high scorers with low scorers, correlates will emerge that relate to these other scales as well as specifically to Pt. While it seems apparent that depressive symptoms are of major importance in differentiating groups of pain patients, it is possible that another method of subgrouping might find other important sources of variance as well. Thus, codetype and cluster analyses were conducted to group patients according to their patterns of scores across scales.

Subgrouping by Codetypes

The most common method of examining subtypes of MMPI profiles is by grouping them according to the pattern of most elevated scales, or code-types. Two major questions were addressed through codetype analyses. The first was whether and how the MMPI-2 differs from the MMPI in this population, and the second was how the MMPI-2 may be useful in providing information about chronic pain patients. Codetype analyses were designed to describe the variety of profile types found in this sample, assess the consistency of MMPI-2 codes with those that would have been found using the original MMPI, and examine correlates of the most common MMPI-2 codetypes.

The pain sample's profiles were broken down by highest clinical scale in the profile, regardless of elevation. Appendix N presents the frequency of profiles with each highpoint using MMPI-2 norms vs. Hathaway and Briggs (1957) norms. Correspondence was measured by the percentage of profiles with a given highpoint using MMPI-2 norms that would have had that same highpoint using the original MMPI norms. It was found that 64% of the men and 78% of the women would have obtained the same highest scale on the original MMPI as they had on the MMPI-2.

Since profiles are interpreted according to elevation and pattern of scales, not just by the highest scale in the profile, all patients' test protocols were assigned a codetype based on the highest clinically elevated scales in the profile. Traditionally, a T-score cutoff of 70 and above has been used to identify clinically elevated scales on the MMPI. Using this criterion, 94% of the men and 90% of the women had at least one clinically elevated scale when scored by original MMPI norms. If a T score of 70 was used for the cutoff on MMPI-2 norms, these percentages dropped to 82% for the men and 83% for the women because of the general effect of new norms and T scores in lowering profile elevation. Using a T score of 65 as the MMPI-2 cutoff resulted in better correspondence with the old MMPI classifications: 93% of the men and 94% of the women were then identified as having clinically elevated profiles. Thus, all further analyses were performed using a cutoff of 65 and above to assign clinical significance to an MMPI-2 scale elevation. Appendix O shows the distribution of all normal limits, spike, and two-point codes in the pain sample, again comparing MMPI-2 scoring with Hathaway-Briggs scoring. Profiles were coded as normal limits if all clinical scales (Hs, D, Hy, Pd, Pa, Pt, Sc, and Ma) were less than 65 for MMPI-2 norms or less than 70 for Hathaway-Briggs norms. Profiles were coded as spikes if only one of the clinical scales was clinically elevated. If more than one scale was elevated, profiles were coded according to the two highest clinical scales in the profile, with those lower in the order taking precedence in case of ties. Using these criteria, 56% of the men and 67% of the women would have obtained exactly the same code if their protocols were scored by old norms as they did when scored by MMPI-2 norms.

Because many of the MMPI-2 codetype groups had only one or two members, the distribution of codes was examined to choose a few common categories for further analyses. An arbitrary cutoff of 5% of the sample was used to decide which codes to retain. In addition, because the men had several small code groups with Sc as one of their highest scales, it was decided to combine these patients into an "Sc Codes" group to see if this was a useful subgrouping. Because there were so many patients in this sample falling into the 1-2/2-1, 1-3/3-1, and 2-3/3-2 groups, these were examined to see whether addition of a third scale (three-point code) would result in sufficiently large subgroups for further analysis. However, in each case the only three-point code groups containing at least 5% of the sample were various combinations of scales 1 (Hs), 2 (D), and 3 (Hy). Thus, it was decided to break down this group of patients into groups based on the relative elevations of these three scales: 1) the "1-2/2-1" group would have clinical elevations on those scales more than 5 T-score points higher than on scale 3; 2) the "neurotic-triad" group would have clinical elevations on 1, 2, and 3, with none of the scales more than 5 points away from the closest of the other two; 3) the "conversion-V" group would have clinical elevations on 1 and 3 with scale 2 at least 5 T-score points lower than either of them; and 4) the "2-3/3-2" group would have clinical elevations on these scales with scale 1 at least 5 T scores lower than both of them.

These grouping procedures resulted in six codetype groups for the men and five for the women each of which contained at least 5% of the sample for their sex. A normal-limits code, a conversion-V code, and a neurotic-

TABLE 5-4. Mean T Scores for Common Codetypes (Men, N = 268)

Scale	Normal Lim. M	S.D.	Spike 1 M	S.D.	1-2/2-1 M	S.D.	Conv. V M	S.D.	Neur. Triad M	S.D.	Sc Codes M	S.D.
L	52.4	7.7	55.4	8.4	49.0	7.9	57.4	12.1	56.2	9.4	46.7	7.3
F	44.1	6.7	49.2	7.2	57.6	12.6	50.9	9.0	54.2	9.4	77.3	20.5
K	51.9	9.0	50.5	11.6	41.6	5.3	53.6	10.2	47.9	9.1	39.8	6.5
Hs	55.9	7.6	68.3	2.4	76.4	8.4	81.8	8.2	76.1	7.9	76.0	11.9
D	48.6	5.0	57.6	5.6	75.1	7.1	64.8	9.4	75.2	7.8	75.0	12.6
Hy	55.8	5.6	57.8	5.2	63.7	7.6	84.3	10.8	77.8	8.6	69.4	12.5
Pd	47.8	9.0	50.2	7.1	56.9	11.6	58.0	9.2	59.3	9.3	66.9	11.4
Mf	40.1	7.9	40.7	12.0	42.7	6.6	46.1	7.3	47.7	8.3	50.2	10.6
Pa	46.9	7.9	46.6	8.2	57.4	10.1	54.5	10.8	57.3	10.3	73.4	18.7
Pt	45.5	4.7	50.3	6.4	62.2	13.3	59.6	10.4	62.2	11.7	79.8	15.1
Sc	44.9	6.1	50.2	5.0	58.7	13.0	58.7	9.8	58.4	10.1	86.9	16.3
Ma	47.2	6.7	50.6	7.5	49.4	6.1	52.5	10.2	46.4	8.0	63.2	8.9
Si	44.5	8.5	49.0	11.2	62.6	9.1	46.4	8.7	56.4	10.3	62.7	13.0
N (%)	18	(7)	18	(7)	14	(5)	79	(30)	45	(17)	18	(7)

Total Classified: 73% of sample.

triad code were retained for both sexes. The codes that were common for men but not for women were a spike 1 code, the 1-2/2-1 code, and the Sc codes group. Codes found to be common for the women were the 2-7/7-2 code and the 3-4/4-3 code. Contrasting these common codetype groups as scored by new and old norms resulted in a higher percentage of matches between MMPI and MMPI-2 norms than when examining all possible groups: the percentages rose to 65% and 84% for men and women, respectively. Tables 5-4 and 5-5 present the clinical scale distributions and the frequency of each common codetype group for men and for women. The mean profiles for each of these codes are then illustrated in Figures 5-10 through 5-20.

It has already been noted that one major effect of the new MMPI-2 norms and uniform T scores is a general lowering of overall profile elevation an average of about 5 T-score points across scales. Comparison of classification rates into a normal-limits code vs. any elevated code supported the prediction that a better match to MMPI codetypes will be achieved if a cutoff of 65 is used to assign codetype memberships on the MMPI-2. However, the degree of change from old to new scoring varies somewhat by scale, resulting in some shifts in relative elevations of scales from the MMPI to the MMPI-2 which cause changes in scale highpoints and codetype memberships. Among the chronic pain population, examination of shifts in highpoint and codetype frequencies revealed that the most frequent changes occur among the relative elevations of the neurotic-triad scales. For both men and women, scale D is scored proportionately lower on new norms than scales Hs and Hy, which can change the configuration of these

TABLE 5-5. Mean T Scores for Common Codetypes (Women, N = 234)

Scale	Normal Lim. M	Normal Lim. S.D.	Conv. V M	Conv. V S.D.	Neur. Triad M	Neur. Triad S.D.	2-7/7-2 M	2-7/7-2 S.D.	3-4/4-3 M	3-4/4-3 S.D.
L	54.5	8.5	57.1	9.6	57.0	9.5	53.3	9.4	49.6	10.3
F	45.0	4.2	49.3	7.6	53.6	9.3	60.1	10.1	56.6	12.5
K	50.5	8.1	54.1	9.6	50.3	11.3	41.2	6.8	50.7	10.3
Hs	57.6	5.0	79.6	9.6	77.9	8.1	67.3	8.5	72.6	9.4
D	53.1	6.8	62.4	9.3	78.0	10.4	86.5	7.7	72.5	12.8
Hy	56.3	6.2	82.4	10.9	79.7	10.4	66.3	9.3	84.5	12.3
Pd	46.8	6.5	54.9	9.4	58.2	10.1	58.7	9.1	77.2	9.6
Mf	54.9	7.1	49.6	9.0	50.7	8.4	51.3	8.4	47.4	9.0
Pa	42.2	5.8	53.8	8.2	54.5	11.6	59.7	9.9	68.2	10.2
Pt	45.8	6.8	58.6	8.9	64.9	9.2	77.7	5.3	68.1	9.7
Sc	43.3	6.5	58.8	9.1	61.2	9.8	64.7	7.9	67.6	12.3
Ma	47.4	7.4	51.7	9.6	47.2	8.9	43.7	7.1	58.2	12.4
Si	46.7	10.1	48.2	8.9	54.7	11.5	66.9	7.9	50.2	10.1
N (%)	14	(6)	81	(35)	47	(20)	15	(6)	17	(7)

Total Classified: 74% of sample.

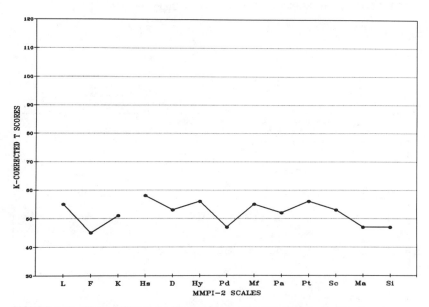

FIGURE 5-10. Mean MMPI-2 Profile for Normal-Limits Codetype (Men)

three scales. Although the majority of profiles are likely to match from old to new forms, one conclusion from these data is that the configuration of scales Hs, D, and Hy should not be automatically assumed to correspond to previous research on these scales. A larger difference between the scales

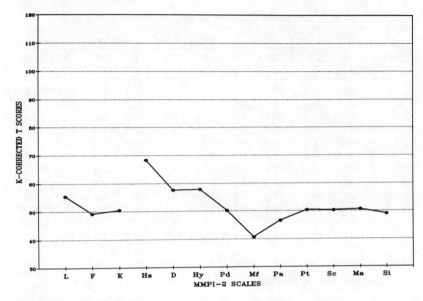

FIGURE 5-11. Mean MMPI-2 Profile for Spike 1 Codetype (Men)

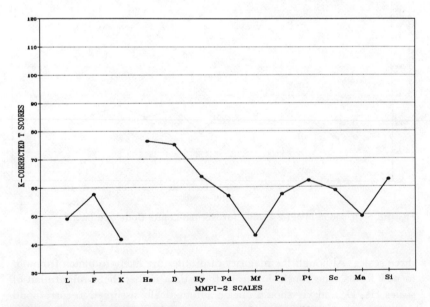

FIGURE 5-12. Mean MMPI-2 Profile for 1-2/2-1 Codetype (Men)

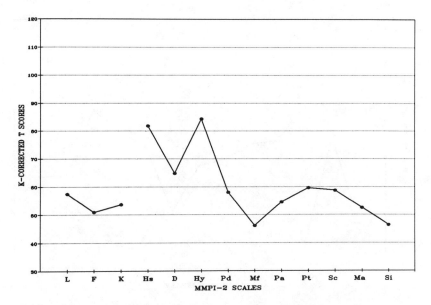

FIGURE 5-13. Mean MMPI-2 Profile for Conversion-V Codetype (Men)

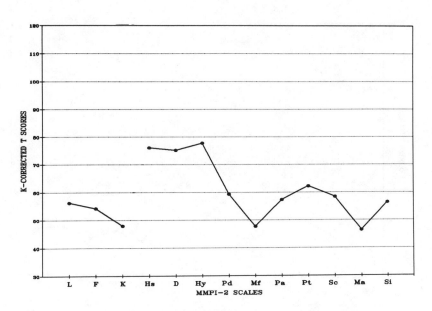

FIGURE 5-14. Mean MMPI-2 Profile for Neurotic-Triad Codetype (Men)

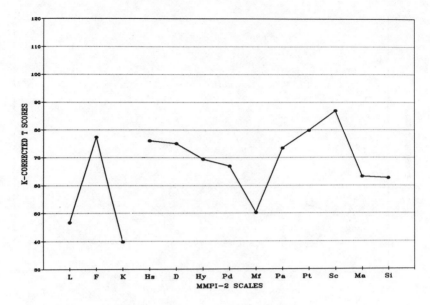

FIGURE 5-15. Mean MMPI-2 Profile for Sc Codetype (Men)

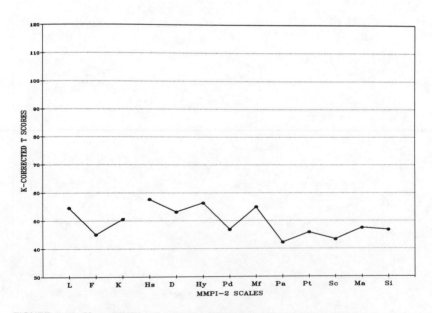

FIGURE 5-16. Mean MMPI-2 Profile for Normal-Limits Codetype (Women)

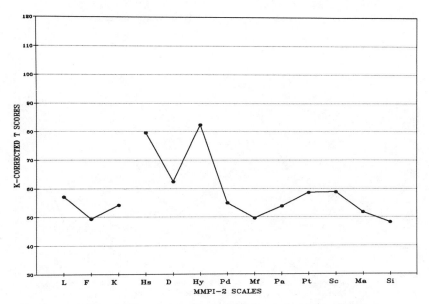

FIGURE 5-17. Mean MMPI-2 Profile for Conversion-V Codetype (Women)

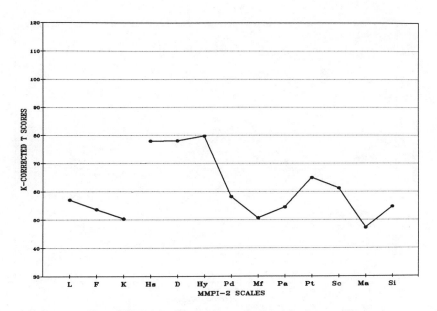

FIGURE 5-18. Mean MMPI-2 Profile for Neurotic-Triad Codetype (Women)

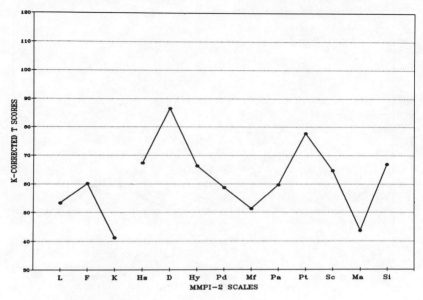

FIGURE 5-19. Mean MMPI-2 Profile for 2-7/7-2 Codetype (Women)

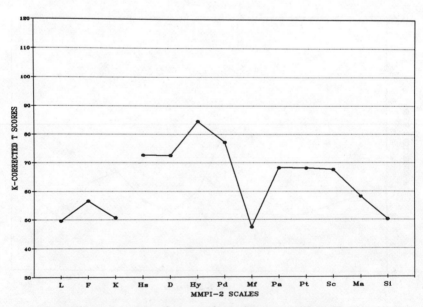

FIGURE 5-20. Mean MMPI-2 Profile for 3-4/4-3 Codetype (Women)

should be required before strong interpretations of conversion-V versus neurotic-triad or reactive-depression profiles are made. In general, patients will look somewhat less depressed and less characterologic (Pd elevations relative to other scales) on the MMPI-2 than on the MMPI. Conversely, patients obtaining elevations on these scales on the MMPI-2 would have had even higher elevations relative to other scales on the MMPI.

A study by Ahles et al. (1986) comparing pain patients' scores on the original MMPI to the scores they obtained using the contemporary Mayo Clinic normalized T scores of Colligan et al. (1984) showed a similar lowering of profiles when contemporary norms are employed. However, Ahles's suggestion that "the incidence of psychopathology in chronic pain patients may be overestimated because of the use of outdated norms" (p. 159) is premature at best. Such conclusions must wait for appropriate correlate data. Indeed, at this point the comparison of pain patients' distribution of scores on scales Hs, HEA (Health Concerns), and Hy to that of the normative sample suggests that using the MMPI cutoff of 70 on the MMPI-2 would *underpathologize* this population, and it is likely the same would be true of the Colligan et al. norms (Graham & Lilly, 1986).

Further support for the comparability of the MMPI and MMPI-2 and for the need to lower interpretive ranges on the latter comes from examination of the relative distributions of codetypes using the two forms. In both cases, the preponderance of 1-2, 1-3, and 2-3 codetypes matches previous literature on this patient population. Obviously, the MMPI-2 is not resulting in major changes in the description of these clients' somatic preoccupation and oft-associated depression. In both cases, the mean profiles for the major codetypes are very similar to those identified in the past (see Figures 2-1 and 2-2 in Chapter 2) by investigators such as Sternbach (1974a, 1974b) and Heaton et al. (1982), and later replicated with MMPI-2 items by Cohen (1987). The method of codetype assignment used here was chosen because of its simplicity, its avoidance of reliance on clinical judgment in sorting profiles, its easy replicability by other researchers, and its ability to classify all patients. The sorting scheme was not selected in advance to match that of Sternbach, Heaton, or Cohen, yet the outcome does with some exceptions match their predictions of important clinical groups. A normal-limits group was found for both sexes, as well as a conversion V (also termed somatization reaction in past research). The hypochondriasis, reactive depression, and somatization reaction with depression groups described by Heaton seem to fall in this study into the 1-2/2-1, Spike 1, and neurotic-triad profiles for the men, with only the women having a significant proportion of profiles with primary elevations on scales D and Pt. The rules used by Heaton for assignment to these groups were based on arbitrary divisions of elevation of the depression scale versus the other scales, and the rules classifying profiles as neurotic triad vs.

conversion V vs. spike and codetype profiles used in the current study were also explicit but arbitrary.

In addition, among the women in the sample a profile was identified that might fit the manipulative reaction groups of past studies, although scale Pd did not occur very frequently in two-point codes among the men. The latter does not rule out the possibility that Pd may have been a frequent additional elevation for the men, since this study examined only one-, two-, and selected three-point codes. Among the men, there was a subgroup of patients with elevations of Sc in combination with various other scales. Their mean profile appears to match the borderline/psychotic, generally elevated profile of Heaton et al. (1982) and probably includes men with elevations on Pd as well.

The prior analyses compared the old and new versions of the MMPI to examine continuity of patterns and subgroups in this population. The codetype analyses indicate that even a relatively simple, easily replicable classification scheme can identify subgroups within a large chronic pain population that share distinctive MMPI-2 profile shapes. The second major question in subgrouping by codetypes is whether these groups are associated with any clinically useful characteristics of the pain patients. To examine this question, analyses were conducted in a similar manner to that described above for single scale elevations, separately for each sex. Patients falling into a particular codetype group were contrasted with all other patients not belonging to that group. Variables examined as possible correlates included all the life events, biographical information, and chart review data used in the prior correlate analyses, and the same adjusted alpha levels were used to identify significant associations. In addition to these comparisons, codetype groups were contrasted on the new content-scale scores by means of t-tests, using an alpha of .003 to determine significance (.05 divided by comparisons on 15 content scales). Tables 5-6 and 5-7 present the distributions of all the content scales by codetype group. Appendixes P and Q summarize the significant correlates of each codetype for each sex.

The correlate analyses provided general support for the distinctiveness of these codetype groups. As might be predicted, the normal-limits codetype patients tended to score less pathologically on content scales reflecting depression, anxiety, somatic preoccupation, and negative work or treatment indicators. They also were less likely to be treated for depression during or after the program, and were less likely to describe their lives as full of stressors. The conversion-V codetype patients were also distinctive in their denial of psychological distress and depression, while endorsing some physical complaints. From these data alone it is not possible to assess whether this reflects an accurate self-appraisal or a pathological denial and conversion of emotional distress to physical symptoms. Another codetype with relatively clear correlates is the group of Sc codes in the men, which

TABLE 5-6. Mean T Scores on Content Scales for Common Codetypes (Men, N = 268)

Scale	Normal Limits		Spike 1		1-2/2-1		Conv. V		Neur. Triad		Sc Codes	
	M	S.D.	M	S.D.	M	S.D.	M	S.D.	M	S.D.	M	S.D.
ANX	48.1	6.6	51.3	7.1	64.2	9.6	56.7	11.0	61.2	9.0	72.4	12.6
FRS	49.6	9.3	49.6	10.9	57.1	13.5	50.7	8.1	51.7	8.8	58.3	11.6
OBS	46.6	8.0	46.4	9.9	57.1	9.5	48.2	8.6	52.7	9.4	68.2	10.7
DEP	46.9	5.9	53.7	7.1	66.3	13.0	56.0	8.5	61.9	9.2	76.8	13.8
HEA	51.1	8.9	64.1	9.0	74.1	9.6	73.5	10.6	71.2	8.8	78.6	12.1
BIZ	46.7	8.2	49.9	9.4	54.9	8.7	49.9	9.2	49.8	7.8	68.7	12.1
ANG	49.8	7.8	51.8	11.6	56.5	10.1	51.1	10.7	54.0	9.9	66.1	10.1
CYN	51.1	9.5	51.1	10.0	58.7	8.5	47.9	9.0	50.1	8.7	62.0	9.3
ASP	49.8	6.2	52.2	10.7	61.5	9.7	48.0	9.4	49.5	8.1	61.1	10.0
TPA	48.5	8.2	48.3	8.5	53.5	6.7	47.0	9.5	47.9	8.9	57.8	10.2
LSE	45.1	7.2	49.3	9.0	63.5	13.9	50.2	8.3	54.2	11.2	71.9	13.8
SOD	46.6	7.8	47.6	10.1	61.1	9.2	45.2	8.3	55.7	10.4	61.7	13.4
FAM	47.9	8.0	46.9	7.4	59.8	11.7	48.3	9.1	49.6	8.9	65.5	11.3
WRK	47.1	5.2	51.2	9.8	65.4	12.3	53.5	9.6	58.6	9.1	73.9	9.8
TRT	46.9	8.1	50.9	8.3	62.6	11.9	50.7	8.3	57.3	11.2	76.1	12.5
N (%)	18	(7)	18	(7)	14	(5)	79	(30)	45	(17)	18	(7)

TABLE 5-7. Mean T Scores on Content Scales for Common Codetypes (Women, N = 234)

Scale	Normal Lim.		Conv. V		Neur. Triad		2-7/7-2		3-4/4-3	
	M	S.D.	M	S.D.	M	S.D.	M	S.D.	M	S.D.
ANX	48.0	7.3	55.3	9.4	61.7	11.8	69.9	10.6	66.6	10.1
FRS	49.3	12.6	51.8	9.8	51.9	12.8	56.7	11.3	48.4	11.0
OBS	45.7	8.4	49.0	8.7	50.5	8.9	64.9	9.1	51.9	10.4
DEP	50.9	4.9	54.9	7.9	61.8	9.9	72.3	9.2	70.3	11.1
HEA	53.3	7.5	71.4	10.7	71.0	10.0	67.3	9.3	65.9	9.9
BIZ	45.2	7.8	50.1	7.9	51.3	8.6	50.6	7.8	54.9	10.9
ANG	49.7	9.1	48.7	9.2	51.9	11.2	57.9	8.7	61.0	12.5
CYN	49.1	9.2	46.0	8.1	49.3	9.9	55.2	7.6	47.2	9.9
ASP	48.3	8.2	45.4	8.3	47.5	8.4	51.3	7.0	51.1	7.3
TPA	48.3	9.4	47.8	8.6	50.3	11.8	55.1	9.5	52.1	11.5
LSE	51.4	8.2	50.9	8.7	57.2	12.0	71.6	10.7	57.5	13.1
SOD	45.6	9.0	47.6	7.8	51.9	10.7	63.6	9.1	49.8	9.7
FAM	46.9	6.7	47.8	9.1	50.9	11.0	55.5	6.6	56.5	11.9
WRK	47.9	9.7	52.9	9.4	59.0	11.3	73.2	9.7	61.6	12.8
TRT	47.6	8.4	50.7	7.8	55.0	10.3	69.5	12.8	59.7	10.8
N (%)	14	(6)	81	(35)	47	(20)	15	(6)	17	(7)

correlated with histories of psychotic problems and elevated levels of distress on most of the content scales, including Bizarre Mentation (BIZ), Family Problems (FAM), Work Interference (WRK), Negative Treatment Indicators (TRT), and Antisocial Practices (ASP).

With the above exceptions, few specific codetype correlates were found in this study. As was noted when discussing the single scale correlates, the lack of codetype correlates does not necessarily mean that grouping pain patients by MMPI-2 profiles has no utility in treatment planning. Since the majority of patients share some degree of elevation on the neurotic-triad scales, comparisons of groups differing only slightly in relative elevation of these scales may not show large differences in correlate variables. Many of the patients within each codetype group probably shared many of the same scale elevations as patients assigned to other codetype groups. It is the more extreme profiles, such as the Sc codetypes among the men, that could be expected to provide information discriminating some of the special needs or characteristics of those patients from those shared by all pain patients. Future studies would probably do well to look at profiles differing more extremely from the group norm, such as by requiring larger differences among the neurotic-triad scales to separate them into primarily depressed, primarily somatically focused, and the modal mixed groups. It might also be useful to separate out the clients with Pd elevations from the general somatically focused group, since the single-scale studies suggested that extremes of characterologic and/or manipulative characteristics can be identified by the MMPI-2 within the larger pain population. While the lack of differences found here may partially result from incomplete or inaccurate correlate data, it seems reasonable to suggest that future codetype studies attempt to define more clearly distinguishable, non-overlapping profile types. This would lower the percentage of patients classified by such schemes, but perhaps increase the usefulness of the MMPI-2 in distinguishing clients with special needs.

In summary, several traditional MMPI clinical scales (D and Pt) and new MMPI-2 content scales (ANX, DEP, LSE) were found to be associated with depressive symptoms. In addition, the Ma and Pd clinical scales, the MAC scale, and the new ASP and ANG content scales were associated with impulse control, characterologic, or "acting out" problems such as alcohol or drug abuse and legal histories. MMPI-2 codetype classification procedures show continuity with the traditional profile classification approach even though the norms are about 5 T-score points lower for the MMPI-2. Thus, the MMPI-2 will give similar codetype patterns to the MMPI with chronic pain patients, and this study shows support for the traditional behavioral correlates of these codetypes even though they are less powerful in discriminating patients within this homogeneous sample than they would be in a more diverse population.

TABLE 5-8. Classification into Costello et al. (1987) Cluster Groups, Original MMPI Norms vs. MMPI-2 Scoring and Norms

A. Men (N = 268)

Group	Frequency Classified			
	MMPI Norms		MMPI-2 Norms	
Type P	45	(17%)	10	(4%)
Type A	16	(6%)	29	(11%)
Type I	26	(10%)	30	(11%)
Type N	13	(5%)	36	(13%)
Unclassified	168	(63%)	163	(61%)
Total matches between classifications:				55%

B. Women (N = 234)

Group	Frequency Classified			
	MMPI Norms		MMPI-2 Norms	
Type P	26	(11%)	8	(3%)
Type A	26	(11%)	30	(13%)
Type I	26	(11%)	23	(9%)
Type N	21	(9%)	24	(10%)
Unclassified	135	(58%)	149	(64%)
Total matches between classifications:				77%

Subgrouping by Cluster Analysis

The use of relatively simple codetyping rules described above resulted in the classification of 73% of the men and 74% of the women into one of several common one-, two-, or three-point codetype groups. In contrast, cluster analysis uses information from all scales in the profile to classify subjects and, by definition, assigns all subjects to a group, resulting in 100% classification. However, if these cluster solutions are to be useful in day-to-day practice, rules need to be developed to assign profiles to appropriate clusters. Costello et al. (1987) suggested a set of sorting rules to assign profiles to one of the four cluster types commonly found throughout pain patient cluster analysis studies: types "P" (corresponding to a general-elevation profile), "A" (a conversion-V profile), "I" (a neurotic-triad profile), and "N" (a normal-limits profile). While Costello et al. suggest each of these types may account for 15-30% of a chronic pain sample, the actual classification rates have not been tested on either the original MMPI or on the MMPI-2. Since their rules are based on elevations and pattern of T scores on validity and clinical scales, it was possible to compare classification rates in the Sister Kenny sample using original MMPI norms and scoring versus new MMPI-2 norms and scoring. Table 5-8 presents the frequencies of each Costello et al. cluster type using these two different methods of scoring.

It can be seen from these tables that the Costello rules allow classification of only about 40% of the sample for either sex. This is not simply due to differences between the new MMPI-2 norms and the original MMPI norms on which the rules were based. Although some shifts in classification occur as a result of the different scoring methods (largely owing to the reduction of profile elevations using MMPI-2 norms), the overall classification rate is just as low using original MMPI scoring. Thus, the Costello rules would need to be adjusted to achieve similar classifications using the MMPI-2 and the MMPI, and even then they cannot be assumed to be equivalent to classifications achieved through a full cluster analysis procedure.

The codetyping scheme used earlier classified patients by the highest one, two, or at most three scales in their MMPI-2 profile. Theoretically, cluster analysis uses information from the entire profile of scores to assign patients to relatively homogeneous groups. On the average, a client within a cluster will have a profile that is more similar to the mean profile of that cluster than to the means of other clusters. However, this does not necessarily mean the client's profile is the same shape as the mean cluster profile: whereas all profiles within a 1-3 codetype group will have highest elevations on those two scales, it cannot be assumed that all profiles within a conversion-V cluster have that profile shape. This is partially illustrated by the rather poor classification rates found when applying the Costello et al. (1987) cluster grouping rules to data from the Sister Kenny sample. These rules attempted to match profiles to the most common mean cluster profiles found in previous studies and as a result left over half the sample unclassified.

To explore the replicability of previous full cluster analysis MMPI results with the MMPI-2, a hierarchical cluster analysis was performed with the Sister Kenny sample. The procedure was chosen to approximate that used by Bradley et al. (1978), since their work has been considered the standard in the field thus far. Analyses were run separately for men and women, and within each sex were run separately for two cohorts for replication purposes. Cohorts were assigned according to those patients who entered in the first half of the study period versus those who entered in the latter half, similar to Bradley's method. The variables used for clustering were the K-corrected T scores on the entire MMPI-2 clinical profile: scales L, F, K, Hs, D, Hy, Pd, Mf, Pa, Pt, Sc, Ma, and Si. To replicate Bradley's study, the SPSS-X Cluster program was run using Ward's method of hierarchical cluster analysis. This method starts with each subject as a separate cluster, computes the means for all variables (scale scores) within the cluster, computes the distance of each case from this cluster mean, and combines those clusters which result in the smallest increase in the overall sum of squared within-cluster distances from the cluster mean (Norusis, 1985). Distance (or similarity) of clusters can be computed several ways, but the most common methods are through Pearson correlation coefficients, which are sensitive to profile shape but not to elevation, or through Euclidean distance (the sum of squared distances between all scales in the two profiles being compared), which confounds both elevation and shape of profile (Morey, Blashfield, & Skinner, 1983). Ward's method uses Euclidean distance as its similarity measure and thus tends to separate clusters according to elevation as well as or in preference to shape (Edelbrock, 1979; Morey et al., 1983; Ward, 1963). This method was chosen as the best one to test similarity of MMPI-2 cluster solutions to previous MMPI studies, and as the best match to traditional MMPI interpretive strategies that take both elevation and profile shape into account.

There is no absolute statistical criterion for the correct number of clusters within a sample. Hierarchical cluster analysis sequentially assigns subjects to larger and larger clusters, starting with one cluster per subject and ending with one cluster encompassing the total sample. One guide to choosing a cluster solution is examination of the distance between the clusters to be combined at the next step of the analysis; if a "jump" occurs at a certain point, it can indicate that dissimilar clusters are being combined after that point and the analysis should have stopped earlier. Applying this criterion to the four separate cluster analyses performed here did not identify a definite jump point, but did indicate a general rise in distance measures around six clusters or so. It was decided to examine all cluster solutions from six to two to find which replicated across the two cohorts within each sample. Six clusters were thought to be enough to identify the four basic clusters found across previous studies plus allow for unique, smaller clusters if present in these data.

Mean profiles were plotted for each cluster found in each cluster solution and compared across cohorts for pattern similarity. Although at each step several of the clusters were similar, for both men and women only the three-cluster solution provided replicability of all clusters across cohorts. Appendix R illustrates the mean profiles for each of these three clusters by cohort and sex.

To provide further replicability and stability of cluster membership, a cluster analysis was run again using the total samples of men and women, respectively, and assigning each subject to one of three clusters. Figures 5-21 and 5-22 present the final mean profiles for the three male clusters and the three female clusters. Cluster 1 in the male sample accounted for 25% of the subjects, and the mean profile for this group could be described as a general-elevation pattern. The mean pattern for Cluster 2 (57% of the men) was an elevated neurotic triad. The third male cluster accounted for 19% of the sample, and the mean profile for this group was entirely within normal limits. For the women, the mean profile of Cluster 1 (37% of the sample) was a neurotic-triad pattern with a subclinical peak on Pt. Cluster 2 included 30% of the women and could be described as having a general-elevation mean profile. The third cluster, including 33% of the women, was within normal limits by MMPI criteria but would be described

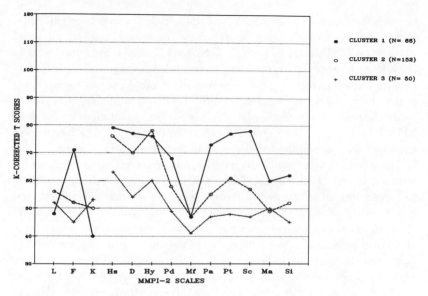

FIGURE 5-21. Mean MMPI-2 Profiles for Male Clusters (Total Group)

as a low conversion-V mean profile using an MMPI-2 clinical T-score cutoff of 65. The mean T scores on all validity and clinical scales for each cluster are presented in Table 5-9.

Examination of the cluster analyses performed on this sample strongly suggested that this method of subgrouping results in separation on the basis of profile elevation rather than profile shape. For both sexes, the three replicated profiles differ primarily in their degree of elevation. Examination of past research indicates this same pattern occurs across studies, with almost all researchers identifying a normal-limits profile, a general-elevation profile, and various combinations of middle-range elevations on the neurotic-triad scales. The only other study to use MMPI-2 items was Cohen's (1987), and his findings showed this same general pattern. Although he found both a neurotic-triad and a conversion-V profile in addition to normal-limits and general-elevation profiles, he did not attempt to replicate patterns across cohorts as was suggested by Bradley (1978) and was done in this study. Thus, the stability of these middle-range profile types remains questionable in Cohen's study. They were not found to be stable across cohorts in the present larger patient sample.

Examination of the 4-, 5-, and 6-cluster solutions for the Sister Kenny sample cohorts, as well as profiles of individual cases, indicated that rather heterogeneous profile types contributed to even the smaller three-cluster solution. For example, among the men included in the normal-limits cluster, only 18 out of 50 actually had profiles with no clinical elevations at

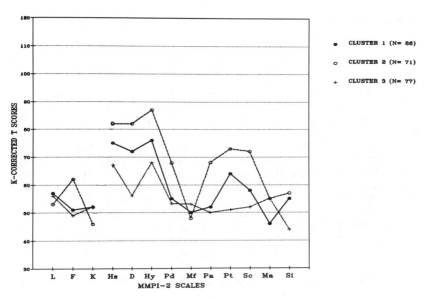

FIGURE 5-22. Mean MMPI-2 Profiles for Female Clusters (Total Group)

TABLE 5-9. Mean T Scores for Chronic Pain Clusters

	Men (N = 268)						Women (N = 234)					
	Cluster 1		Cluster 2		Cluster 3		Cluster 1		Cluster 2		Cluster 3	
Scale	M	S.D.	M	S.D.	M	S.D.	M	S.D.	M	S.D.	M	S.D.
L	47.7	7.5	56.5	10.6	52.5	7.6	56.8	7.5	52.5	10.5	55.6	10.4
F	70.8	13.9	51.7	8.0	45.2	5.9	50.7	6.7	61.5	13.3	48.5	8.2
K	39.6	6.8	50.0	10.2	53.0	9.9	51.7	10.3	45.6	9.1	51.9	10.6
Hs	78.5	11.7	76.4	8.5	63.0	8.1	74.9	9.5	81.6	9.8	66.9	8.8
D	77.3	13.3	69.5	7.9	53.9	8.2	71.6	9.4	81.6	11.8	55.6	6.7
Hy	75.8	14.1	78.0	11.8	59.6	7.4	76.5	10.0	87.1	11.7	68.5	10.3
Pd	68.2	11.2	58.5	10.4	49.4	8.8	55.4	9.2	68.3	11.5	52.6	8.7
Mf	47.2	9.7	47.4	8.6	41.4	7.7	49.9	9.0	48.1	9.2	52.7	8.6
Pa	72.8	14.1	55.0	9.2	47.3	8.3	52.3	7.7	68.3	9.3	50.3	10.4
Pt	77.2	13.4	61.1	9.5	47.8	6.5	63.6	8.2	73.0	9.1	51.1	7.2
Sc	77.6	13.9	57.2	8.0	47.2	6.4	58.1	7.6	72.2	8.3	52.0	8.8
Ma	59.9	13.1	49.2	8.9	49.6	7.6	45.6	6.4	54.9	12.4	55.0	11.5
Si	61.9	11.2	52.1	10.2	44.7	8.2	55.0	9.4	56.9	11.2	44.4	9.4
N (%)	66	(25)	152	(57)	50	(19)	86	(37)	71	(30)	77	(33)

65 or above. For the general-elevation cluster, two-point codetypes varied across almost all possible combinations of scales. Thus, although these general profile types do match clusters found in previous studies, the heterogeneity within such statistically derived groups, as well as the

TABLE 5-10. Mean Content Scale T Scores for Chronic Pain Clusters

	Men (N = 268)						Women (N = 234)					
	Cluster 1		Cluster 2		Cluster 3		Cluster 1		Cluster 2		Cluster 3	
Scale	M	S.D.	M	S.D.	M	S.D.	M	S.D.	M	S.D.	M	S.D.
ANX	73.1	10.3	59.0	9.4	49.2	6.9	58.3	9.6	71.2	9.9	52.2	8.4
FRS	57.1	12.6	51.5	8.7	48.1	9.7	52.2	10.4	54.6	12.5	48.8	9.2
OBS	65.8	9.3	50.5	9.0	46.1	8.1	51.6	9.4	57.2	10.8	46.9	8.1
DEP	75.3	10.5	59.4	8.0	49.5	6.5	59.4	8.4	70.6	9.6	52.5	7.0
HEA	79.3	11.1	70.7	8.2	57.3	9.1	67.9	9.0	77.2	10.2	61.1	9.2
BIZ	63.5	11.4	49.1	8.3	48.0	8.1	49.8	7.9	56.4	10.7	49.8	8.6
ANG	65.1	10.9	53.8	11.0	48.4	7.9	48.6	9.2	59.2	11.1	50.3	8.7
CYN	60.3	10.2	49.8	9.7	50.0	9.1	47.7	9.6	51.5	9.4	48.2	9.3
ASP	60.7	12.0	49.7	9.7	50.4	8.7	45.4	7.7	50.5	9.3	48.5	8.9
TPA	59.1	10.8	48.5	9.3	47.5	7.5	47.4	9.6	55.4	11.2	47.5	7.3
LSE	67.9	10.4	53.2	9.9	46.0	7.9	56.3	10.3	63.3	12.0	48.5	7.3
SOD	59.6	12.2	50.5	10.3	45.3	7.5	53.1	9.0	53.5	10.3	45.4	8.7
FAM	64.6	10.7	50.0	9.3	45.8	6.6	48.4	8.1	59.0	10.5	47.9	9.3
WRK	71.8	8.8	56.9	9.1	47.5	6.4	57.2	9.8	67.2	11.4	49.9	8.4
TRT	70.2	11.0	53.9	8.7	47.4	7.3	54.3	8.7	62.3	12.6	48.9	7.8
N (%)	66	(25)	152	(57)	50	(19)	86	(37)	71	(30)	77	(33)

arbitrary and somewhat subjective nature of cluster analysis, makes both replication and interpretation of clusters quite difficult. While these results again support comparability of the MMPI-2 to the MMPI, the usefulness of cluster approaches to MMPI-2 interpretation is not demonstrated as clearly.

Once the replicability of a cluster solution has been established, the usefulness of such a subgrouping must be established by demonstrating clinical utility. As in the previous subgrouping methods, this was examined by searching for correlates of cluster group membership among the life events, biographical information, chart review, and content-scale data. The same methods were employed as in the codetype analyses: within each sex, those subjects belonging to a particular cluster group were contrasted with those who belonged to either of the other two groups. The same adjusted alpha levels were used to identify significant associations as those reported earlier. Table 5-10 contrasts the mean T scores for all the content scales across cluster groups. Appendixes S and T summarize which of these scales were significantly associated with particular clusters, as well as presenting correlate data from the other measures.

The pattern of correlates found in this study for the cluster types, with some exceptions, supports the view that the clusters represent a continuum of generalized distress or pathology rather than specific patterns of problems. While this is certainly an endorsement of the ability of the MMPI-2 to reflect such difficulties, particularly degree of depression, it does not seem enough to justify extensive statistical analyses in order to identify groups that could as easily be classified simply by profile elevation. While the differentiation by elevation is partially a result of the method of cluster analysis used here and by Bradley et al. (1978), even the cluster research by other investigators using different methods has not resulted in uniquely different profiles from those suggested as clinically useful by clinicians using codetype sorting strategies. It is suggested here that the use of well-defined codetype sorting schemes that take scale elevation into account as well as incorporating checks for elevations on scales Pd, Pt, and Sc would allow for better replicability of research efforts and simpler transfer of results to clinical practice.

Summary of Major Findings and Conclusions

The analyses presented in this monograph were designed to address two major areas. The first was the comparability of the MMPI-2 to the original MMPI, and the second was the provision of preliminary clinical data on the usefulness of the MMPI-2 among chronic pain patients. In addition to these overarching goals, the clinical data collected for MMPI-2 validation purposes provided a good general description of the characteristics of pain patients participating in a multidisciplinary treatment program.

Sample description was addressed first to provide future researchers with the information needed to compare this sample to their own, and to provide a picture of the average pain patient which could be used to assess the accuracy of the average MMPI-2 profile produced by this group. Non-MMPI information used in this study included patient self-report responses to biographical information and life events forms, and information abstracted from the patients' charts. Where possible, the responses of pain patients were compared with those of the national normative sample used in restandardizing the MMPI, and to a large group of hospitalized psychiatric patients who had also completed the restandardization research forms.

Results of these analyses supported the descriptions of modal pain patients reported in many previous studies, including such characteristics as blue-collar background, back pain blamed on a job injury, multiple pain complaints, availability of compensation for their injury, extensive prior treatment histories, and prominent symptoms of depression along with somatic preoccupation. In many measures reflecting degree of life disruption and disability, the pain sample tended to fall between the normative and psychiatric samples. The only area in which they tended to outscore both groups was on complaints of physical disability and illness, and they also complained of a degree of depression that largely overlapped with the psychiatric group.

These characteristics were reflected in the mean MMPI profiles of the chronic pain population as well. For both men and women, primary scale elevations compared to the normative sample occurred on scales reflecting preoccupation with physical illness and disability, and on the depression scale. Anxiety was also reflected in somewhat lower scale elevations. Compared to the psychiatric sample, the pain patients' scores reflected less distress or disturbance except on scales measuring concerns about physical health, where they scored higher than the psychiatric sample, and on depression, where they scored similarly. Thus, the mean MMPI profile for the chronic pain sample fit the characteristics of this clinical group very well.

The same general MMPI profile shape was maintained when the patients' tests were scored by MMPI-2 norms rather than original MMPI norms, although the overall elevation of the profile dropped by an average of about 5 T-score points. The MMPI Restandardization Committee (Butcher, Dahlstrom et al., 1989) has recommended that interpreters of the MMPI-2 should use a T-score cutoff of 65 and above to indicate clinical significance instead of the traditional T score of 70; this study supported that recommendation. Comparison of score frequency distributions between the normative and pain samples suggested that a T score of 65 provides a much better separation of the two samples on the somatic preoccupation scales, for which the pain sample seems to be an appropriate clinical criterion group.

Comparisons of codetype classifications assigned by MMPI vs. MMPI-2 scoring systems again suggested that a better match between the two forms could be achieved if a cutoff of 65 is used for the MMPI-2 classification rules. Although the majority of pain patients will have two-point codes on the MMPI-2 identical to the codes they would have had on the MMPI, some changes in relative scale elevation will result in codetype differences. These are unlikely to result in major interpretive differences clinically, although the changes would be more significant for research studies using very tightly defined codetype criteria. It was suggested that the relative elevations of scales Hs, D, and Hy not be interpreted too rigidly on the MMPI-2, since scale D will be lower relative to the other two scales. Scale Pd will also be somewhat lower relative to the other scales than it would have been on the original MMPI.

These analyses supported the continuity of research using the MMPI to the revised form of this test, as long as clinicians and researchers adjust the level of scale elevation at which they make interpretations and as long as small differences among scales Hs, D, and Hy are not overinterpreted. The distinctiveness of this sample's mean performance on the MMPI-2 as compared to normative or psychiatric patients was also demonstrated, suggesting that the test may be a useful screening measure for identifying chronic pain patients. This study did not directly address the ability of the MMPI-2 to distinguish current or potential chronic pain patients from general medical patients or from pain patients who will respond to less intensive treatment. Further studies with appropriate control groups will be necessary to assess the usefulness of the MMPI-2 at such screening points.

This project presented data addressing the ability of the MMPI-2 to identify clinically relevant subgroups among a group of pain patients who had already been selected as appropriate for a multidisciplinary treatment program. This is a more difficult test of a general measure of psychopathology such as the MMPI-2 than differentiating such patients from other patient populations. Patients were grouped according to single scale elevations, codetypes based on clinically elevated patterns of one, two, or three scales, and by groups identified through cluster analysis. These groups were then contrasted on their responses to the life events and biographical information forms, and on the data collected from reviews of their charts. In general, results supported the validity of the MMPI-2 as a measure of general level of distress and disability, largely through its ability to reflect patients' level of depression. Within this somewhat homogeneous sample, depression emerged as the major source of variability across MMPI-2 results and correlates from the extra-test information. Other important correlates identified were the association of characterologic histories (arrest records, anger problems, chemical abuse problems) with scales Pd and ASP (Antisocial Practices), and the association of psychotic symptom histories with Sc elevations. In general, higher profile elevations were associated with greater levels of distress, prior psychiatric histories, and life stress.

Overall, however, there were relatively few specific correlates of any of these subgroups considering the large amount of patient data that had been collected. There are several possible explanations for this finding. One, of course, is that the MMPI-2 is not particularly useful in identifying treatment-relevant groups within a preselected chronic pain population. It could be expected to be more useful as part of an earlier screening process where a greater variety of patient problems were encountered. A second possibility is that the data collected here were not accurate reflections of true patient characteristics. This is certainly true to some extent; self-report data cannot be assumed to be accurate, and the chart reviews were limited by incomplete and inconsistent data at times. No systematic follow-up evaluation was undertaken, so the lack of treatment outcome correlates should certainly not be taken as definitive. The outcome rating data were the weakest of the study, and were not available on the majority of patients. In addition, the strict significance level required because of multiple comparisons may have resulted in overlooking important relationships, and the definitions of subgroups may not have been sufficiently strict to provide truly homogeneous profile types.

In all probability, the small number of correlates resulted from a combination of these factors. Future research could correct some of these problems by designing specific research forms to be completed during the patients' program rather than using retrospective chart reviews, by choosing fewer variables to study in order to allow less stringent significance levels, by delineating specific outcome criteria and incorporating these into the follow-up evaluation, and by using more sophisticated codetyping strategies. It was suggested in this study that the use of cluster analysis techniques with the MMPI and MMPI-2 has not identified profile patterns that differ substantially from those proposed in codetyping studies, and indeed this method results in more heterogeneous groups than a codetyping system that takes profile elevation into account. While cluster analyses incorporating other data in addition to MMPI scales might identify some interesting interactions or combinations of variables, it seems unlikely that MMPI cluster analyses alone will discover any new patterns among the chronic pain population at this point. Future research might do well to concentrate on developing clearly defined, replicable codetype rules and exploring their relationship to variables specifically chosen to relate to treatment planning, such as level of depression, psychotic symptoms, manipulativeness, chemical dependency proneness, anxiety, and suggestibility. While such strictly defined codetype systems will result in fewer patients being classified, this seems compatible with a goal of identifying the patients within a chronic pain population who do not quite fit the modal profile and thus may have somewhat different treatment needs than the majority group.

In recent years, assessment strategies used with chronic pain patients have moved away from single-measure studies and instead have begun to parallel multidimensional treatment strategies by employing multidimensional assessment approaches. Self-report measures have often proven inadequate in predicting actual pain behaviors such as activity level, medication use, health care utilization, etc. (Fordyce et al., 1984; Kremer, Block, & Atkinson, 1983; Kremer, Block, & Gaylor, 1981). More comprehensive assessment strategies now supplement self-report personality measures and pain reports with measures of the impact of pain on the patients' life, interviews with significant others to determine their responses to pain, physiological data and physical ability measures, and observations of patients' pain behaviors including such things as medication intake, level of activity, guarding behaviors, and complaints of pain (Duncan, Gregg, & Ghia, 1978; Follick, Smith, & Ahern, 1985; Getto, Heaton, & Lehman, 1983; Hoon, Feuerstein, & Papciak, 1985; Kerns, Turk, & Rudy, 1985; Naliboff et al., 1985).

The MMPI-2 may prove most useful in combination with a variety of other measures that can be used to aid and expand its interpretation with chronic pain patients. Such a multifactorial approach would come closer to meeting criteria described by Turk and Kerns (1983-84) for comprehensive pain assessment: 1) description of pain characteristics such as location, intensity, quality, and chronology; 2) evaluation of the physical, emotional, cognitive, and behavioral responses occurring with pain; 3) evaluation of the patient's perception of the meaning of pain; 4) evaluation of the impact of pain on different aspects of the patient's life (physical, marital, social, vocational, recreational); and 5) evaluation of the adaptive and maladaptive mechanisms used to cope with pain. At this point there are few widely used, standardized measures that can be incorporated into such an assessment battery. It is hoped that this study and future research will continue to help define the usefulness and validity of one potential component of such a comprehensive assessment approach, the revised Minnesota Multiphasic Personality Inventory (MMPI-2).

Chapter 6

**Case Examples and
Suggestions for
Clinical
Interpretation**

The primary goal of this chapter is to illustrate the use of the MMPI-2 with clinical cases and present some suggestions for interpretive strategies. We will present detailed information on several cases from the Sister Kenny Institute chronic pain study sample to show how the MMPI-2 clinical and content scales can be used to view the individual's symptom expression and personality characteristics. For each case, a computer-generated narrative report, The Minnesota Clinical Report for the MMPI-2 (Butcher, 1989), will be included to give an objective appraisal of the individual's MMPI-2 profile pattern. However, before proceeding with the case illustrations, we will discuss an MMPI-2 interpretation strategy with particular relevance for chronic pain patients.

Interpretation of MMPI-2 Profiles with Chronic Pain Patients

As was discussed earlier in this volume, there are relatively few empirical studies of specific correlates of various MMPI profile patterns among chronic pain patient populations, and the present research is the first to look at correlates of the MMPI-2. Thus, interpretation of MMPI profiles has largely been based on correlates found among psychiatric patients and summarized in various "cookbooks." It will be assumed here that the reader is fairly familiar with MMPI interpretation and is aware of such helpful MMPI interpretive resources as Dahlstrom, Welsh, and Dahlstrom (1972, 1975) and Graham (1987), as well as the many other books available. Interpretive resources geared to the MMPI-2 include the MMPI-2 manual and the content scale monograph published by University of Minnesota Press (Butcher, Dahlstrom, Graham, Tellegen, & Kaemmer, 1989; Butcher, Graham, Williams, & Ben-Porath, 1989) as well as Graham's text (1990) and Butcher's 1990 text on using the MMPI-2 in treatment planning. We refer readers to those books to review a general MMPI/MMPI-2 interpretive strategy which will not be repeated here.

Modifying such an interpretive approach for application to chronic pain patients requires keeping different base rates in mind as well as somewhat different treatment questions than are of most interest with psychiatric patients. Henrichs (1981) notes that an "important factor in developing skill in interpreting a patterning of scores is to have, whenever possible, some a priori conceptualization or actual representation of various 'expected' patterns from individuals in a medical setting" (p. 4). The interpretive question of most interest concerning pain patients is not so much whether they differ from the normative population—they do, they endorse more somatic symptoms. Thus, correspondence to the "mean pain patient profile" or that of the "mean medical patient" does not offer much treatment-relevant information. Instead, "the central role of devices such as the MMPI is to shed light on why pain behaviors are persisting in the individuals to be evaluated. Since, in chronic pain, physical findings by themselves are often unsure bases for explaining persisting pain behaviors, to what extent can other potential explanations be derived?" (Fordyce, 1979, p. 3).

Fordyce (1979) suggests using the MMPI to assess the patient's readiness to signal pain, the response cost of pain behaviors to the patient, other problems that may make continued disability rewarding to the patient such as possible intellectual deficits or psychiatric problems, and specific contributors to continued pain problems including depression, tension, and "traumatic neurosis." Thus, assessment is not aimed at determining whether the patient's problems are organic versus functional: rather, the clinician can use the MMPI or MMPI-2 to generate hypotheses about the degree of "excess disability" associated with the patient's condition and the multiple factors that may be contributing to maintenance of pain behaviors. Fordyce suggests searching for either direct reward for pain behaviors or avoidance learning, i.e., ways in which the patient's disability provides time out from more aversive events or activities. He, along with others such as Sternbach and Bradley, reviewed earlier, have shown there are a variety of MMPI profile patterns to be found among chronic pain patients; we are beginning to have empirical support for their predictions that these patterns will have differential clinical and treatment outcome correlates. Some of the research results and clinical impressions reviewed in Chapter 2 as well as in Costello et al. (1987), Fordyce (1979), Love and Peck (1987), and Snyder (in press) are incorporated into the brief interpretive suggestions below. Henrichs (1981) has provided a table summarizing correlates of the basic MMPI scales and two-point codetypes among general medical patients.

Validity Scale Pattern

Careful evaluation of the validity scales is particularly important with chronic pain patients because of extraneous variables such as the need to claim excessive personal virtue in an effort to emphatically assert physical injury in a compensation case, or the need to present oneself as having severe psychological problems to justify a stress-based psychological damages claim. With the elevation and pattern of the rest of the profile, the validity scales can indicate possible drug or alcohol toxicity or cognitive impairment to be evaluated further. The validity configuration helps in assessing how "comfortable" the patient is with his or her current lifestyle and problems. The validity scales together with the rest of the profile can also provide clues to the patient's typical defense mechanisms (denial and minimization of psychological problems are particularly typical of pain patients) and view of his or her own resources to deal with problems. Fordyce (1979) suggests that for a subset of patients, high K and L with high Hy can suggest the use of hysteroid defenses and possible extreme suggestibility as part of the patient's problem. He suggests evaluating whether the patient may be "simply over-responding to modest levels of nociception (i.e., pain stimuli) or to information about the nature of an illness or injury received from physicians, family members, or others" (p. 10). If so, group support, re-education, and alteration of reinforcement contingencies in the patient's social support network might be particularly helpful. Fordyce also suggests this configuration together with Pt elevations may be indicative of phobic-like behavior, indicating that detailed assessment of stimuli which elicit pain behaviors should be explored and desensitization may be a treatment of choice.

One of the strengths of the MMPI-2 is that it provides several validity scales to assess the test-taking attitudes of the client. In addition to the original validity indicators and profile patterns indicative of invalid protocols, two new validity scales have been added (TRIN and VRIN) which assess acquiescent and random response styles (Tellegen, 1988a; Butcher et al., 1989). In assessing chronic pain patients the validity pattern may prove to be some of the most valuable information available from the MMPI-2 (Butcher & Harlow, 1987).

Profile Elevation and Pattern

After examining the validity of a profile, looking at its overall elevation can provide important information about the client's degree of distress, disability, and the "cost" of the condition in his or her life. Cluster analytic research, including our own, has generally shown that increasing profile elevation is associated with increasing disability in many areas of a client's life, as well as with poorer outcome from traditional or single-mode treatments. Fordyce (1979) notes that high elevations on scales Hs and Hy indicate a great readiness to signal pain and discomfort to others, thereby increasing the probability that such behaviors are or will be maintained by social reinforcement contingencies. In contrast, the individual who does not exhibit or complain of somatic problems is unlikely to have these behaviors maintained by social contingencies.

Determining the empirical descriptors that are most appropriate for the particular client is the next step in performing a profile interpretation. The most efficient approach to prototype selection is the use of clinical scale peaks or codetypes. For the MMPI-2, this will involve taking the most prominent scale or combination of scales elevated above a T score of 65. The appropriate symptom descriptors, personality characteristics, and so forth for this codetype would be obtained by consulting a basic interpretive text summarizing empirical research in various patient populations (Butcher, 1990; Graham, 1990; Greene, 1980; Lachar, 1974).

As we have noted, relatively few distinct codetypes are typically found with any frequency in chronic pain samples. Our own research confirmed this with the MMPI-2. The most common codes with both the MMPI and the MMPI-2 are various combinations of scales 1, 2, and 3, such as 1-2/2-1, 1-3/3-1, and 2-3/3-2. Codes including scales 7, 4, and 8 are also found but with less frequency, such as the 2-7/7-2 or 3-4/4-3 combination, or various codes including the Sc elevation (see Table 5-7). The fact that relatively few profile codes occur can simplify the application of MMPI-2 correlates even though it may become a bit redundant across cases. This commonality in personality characteristics and symptoms in chronic pain patients can be seen as reflecting strengths of objective personality testing: individuals with similar problems tend to respond the same and to be viewed by others as having similar problems. Profiles obtained in other settings, for example prisons, show rather different patterns from pain patients but can be rather homogeneous in their own right: individuals in correctional settings typically show high Pd and Ma elevations in combination with other scales: 4-9/9-4, 4-6/6-4, 4-8/8-4, 8-9/9-8.

Despite the relative homogeneity in pain patient codetype patterns, our study along with others in the literature indicates that there is some variability among pain patients which is reflected in variations in MMPI and MMPI-2 profiles. We have suggested that the most interesting and useful MMPI-2 patterns among pain patients will be those that differ from the "norm" for this group in some important way, potentially offering differential treatment and outcome indicators. Although our study did not provide large numbers of unique correlates for different profile patterns, it did suggest the importance of evaluating the level of scales related to depression to assess whether treatment focused on that psychiatric disorder is appropriate. It also suggested that examining codetypes containing Pd elevations will be important in indicating possible substance abuse and characterologic problems. Codetypes with elevations on Sc were associated with histories of complex psychiatric problems that could impede the patient's ability to function in a non-disabled role even if the patient's pain was suddenly relieved.

Snyder (in press) has summarized other codetype interpretive suggestions relevant to pain patients. He notes that increasing elevations on Hs and Hy are associated with increased chronicity and intensity of pain complaints, more functional limitations, reduced activity, and poor response to traditional medical or psychological treatment. He cautions that these elevations are more useful in evaluating appropriateness of disability than degree of organic impairment. Elevations on D may indicate reactive depression, but prognosis may be better for 2-7 combinations than for those more focused on somatic concerns and utilizing more defenses such as the 2-3 combinations.

Fordyce (1979) suggests several codetypes that may have differential implications for assessment of a pain patient. He notes that the relative elevation of scale 2 compared to scales 1 and 3 can suggest the response cost of ongoing disability for the patient, i.e., how "comfortably sick" the patient feels. The classical conversion-V pattern could describe someone who finds the illness role reinforcing in some way. However, even when 2 is high along with 1 and 3, Fordyce suggests that a low Pd scale possibly accompanied by elevated Si and/or a score deviating strongly in the "feminine" direction on Mf can suggest a person who might have difficulty coping with the interpersonal demands of the non-disabled role and illness "can serve as a reinforcing buffer against environmental pressures." With an elevation on Pd as well as on Hy, it may become more likely that the patient will use illness and pain behaviors to manipulate others into meeting his or her needs.

Fordyce also suggests evaluating for other problems that could make the illness role reinforcing. Elevations on the right side of the profile, i.e., scales Pa and Sc, can suggest chronic psychiatric problems that could make illness an acceptable "out" for someone who has difficulty coping with the demands of daily life. Extreme D or Pt elevations can also indicate intense depression or anxiety disorders, and an 8-9 combination could suggest cognitive problems and confusion owing to drug toxicity or organic problems that should be evaluated further. In a subset of the elderly population, chronic pain may serve as a more acceptable rationale for increasing disability than acknowledgment of cognitive deterioration. Scale 7 can suggest possible tension contributors to ongoing pain problems, particularly in back, neck, and shoulder pain, and might also suggest the appropriateness of desensitization strategies in treatment. Finally, although out-and-out malingering is not very common among chronic pain patients, the 4-9 combination in this context should alert the clinician to assess the degree to which the client is "using" his or her symptoms to obtain financial reinforcement, drugs, or other secondary gain.

Correlate information related to pain patient cluster groups is even more limited than with codetypes. Although Costello et al. (1987) presented a classification scheme to group patients into the four most common cluster types found by several different researchers, we have shown that these rules failed to classify more than half of our sample and there were significant shifts in classification when the MMPI-2 is used instead of the MMPI. We also failed to find four distinctive cluster types in our sample, and at this point do not suggest making strong interpretive statements based on cluster membership. Our view is that paying attention to overall profile elevation and the codetype configuration will provide as much or more information as can be obtained from cluster membership. However, the interested reader is referred to Costello et al. (1987) and our own review in Chapter 2 for more details of cluster correlates obtained so far in the research literature.

Analysis of Content Themes and Supplementary Scales

The next step in MMPI or MMPI-2 interpretation is to modify and augment the codetype interpretation with appraisal of the specific content themes or attitudes endorsed by the individual and examination of supplementary scales relevant to assessing pain patients. The Harris-Lingoes subscales are often helpful in highlighting specific problems underlying a particular scale elevation (see Graham, 1990). For example, a high elevation on Pd might mean one thing (e.g., antisocial attitudes) if the Authority Conflict Subscale is most prominent but something different, such as situational problems, if the Family Problems Subscale is most prominent. The evaluation of homogeneous subscale item groups using the Harris-Lingoes subscales can give the clinician clues to refining scale interpretation. However, since many of the subscales are short—as few as six items—their value as a psychometric measure is limited. Caution should be exercised in employing these subscales.

The new MMPI-2 content scales (Butcher, Graham, Williams, & Ben-Porath, 1989) are psychometrically sound measures that provide the clinician with information about the important themes the client has presented. Content scales can be interpreted according to the themes or attitudes reflected in the item meanings. For example, a high score on OBS reflects indecisiveness, inability to concentrate, and the intrusion of obsessive thoughts. In addition to possessing homogeneous, easily interpreted content, the MMPI-2 content scales have been found to have external validities that are equal to or that surpass those of the clinical scales (Butcher et al., 1989). Although our study is the first to examine their utility within a pain patient population, we predict that the clinician working with chronic pain patients will find that the content scales provide an added source of useful hypotheses for this population. Our research indicated that the HEA scale is likely to function almost as a marker of somatic preoccupation and concerns, and is certainly valid in differentiating pain patients from the normal population on this dimension. The other content scales are more likely to be useful in differentiating different treatment needs among pain patients. The WRK and TRT scales seem particularly promising in identifying problematic treatment and work attitudes.

Supplementary scales developed for the MMPI over the years and included in MMPI-2 are also likely to be useful with pain patients. A common problem for many chronic pain patients is the reliance on addictive substances to relieve perceived pain. Consequently, careful appraisal of the tendency for some individuals in pain programs to become addicted to drugs or alcohol should be conducted. The MAC scale has been shown to be a useful indication of substance abuse potential in past MMPI research, and our study indicated it is associated with substance abuse histories among pain patients tested with the MMPI-2 as well.

Case Illustrations

As noted earlier, the case descriptions in the following section will include a computer-based MMPI-2 report along with personal history and treatment information to illustrate how an objective evaluation of the MMPI-2 describes the particular patient. The cases were chosen to illustrate a variety of profile patterns and elevation levels. The Minnesota Clinical Report was chosen because it is the system most familiar to the authors (the second author wrote this interpretive system) and it was designed to include interpretive statements written with the chronic pain patient in mind. Further details of the structure of this system and the interpretive information included in it can be found in the *User's Guide to the Minnesota Clinical Report for the MMPI-2* (Butcher, 1989). It is a codetype-based system which provides an overall interpretive report based on the individual's clinical scale profile pattern, then adds modifying and supplementary statements based on supplementary and content scale elevations. The range of T scores at which interpretive statements are made is lower in this report by about 5 T-score points than in the original interpretive report for the MMPI. (The reader will note that on the clinical profile page plotted by the computer, a comparison of the client's MMPI-2 performance versus the profile they would have obtained on the original MMPI can be made by looking at the Welsh codes presented at the bottom of the page.) Within the narrative report, statements based on the new content scales are clearly prefaced with an indication that these interpretive suggestions do come from content of the client's responses.

This computerized scoring and interpretive system has been designed to classify pain patients' profiles according to the Costello et al. (1987) four-cluster classification rules and to offer interpretive possibilities based on their summary of cluster correlates. However, as noted earlier in this volume (see Table 5-8), these rules tend to leave over 60% of an inpatient chronic pain sample unclassified. With the shift from MMPI to MMPI-2 norms, using the Costello clustering rules will also result in fewer individuals being classified in the most pathological cluster type (Type "P") and more being classified in the least pathological type (Type "N"). Thus, the reader will note that most of the cases illustrated in this chapter do not have any interpretive statements related to a Costello cluster type. Our own research tends to question the reliability and discriminability of their two middle-range clusters, types "A" and "I," and instead suggests overall elevation of the profile (normal limits, middle elevation, or general elevation) may be a more reliable and treatment-relevant classification system. Thus, in presenting these cases we note in the case description what cluster type the client fell into in the Keller-Butcher study, to supplement information presented in the interpretive report. As more research and clinical data accumulate on the use of the MMPI-2 with chronic pain patients, it is likely the MMPI-2 automated report will need to be updated to include a different clustering system or to drop such a system entirely in favor of more differentiated codetype descriptors specific to pain patients. For now, the Costello statements should be viewed as hypotheses about the client's functioning to be tested against other sources of data, as is true of other interpretations based solely on the MMPI-2 or any other single uncorroborated source of information.

The following six cases were chosen to illustrate a variety of MMPI-2 profile types. As part of the editorial process in developing the revised Minnesota Report for the MMPI-2, a randomly selected subset of the chronic pain patients' MMPI-2 data were run through this computer system and reports were generated for each. The second author selected several of these reports representing a range of profile types and elevations. The first author then matched these profiles with data from clients' life events, biographical information, and chart review forms. Thus, these case examples were not pre-selected because of any particular correspondence between MMPI-2 scores and correlate information. Naturally, test misses will occur with the MMPI-2 as well as with any single source of data. We present these cases as illustrative of speculations and hypotheses that may be made using the MMPI-2, but strongly advocate using it as only one component of a multidimensional assessment strategy.

CASE STUDY #1: CHRONIC PAIN PATIENT #25158

Setting: Inpatient Chronic Pain Treatment Program

Patient: Single Caucasian Female, Age 39

Education: Associate of Arts Degree, Registered Nurse

Employment Status: Registered Nurse, on Disability Leave

MMPI-2 Welsh Code: 35/19 80 2467: K/LF:

MMPI-2 Cluster Type (Keller & Butcher): Low-elevation, normal-limits profile

Case History

This 39-year-old woman had a history of chronic back pain since 1982, when she had slipped and fallen in the bathtub. She continued to work and apparently did not let her back pain significantly interfere with her life activities despite gradually worsening pain problems. In 1985 she went on medical leave to undergo lumbar decompression surgery and was recovering until she had a recurrence of low back and leg pain when lifting a garage door in 1986. She had received some treatment through passive physical therapy but did not have the extensive, multi-modal treatment history seen with many pain patients. She was admitted to the Sister Kenny program in early 1987 with primary complaints of back and leg pain, and was receiving Workers' Compensation wage loss payments at the time which were somewhat less than her premorbid income. She was not involved in any litigation related to her pain and was not taking any narcotic medications from which she needed to be weaned. The client was not seen as significantly depressed either by herself or by staff, but was noted to be overweight and deconditioned as well as experiencing some anxiety related to her continuing disability as well as the possible stress of returning to her job as an emergency room nursing supervisor.

The client had never been married, had no children, and lived alone in a home she owned herself. She had no history of mental health or chemical dependency problems or treatment, and denied any history of mental illness, chemical dependency problems, or chronic medical problems in her family.

Treatment and Aftercare Information

The client completed the full three-week inpatient program and participated in the six monthly aftercare sessions. Staff concentrated on helping her with physical reactivation, exercise, and stress management techniques along with weight reduction. The client's compliance with treatment recommendations was rated as very good during both the inpatient and aftercare portions of the program; she was seen as highly motivated to return to her previous level of functioning. She was felt to be capable of returning to her previous employment, and by six months after her discharge from the program she was back to work full-time and seemed to be doing very well at applying the pain management techniques she had learned.

Comments

See Figure 6-1 for automated interpretation. This profile type fits the normal-limits codetype and cluster patterns that have been found to be associated with better outcome and fewer complicating life factors among chronic pain patients. There were no indications from the MMPI-2 in this case of unusual readiness to communicate pain or to use pain symptoms to manipulate others, nor were there indications of psychological or personality factors that might make appropriate functioning in daily life difficult for this client. Thus, one might predict she would benefit from a reactivation program without inordinate attention being paid to mood disturbance, chemical abuse issues, family reinforcement patterns, vocational issues, etc., and in this particular case that prediction seemed justified.

CASE STUDY #2: CHRONIC PAIN PATIENT #37041

Setting: Inpatient Chronic Pain Treatment Program

Patient: Married Caucasian Male, Age 56

Education: Eighth Grade

Employment Status: Former Heavy Labor, now on Disability

MMPI-2 Welsh Code: 1'2-38 09 74/5:6# F/L:K#

MMPI-2 Cluster Type (Keller & Butcher): Middle-elevation profile

Case History

This 56-year-old man had a history of chronic low back pain since a work-related incident in 1986. He had been employed in a heavy labor position and noted the onset of acute back pain with radiation down both legs after assisting in turning a large storage tank. He also complained of groin and testicular pain. Medical impression was chronic musculoligamentous strain to the lumbar spine and degenerative facet disease. Prior treatments included both narcotic and non-narcotic pain medications, passive and active physical therapy, and trigger point injections. The client had not received surgical intervention for his pain problems. The client had a hemorrhoidectomy in the past, suffered from diverticulitis, and had a history of anginal pain; he was taking Inderal, Tagamet, and Xanax at the time of his admission. Both he and his wife had been treated for chemical dependency (alcoholism) in the past and had maintained their sobriety for the past ten years. The client had not returned to work since his injury and expressed considerable anxiety about his ability to work in the future.

The patient had been married for 19 years to his first wife and their relationship seemed stable and supportive. The couple had no children and lived together in a rented home. The patient denied any history of psychiatric problems in himself or his family members but acknowledged that he, his wife, and his father had all been in treatment for alcoholism. The patient's father had suffered from chronic pain problems and a sibling had died of a heart attack.

Treatment and Aftercare Information

The client completed the full three-week inpatient program and participated in the entire six-month aftercare program. Staff saw him as a rather passive-dependent man with a great deal of anxiety focused on his physical symptoms and the possibility he would be unable to work again or that he would have the severe physical problems others in his family had suffered. Treatment was focused on supporting him in vocational planning, working on stress management and relaxation skills, and a behavioral approach to physical reactivation. He was taken off Xanax and at discharge was not taking medications other than Tylenol, Inderal, and Tagamet. He was also felt to be mildly depressed but this was treated indirectly through vocational support and reactivation. Although the patient continued to complain of significant pain, his compliance with treatment recommendations was rated as good during the program and very good during aftercare. He did reach his goal of returning to full-time employment by six months after discharge.

Comments

See Figure 6-2 for automated interpretation. This profile illustrates the potential usefulness of the MacAndrew Alcoholism Scale as well as ASP in suggesting characterologic and addiction problems which must be evaluated carefully. In this case, they were more useful in picking up past history than current active problems, but could alert the clinician to evaluate for substance abuse and for other potential secondary gain or manipulative components of the client's problems. It is interesting that despite the somewhat negative treatment predictions one might make for a spike 1 profile with this degree of somatic preoccupation, this client's WRK and TRT scales were not significantly elevated, suggesting that he did not endorse large numbers of items associated with negative treatment and work attitudes. One might speculate, given the client's background, that his somatic preoccupation was certainly influenced by concerns over repeating family patterns of disability and by his own uncertainty about "having what it takes" to get back to work. When these concerns were addressed supportively with a behavioral reactivation program and vocational help, the "meaning" of his continued pain seemed to have become less frightening and all-consuming to him, and he was able to get back to work.

CASE STUDY #3: CHRONIC PAIN PATIENT #15211

Setting: Inpatient Chronic Pain Treatment Program

Patient: Single Caucasian Male, Age 25

Education: High School Graduate plus 3 years Vo-Tech

Employment Status: Laborer for Meat Packing Plant, on Disability Leave

MMPI-2 Welsh Code: 3''1'24-796/580 KF:L

MMPI-2 Cluster Type (Keller & Butcher): Middle-elevation profile

Case History

This 25-year-old man had been working at a meat packing plant for three months when he began to experience pain in both wrists. He had one surgery for an early carpal tunnel syndrome, but his pain did not abate; instead he developed arm, shoulder, and back pain in addition to the gradually worsening wrist pain. Previous treatments included passive physical therapy, nerve blocks, and chiropractic treatments as well as the surgery. He had not worked for the year prior to his pain clinic admission and was receiving Workers' Compensation wage loss payments. At the time of admission he was living in a rented apartment with a steady girlfriend who also had back pain problems.

The client had never been married and had no children. He came from a family of six children born to parents who were both laborers themselves. There was an extensive family history of chronic disease and chronic pain. Grandparents on both sides had diabetes, cancer, and back problems. The client's father was receiving disability payments for problems with his shoulder, his mother had chronic back pain for which she'd had several surgeries, and he had one brother with a "bad back." The client also acknowledged that several family members had chemical dependency problems. He himself admitted to occasionally heavy alcohol and marijuana use, but denied this was a problem for him. In addition to his other difficulties, the client had a history of chronic gastrointestinal distress and ulcers.

Treatment and Aftercare Information

The client completed the full three-week inpatient program and participated in the six monthly aftercare sessions. Staff concentrated on helping him with physical reactivation, exercise, and stress management techniques along with weight reduction. He was not seen as particularly depressed and thus mood problems were not a major focus of treatment. The client's compliance with treatment recommendations was rated as fair during the inpatient program and poor during aftercare. Although staff felt he was capable of returning to work, he had made no efforts to do so by the end of the six-month follow-up period. Primary contributors to his continuing disability were felt to be family models and reinforcement of disability, continued monetary compensation for disability through his Workers' Compensation payments, and alcohol and drug abuse. His final evaluation noted that prognosis seemed poor unless he were to lose his Workers' Compensation payments and was forced to seek employment again for financial reasons.

Comments

See Figure 6-3 for automated interpretation. Like the profile in case #2, this patient's profile is a relatively common pattern for pain patients in having primary elevations on one or more of the first three scales and falling into the middle-elevation cluster type. The 1-3 pattern illustrated here should signal the clinician to check for secondary gain factors and suggestibility possibly contributing to pain problem maintenance, and in this case there were many pain models for this client as well as secondary gain through financial compensation and avoidance of work he did not enjoy. The ANG scale elevation might be explored further as a possible indicator of problematic interpersonal attitudes or authority problems that might also be working against his performing adequately in the work world.

CASE STUDY #4: CHRONIC PAIN PATIENT #37038

Setting: Inpatient Chronic Pain Treatment Program

Patient: Married Caucasian Female, Age 51

Education: High School Graduate

Employment Status: Laborer, on Disability Leave

MMPI-2 Welsh Code: 20'-365/174:89# L/F:K#

MMPI-2 Cluster Type (Keller & Butcher): Middle-elevation profile

Case History

This patient had problems with back and right leg pain since a work-related injury in 1986. She slipped and fell on her back, resulting in pain which gradually worsened over time and eventually prevented her from returning to work for the six months before her admission in 1987. She had received numerous forms of treatment including analgesic medication, physical therapy modalities, and steroid injections with no significant relief. She was felt to have pain from a soft-tissue injury and possible neuritis of the sciatic nerve. The client acknowledged being quite anxious and depressed about the family financial situation and her own difficulty returning to work. Although she was receiving Workers' Compensation payments, this income was lower than when she had been employed. The client had no history of psychiatric or chemical dependency problems or treatment, and denied any other significant health problems. At admission she had been experiencing severe sleep and appetite disturbance as well as acknowledging dysphoric mood.

The patient was living in a rented home with her husband of 25 years; they had two grown children who were living on their own. Financial difficulties were causing some stress in the marriage but she generally considered it stable and supportive. The patient had lived most of her life in rural areas and came from a family of laborers who had not completed much education. Her mother had a history of three major depressive episodes; she denied any other family history of mental illness or chemical dependency. Both parents had died of heart problems, but the patient had no history or specific concerns about heart problems herself. She denied ever using alcohol or any illicit drugs.

Treatment and Aftercare Information

The client completed the full three-week multidisciplinary pain program as well as the six-month aftercare program. Her compliance with treatment recommendations was rated as good during the inpatient program and fair during aftercare. Staff saw her as depressed and quite anxious about financial problems and that these concerns were complicating her recovery from her soft-tissue injury. She was treated with antidepressant medication and thyroid replacement medication as well as physical reactivation and stress management training. Although her depression remitted somewhat, she was also seen as unhappy with her job situation and not particularly motivated to seek new employment despite her financial concerns. Although staff felt she was capable of returning to work, she had not done so by the end of six-month followup. Her progress in incorporating stress management and relaxation skills in her life was rated as only fair, as was her incorporation of physical exercise and reactivation into her daily life.

Comments

See Figure 6-4 for automated interpretation. This profile illustrates a pattern that is less common than the Hs and/or Hy codetype combinations among pain patients but is an important subgroup, i.e., those patients presenting with a major depressive disorder. Staff appropriately treated the psychiatric illness and the client did apparently experience some improvement in her mood, possibly related to medication, but in this individual's case exploration of the precipitants of her depression suggests rather chronic unhappiness with her life situation even outside of the pain problem she was experiencing. The WRK scale seems helpful with this particular client in capturing her negative attitudes toward her employment. With such a client, it might be appropriate to concentrate on looking at wider life-style issues and goals rather than focusing exclusively on physical reactivation. Indeed, cognitive-behavioral treatment of depression along with vocational counseling and possibly marital counseling might prove more useful than treatment focused on the pain problem per se.

CASE STUDY #5: CHRONIC PAIN PATIENT #14026

Setting: Inpatient Chronic Pain Treatment Program

Patient: Divorced Caucasian Female, Age 42

Education: High School Graduate

Employment Status: Sales Manager, on Disability Leave

MMPI-2 Welsh Code: 4*326" 197'8-0/:5 FK:L

MMPI-2 Cluster Type (Keller & Butcher): General-elevation profile

Case History

This client had experienced back pain since a car accident three years before her admission. She did not complain of pain in any other part of her body, but felt the back pain had gradually worsened with time. She brought a lawsuit as the result of the accident, litigation was still pending at the time of admission, and her current source of income was disability payments through a private insurance company. Past treatments for her pain included non-narcotic medications and physical therapy. She had trouble with back pain before the accident but denied that it had ever interfered with her daily life. She had stopped working as a result of her pain complaints since the accident.

The client had a long history of problems with depression and compulsive behaviors including an eating disorder, compulsive gambling, shoplifting and overspending, and dependence on anti-anxiety medications. She had been hospitalized for psychiatric treatment at least three times and had also been in treatment for dependence on prescription anti-anxiety medications, although she denied any history of problems with alcohol or illicit drugs. Her mother carried a diagnosis of schizophrenia and committed suicide. Information on the mental health of other family members was not available in the chart, although the client noted a great deal of distress around poor relationships with her brothers whom she said constantly undermined her self-confidence by bringing up her past behaviors and psychiatric problems. One brother apparently had been treated for alcoholism. The client had been divorced twice, had no children, and lived alone in a rented apartment. She drove by herself from Texas to enter the inpatient program. Other medical problems at the time of admission included obesity, ulcers, and dependence on Ativan. Physical examination did not reveal any major organic problems contributing to the patient's experience of pain.

Treatment and Aftercare Information

The client completed the full three-week multidisciplinary pain program and her compliance with treatment recommendations during that time was rated as good. Staff concentrated on medication weaning, physical rehabilitation and weight loss, and incorporation of stress management techniques. Drug dependence, physical deconditioning, lack of family support, and psychiatric problems were seen as important contributors to her disability. She cooperated fully in being weaned from Ativan, participated actively in the exercise component of the program, and managed to lose 12 pounds during her three-week stay. In counseling sessions she was described as very insightful about the contribution of her psychiatric problems to her chronic pain disability and seemed ready to work on changing her behavior, not just her attitudes. By the time of discharge, she had agreed to a referral for treatment at a compulsivity clinic in California and was planning to move out there for a new job opportunity. No further aftercare information was available because she lived too far away to return for the monthly sessions.

Comments

See Figure 6-5 for automated interpretation. This profile illustrates the general-elevation cluster type as well as a 4-3 codetype with several other clinically significant elevations. Note that the content scales support the clinical profile in indicating a wide variety of characterologic, psychiatric, and somatic problems: of the fifteen MMPI-2 content scales, five are in the clinically significant range for this patient (ANX, DEP, HEA, ANG, and FAM) and a large number of the narrative report's interpretive statements are based on content scale themes. The MMPI-2 generally indicates that pain problems are just one aspect of numerous life problems experienced by this individual, and effective treatment will need to take a highly multidimensional approach with such a person. Compared to the rest of her profile, her TRT and WRK scores are not elevated into the "clinically significant" range, which seems somewhat surprising given the degree of anger and characterologic problems indicated elsewhere in the profile but was consistent with her non-defensive, possibly help-seeking approach to the test noted in the validity scale pattern. In this case these scales seem to have accurately reflected her willingness to address her multiple problems during treatment, although one might expect that long-term prognosis would remain guarded.

CASE STUDY #6: CHRONIC PAIN PATIENT #13471

Setting: Inpatient Chronic Pain Treatment Program

Patient: Married Caucasian Male, Age 41

Education: Ninth Grade

Employment Status: Construction Worker, on Disability Leave

MMPI-2 Welsh Code: 689"74'123-0/5 F'-L/:K

MMPI-2 Cluster Type (Keller & Butcher): General-elevation profile

Case History

This 41-year-old client from Manitoba had a history of chronic back and leg pain dating back to a work-related accident five years before his pain program admission. He was standing in a labor union picket line at a quarry site when he was struck in the back by a pickup truck. He suffered a fractured spine and fractured pelvis from that accident and had surgery as a result. Over time he also received numerous conservative treatments for pain including nerve blocks, non-narcotic medications, physical therapy, transcutaneous electrical stimulation (TENS), a back brace, and a previous inpatient pain management program. He reported that his pain had gradually worsened over time, and had been aggravated by slipping on ice and falling on his back one year before admission. Impressions on physical exam included persistent muscle spasms and marked guarding behavior, no major objective findings.

The patient brought a lawsuit as a result of his injury and litigation was still pending at the time of his admission. He had not worked in five years and was receiving Social Security Disability Income payments; he reported his current income was much lower than he had been making as a laborer. He had a brother who was also receiving disability payments for back problems, had had three back surgeries, and had been in alcohol treatment. The client had a history of ulcer problems and also had knee surgery ten years ago. He was hospitalized in the mid-70s because of headache complaints and his physician's concern that he was abusing prescription pain medications. He had an extensive history of psychiatric treatment for affective, anxiety, and psychotic symptoms and had been assaultive at times in the past. He was hospitalized once after a suicide attempt. He denied any history of psychiatric problems in other family members, and denied any personal problems with alcohol or illicit drugs. The client had been married to his first wife for sixteen years and had one child who lived with them in a rented house.

Treatment and Aftercare Information

The client completed the full three-week multidisciplinary pain program and his compliance with treatment recommendations during that time was rated as good. A psychiatric evaluation was requested early in treatment and the psychiatrist felt the diagnostic possibilities to be considered included bipolar disorder, schizoaffective disorder, major depressive disorder, or paranoid schizophrenia. An underlying paranoid personality disorder was felt to be present. Although the psychiatrist recommended treatment with antipsychotic medications, during the program the client was put on anti-depressant medication and lithium, and staff concentrated on helping him with physical conditioning and anxiety management. He continued to exhibit extensive guarding behaviors and to make frequent pain complaints throughout the program, and his Beck Depression Inventory score went from 16 to 20 over the three-week period. He was noted to maintain a very high degree of illness conviction in spite of participating in all components of the program.

After discharge, the client returned for a few aftercare sessions but then failed to show up for the rest. His compliance with discharge recommendations was rated as poor. Although staff felt he was capable of returning to work, he had not made efforts to do so by the time of last follow-up. He remained quite depressed, anxious, and angry, and did not seem to have given up his illness conviction or taken personal responsibility for making changes. It was noted that in addition to his psychiatric problems, his family tended to reinforce continued disability by their own example and their lack of support for him moving on with his life.

Comments

See Figure 6-6 for automated interpretation. This profile and case description clearly illustrate the type of case where psychiatric history is extremely important in understanding a client's ongoing difficulties performing adequately in "well" roles in his life. Consistent with the multiple elevations on the client's MMPI-2 clinical and content scales, there seemed to be numerous factors in his life all of which could be contributing to the maintenance of chronic disability: his severe psychiatric problems, his family's reinforcement of disability, etc. The profile fits the most pathological of codetypes (the "Sc Codes") identified in our study as well as the most elevated cluster type. It might be expected that treatment of this client would have to address numerous life problems and even then he is likely to have ongoing factors militating against him performing responsibly and adequately in adult roles. This particular individual seems to have fulfilled those rather negative expectations, and it seems likely ongoing psychiatric treatment will be needed as well as intensive work with his social reinforcement system before any significant changes could be expected.

```
                              TM
                            MMPI-2
                                          TM
           MINNESOTA MULTIPHASIC PERSONALITY INVENTORY-2

           By Starke R. Hathaway and J. Charnley McKinley


                                 TM
                    THE MINNESOTA REPORT:
                    ADULT CLINICAL SYSTEM
                    INTERPRETIVE REPORT

                    By James N. Butcher




                  Client ID:     0025158
                Report Date:     23-AUG-89
                       Age:      39
                       Sex:      Female
                    Setting:     Chronic Pain
                  Education:     12
             Marital Status:     Never Married




            MINNESOTA MULTIPHASIC PERSONALITY INVENTORY-2
       Copyright (c) by THE REGENTS OF THE UNIVERSITY OF MINNESOTA
          1942, 1943 (renewed 1970), 1989.  This Report 1989.
                         All Rights Reserved.
       Distributed Exclusively by NATIONAL COMPUTER SYSTEMS, INC.
              Under License from The University of Minnesota.

          "MMPI-2," "Minnesota Multiphasic Personality Inventory-2," and
       "The Minnesota Report" are trademarks owned by The University of Minnesota.
                    Printed in the United States of America.
```

FIGURE 6-1. Computer-Generated MMPI-2 Interpretive Report for Case Study #1

```
         TM                                                     page 1
MMPI-2              TM
THE MINNESOTA REPORT:               ID: 0025158    REPORT DATE: 23-AUG-89
ADULT CLINICAL SYSTEM
INTERPRETIVE REPORT


PROFILE VALIDITY

This client's approach to the MMPI-2 was open and cooperative.  The
resulting MMPI-2 profile is valid and probably a good indication of her
present level of personality functioning.  This may be viewed as a positive
indication of her involvement with the evaluation.


SYMPTOMATIC PATTERNS

This MMPI-2 clinical profile is within normal limits.  The client did not
report psychological conflicts or situational stresses that are producing
great difficulty for her at this time.  She appears to be dealing
effectively with her life situation, and seems to be obtaining sufficient
satisfaction out of life at this point.

Her sex role identity is not limited to a traditionally feminine pattern and
she appears to have no sex-role conflicts.  Her range of interests includes,
but is not limited to, homemaking and cultural activities.

In addition, the following description is suggested by the content of this
client's responses.  The client does not appear to be an overly anxious
person prone to developing unrealistic fears.  Any fears she reports are
more likely to be reality-based than internally generated.  Her responses
suggest that she has a very trusting attitude toward the world, respects the
law, is honest, and is sensitive to others' needs.  She is rather
conservative and dislikes taking risks.  She reports that her work situation
is generally satisfactory.  No significant negative work attitudes requiring
treatment attention were noted in her item content.


INTERPERSONAL RELATIONS

She has an average interest in being with others and is not socially
isolated or withdrawn.  She appears to meet and talk with other people with
relative ease and is not overly anxious when in social gatherings.


DIAGNOSTIC CONSIDERATIONS

This profile is within normal limits and no clinical diagnosis is provided.

Her MMPI-2 profile most closely matches the "N" Type of pattern found in
cluster analytic studies of chronic pain patient MMPI profiles.  A defining
feature of this chronic pain subtype is the relative absence of clinical
scale elevations.
```

FIGURE 6-1. Continued

```
          TM                                                       page 2
MMPI-2                        TM
THE MINNESOTA REPORT:                    ID: 0025159     REPORT DATE: 23-AUG-89
ADULT CLINICAL SYSTEM
INTERPRETIVE REPORT


The patients matching this subtype typically are thought to have the best
prognosis of chronic pain patient subgroups.  They tend to report fewer
psychological problems and appear to be more emotionally stable than other
pain patients.


---------------------------------------------------------------------------
NOTE:  This MMPI-2 interpretation can serve as a useful source of hypotheses
about clients.  This report is based on objectively derived scale indexes
and scale interpretations that have been developed in diverse groups of
patients.  The personality descriptions, inferences and recommendations
contained herein need to be verified by other sources of clinical
information since individual clients may not fully match the prototype.  The
information in this report should most appropriately be used by a trained,
qualified test interpreter.  The information contained in this report should
be considered confidential.
---------------------------------------------------------------------------
```

FIGURE 6-1. Continued

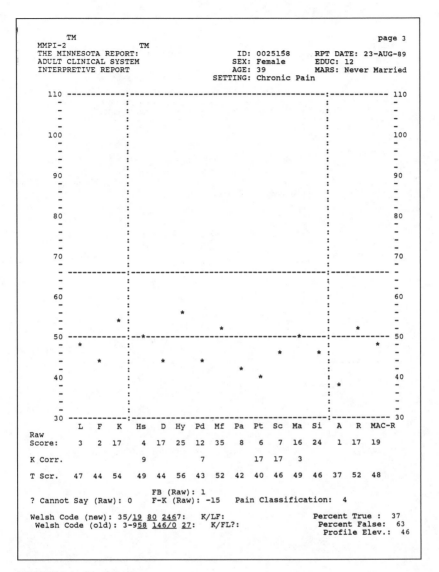

```
        TM                                                    page 3
MMPI-2                  TM
THE MINNESOTA REPORT:                   ID: 0025158    RPT DATE: 23-AUG-89
ADULT CLINICAL SYSTEM                   SEX: Female    EDUC: 12
INTERPRETIVE REPORT                     AGE: 39        MARS: Never Married
                                    SETTING: Chronic Pain

   110 ------------:---------------------------------------:------------ 110
    -               :                                        :            -
    -               :                                        :            -
    -               :                                        :            -
   100              :                                        :           100
    -               :                                        :            -
    -               :                                        :            -
    -               :                                        :            -
    90              :                                        :            90
    -               :                                        :            -
    -               :                                        :            -
    -               :                                        :            -
    80              :                                        :            80
    -               :                                        :            -
    -               :                                        :            -
    -               :                                        :            -
    70              :                                        :            70
    - -------------:---------------------------------------:------------  -
    -               :                                        :            -
    -               :                                        :            -
    60              :                                        :            60
    -               :                                        :            -
    -              *:                     *                  :            -
    -             * :                                        :     *      -
    50 ------------:--*----------------------*-----:------------- 50
    -        *      :                                        :    *       -
    -               :                           *      *    :            -
    -         *     :     *      *                          :            -
    40              :                *      *                :            40
    -               :                                        :  *         -
    -               :                                        :            -
    -               :                                        :            -
    30 ------------:---------------------------------------:------------ 30
         L    F    K   Hs   D   Hy  Pd  Mf  Pa  Pt  Sc  Ma  Si   A    R   MAC-R
Raw
Score:   3    2   17    4  17   25  12  35   8   6   7  16  24  17   17   19

K Corr.             9           7          17  17   3

T Scr.  47   44   54   49  44   56  43  52  42  40  46  49  46  37   52   48

                        FB (Raw): 1
? Cannot Say (Raw): 0   F-K (Raw): -15   Pain Classification:  4

Welsh Code (new): 35/19 80 2467:   K/LF:              Percent True :  37
  Welsh Code (old): 3-958 146/0 27:   K/FL?:          Percent False: 63
                                                      Profile Elev.:  46
```

FIGURE 6-1. Continued

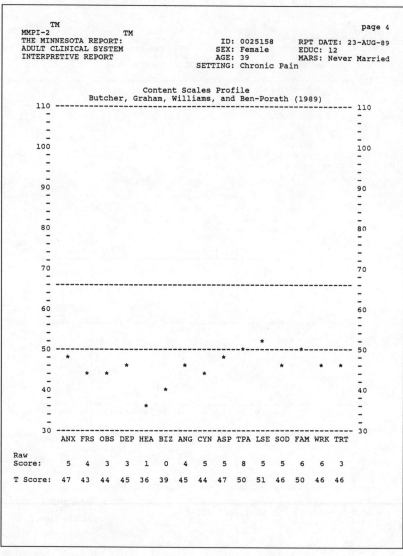

FIGURE 6-1. Continued

```
        TM                                                      page 5
MMPI-2                  TM
THE MINNESOTA REPORT:               ID: 0025158    REPORT DATE: 23-AUG-89
ADULT CLINICAL SYSTEM
INTERPRETIVE REPORT


                        SUPPLEMENTARY SCORE REPORT


                                    Raw Score         T Score

        Ego Strength (Es)               43               68
        Dominance (Do)                  17               53
        Social Responsibility (Re)      23               56
        Overcontrolled Hostility (O-H)  10               37
        PTSD - Keane (PK)                3               42
        PTSD - Schlenger (PS)            4               41
        True Response Inconsistency (TRIN)   8           58F
        Variable Response Inconsistency (VRIN)  2        38


Depression Subscales (Harris-Lingoes):

        Subjective Depression (D1)       3               39
        Psychomotor Retardation (D2)     5               46
        Physical Malfunctioning (D3)     4               56
        Mental Dullness (D4)             3               52
        Brooding (D5)                    1               42


Hysteria Subscales (Harris-Lingoes):

        Denial of Social Anxiety (Hy1)   6               61
        Need for Affection (Hy2)         8               55
        Lassitude-Malaise (Hy3)          4               55
        Somatic Complaints (Hy4)         1               41
        Inhibition of Aggression (Hy5)   4               54


Psychopathic Deviate Subscales (Harris-Lingoes):

        Familial Discord (Pd1)           0               38
        Authority Problems (Pd2)         2               47
        Social Imperturbability (Pd3)    4               54
        Social Alienation (Pd4)          2               40
        Self-Alienation (Pd5)            3               48


Paranoia Subscales (Harris-Lingoes):

        Persecutory Ideas (Pa1)          1               45
        Poignancy (Pa2)                  0               34
        Naivete (Pa3)                    5               50
```

FIGURE 6-1. Continued

```
     TM                                                             page 6
MMPI-2                   TM
THE MINNESOTA REPORT:                  ID: 0025158      REPORT DATE: 23-AUG-89
ADULT CLINICAL SYSTEM
INTERPRETIVE REPORT


                                              Raw Score      T Score

Schizophrenia Subscales (Harris-Lingoes):

        Social Alienation (Sc1)                   3            50
        Emotional Alienation (Sc2)                1            49
        Lack of Ego Mastery, Cognitive (Sc3)      1            49
        Lack of Ego Mastery, Conative (Sc4)       2            49
        Lack of Ego Mastery, Def. Inhib. (Sc5)    1            46
        Bizarre Sensory Experiences (Sc6)         1            45


Hypomania Subscales (Harris-Lingoes):

        Amorality (Ma1)                           1            45
        Psychomotor Acceleration (Ma2)            7            60
        Imperturbability (Ma3)                    4            56
        Ego Inflation (Ma4)                       2            43


Social Introversion Subscales (Ben-Porath, Hostetler, Butcher, & Graham):

        Shyness / Self-Consciousness (Si1)        2            41
        Social Avoidance (Si2)                    2            47
        Alienation--Self and Others (Si3)         3            44


Uniform T scores are used for Hs, D, Hy, Pd, Pa, Pt, Sc, Ma, and the Content
Scales; all other MMPI-2 scales use linear T scores.
```

FIGURE 6-1. Continued

```
        TM                                                      page 7
MMPI-2                  TM
THE MINNESOTA REPORT:                ID: 0025158    REPORT DATE: 23-AUG-89
ADULT CLINICAL SYSTEM
INTERPRETIVE REPORT


                        CRITICAL ITEMS

The following critical items have been found to have possible significance in
analyzing a client's problem situation.  Although these items may serve as a
source of hypotheses for further investigation, caution should be taken in
interpreting individual items because they may have been inadvertently
checked.


Acute Anxiety State  (Koss-Butcher Critical Items)

    3. I wake up fresh and rested most mornings.  (F)
   10. I am about as able to work as I ever was. .(F)
   15. I work under a great deal of tension.  (T)


Depressed Suicidal Ideation  (Koss-Butcher Critical Items)

    9. My daily life is full of things that keep me interested.  (F)
  130. I certainly feel useless at times.  (T)
  518. I have made lots of bad mistakes in my life.  (T)


Threatened Assault  (Koss-Butcher Critical Items)

   37. At times I feel like smashing things.  (T)


Situational Stress Due to Alcoholism  (Koss-Butcher Critical Items)

  518. I have made lots of bad mistakes in my life.  (T)


Mental Confusion  (Koss-Butcher Critical Items)

  299. I cannot keep my mind on one thing.  (T)


Antisocial Attitude  (Lachar-Wrobel Critical Items)

  266. I have never been in trouble with the law.  (F)


Somatic Symptoms  (Lachar-Wrobel Critical Items)

  224. I have few or no pains.  (F)
```

FIGURE 6-1. Continued

```
            TM                                                   page 8
     MMPI-2              TM
     THE MINNESOTA REPORT:              ID: 0025158      REPORT DATE: 23-AUG-89
     ADULT CLINICAL SYSTEM
     INTERPRETIVE REPORT


     Anxiety and Tension  (Lachar-Wrobel Critical Items)

       15. I work under a great deal of tension.  (T)
      299. I cannot keep my mind on one thing.  (T)
      320. I have been afraid of things or people that I knew could not hurt
           me.  (T)


     Deviant Thinking and Experience  (Lachar-Wrobel Critical Items)

      122. At times my thoughts have raced ahead faster than I could speak
           them.  (T)


     Depression and Worry  (Lachar-Wrobel Critical Items)

        3. I wake up fresh and rested most mornings.  (F)
       10. I am about as able to work as I ever was.  (F)
      130. I certainly feel useless at times.  (T)


     Deviant Beliefs  (Lachar-Wrobel Critical Items)

      106. My speech is the same as always (not faster or slower, no slurring or
           hoarseness).  (F)
```

FIGURE 6-1. Continued

```
                              TM
                            MMPI-2
                                                      TM
             MINNESOTA MULTIPHASIC PERSONALITY INVENTORY-2

             By Starke R. Hathaway and J. Charnley McKinley


                                          TM
                         THE MINNESOTA REPORT:
                         ADULT CLINICAL SYSTEM
                         INTERPRETIVE REPORT

                         By James N. Butcher




                      Client ID:   0037041
                    Report Date:   23-AUG-89
                            Age:   56
                            Sex:   Male
                        Setting:   Chronic Pain
                      Education:   12
                 Marital Status:   Married




               MINNESOTA MULTIPHASIC PERSONALITY INVENTORY-2
            Copyright (c) by THE REGENTS OF THE UNIVERSITY OF MINNESOTA
               1942, 1943 (renewed 1970), 1989.  This Report 1989.
                            All Rights Reserved.
             Distributed Exclusively by NATIONAL COMPUTER SYSTEMS, INC.
                 Under License from The University of Minnesota.

             "MMPI-2," "Minnesota Multiphasic Personality Inventory-2," and
         "The Minnesota Report" are trademarks owned by The University of Minnesota.
                       Printed in the United States of America.
```

FIGURE 6-2. Computer-Generated MMPI-2 Interpretive Report for Case Study #2

```
      TM                                                              page 1
MMPI-2                    TM
THE MINNESOTA REPORT:                 ID: 0037041      REPORT DATE: 23-AUG-89
ADULT CLINICAL SYSTEM
INTERPRETIVE REPORT


PROFILE VALIDITY

This is a valid MMPI-2 profile.  The client was quite cooperative with the
evaluation and appears to be willing to disclose personal information.
There may be some tendency on the part of the client to be overly frank and
to exaggerate his symptoms in an effort to obtain help.  He may be open to
the idea of psychological counseling if his clinical scale pattern reflects
psychological symptoms in need of attention.


SYMPTOMATIC PATTERNS

Although the client complains excessively of pain and somatic problems and
organizes his life around what he perceives to be a physical illness, his
complaints probably cannot be explained by actual physical findings.  He
appears to be very dissatisfied with life and pessimistic about the future.
He tends to react to even minor stress with vague physical complaints.
Because of this somatic preoccupation, he probably receives much secondary
gain from the attention of others or from services he receives.


INTERPERSONAL RELATIONS

Somewhat passive-dependent, he tends to be a demanding person who attempts
to dominate relationships through physical complaints.  He becomes hostile
when his needs are not met to his satisfaction.  He seems to require an
excessive amount of emotional support from his spouse.  Many married people
with this profile have difficulties with their marriage.  They are so overly
concerned with their health and preoccupied with bodily problems that they
are unable to show interest in their spouse.

He has an average interest in being with others and is not socially isolated
or withdrawn.  He appears to meet and talk with other people with relative
ease and is not overly anxious when in social gatherings.

The content of this client's MMPI-2 responses suggests the following
additional information concerning his interpersonal relations.  He feels
some family conflict at this time.  However, this does not appear to him to
be a major problem in his life.


BEHAVIORAL STABILITY

Somatic reactivity may be somewhat exaggerated here; he may be reacting to
some stress in his present situation.  If stress is minimal, or if he has
many previous visits to physicians, his personality pattern may suggest a
persistent character problem.  Individuals with this pattern typically have
personality features that persist over time.  His interpersonal style is not
likely to change significantly if retested at a later date.
```

FIGURE 6-2. Continued

```
        TM                                                              page 2
MMPI-2              TM
THE MINNESOTA REPORT:                ID: 0037041      REPORT DATE: 23-AUG-89
ADULT CLINICAL SYSTEM
INTERPRETIVE REPORT


DIAGNOSTIC CONSIDERATIONS

Many individuals with this pattern are described as chronically maladjusted.
If extensive stress and actual multisystem physical disorders are ruled out,
the client would probably be diagnosed as having a Somatoform Disorder.
There is a strong possibility that an Axis II diagnosis of
Passive-Aggressive or Dependent Personality would also be appropriate.

There is a strong possibility that this client has some difficulty with
substance use or abuse.  His personality pattern and score on the MacAndrew
Alcoholism Scale - Revised suggest that possible addiction problems may
warrant further evaluation.


TREATMENT CONSIDERATIONS

He has a poor prognosis for gaining from psychological treatment, since he
holds to a physical explanation of his condition and does not accept
psychological causes for his problems.  Moreover, his cynicism and lack of
introspection make insight-oriented psychotherapy a difficult process.

The possibility that he abuses prescription medications to treat his
discomfort should be evaluated.  Some individuals with this profile who
experience chronic pain respond to behavioral management techniques.


--------------------------------------------------------------------------
NOTE:  This MMPI-2 interpretation can serve as a useful source of hypotheses
about clients.  This report is based on objectively derived scale indexes
and scale interpretations that have been developed in diverse groups of
patients.  The personality descriptions, inferences and recommendations
contained herein need to be verified by other sources of clinical
information since individual clients may not fully match the prototype.  The
information in this report should most appropriately be used by a trained,
qualified test interpreter.  The information contained in this report should
be considered confidential.
--------------------------------------------------------------------------
```

FIGURE 6-2. Continued

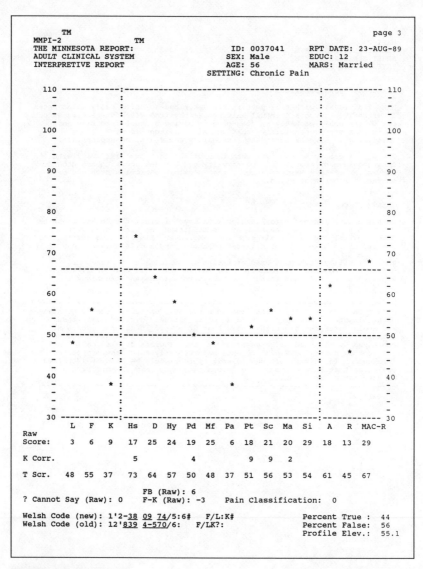

FIGURE 6-2. Continued

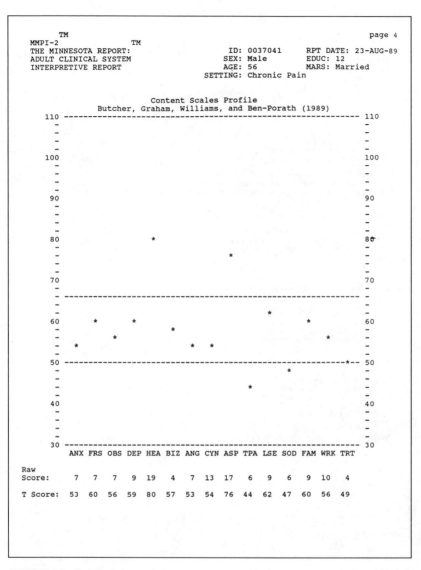

FIGURE 6-2. Continued

```
           TM                                                              page 5
MMPI-2                TM
THE MINNESOTA REPORT:                    ID: 0037041      REPORT DATE: 23-AUG-89
ADULT CLINICAL SYSTEM
INTERPRETIVE REPORT


                        SUPPLEMENTARY SCORE REPORT


                                          Raw Score        T Score

       Ego Strength (Es)                       34             42
       Dominance (Do)                          13             38
       Social Responsibility (Re)               9             30
       Overcontrolled Hostility (O-H)          12             48
       PTSD - Keane (PK)                       11             55
       PTSD - Schlenger (PS)                   17             58
       True Response Inconsistency (TRIN)      12             72T
       Variable Response Inconsistency (VRIN)   9             65


Depression Subscales (Harris-Lingoes):

       Subjective Depression (D1)               9             56
       Psychomotor Retardation (D2)             5             48
       Physical Malfunctioning (D3)             7             83
       Mental Dullness (D4)                     5             62
       Brooding (D5)                            4             62


Hysteria Subscales (Harris-Lingoes):

       Denial of Social Anxiety (Hy1)           3             45
       Need for Affection (Hy2)                 4             40
       Lassitude-Malaise (Hy3)                  6             66
       Somatic Complaints (Hy4)                 6             67
       Inhibition of Aggression (Hy5)           3             48


Psychopathic Deviate Subscales (Harris-Lingoes):

       Familial Discord (Pd1)                   3             58
       Authority Problems (Pd2)                 6             68
       Social Imperturbability (Pd3)            2             40
       Social Alienation (Pd4)                  5             57
       Self-Alienation (Pd5)                    4             53


Paranoia Subscales (Harris-Lingoes):

       Persecutory Ideas (Pa1)                  1             46
       Poignancy (Pa2)                          1             41
       Naivete (Pa3)                            2             36
```

FIGURE 6-2. Continued

```
     TM                                                      page 6
MMPI-2              TM
THE MINNESOTA REPORT:              ID: 0037041      REPORT DATE: 23-AUG-89
ADULT CLINICAL SYSTEM
INTERPRETIVE REPORT


                                    Raw Score      T Score
Schizophrenia Subscales (Harris-Lingoes):

        Social Alienation (Sc1)              5             59
        Emotional Alienation (Sc2)           0             40
        Lack of Ego Mastery, Cognitive (Sc3) 3             60
        Lack of Ego Mastery, Conative (Sc4)  3             55
        Lack of Ego Mastery, Def. Inhib. (Sc5) 3           61
        Bizarre Sensory Experiences (Sc6)    9             85


Hypomania Subscales (Harris-Lingoes):

        Amorality (Ma1)                      4             66
        Psychomotor Acceleration (Ma2)       8             63
        Imperturbability (Ma3)               2             41
        Ego Inflation (Ma4)                  2             43


Social Introversion Subscales (Ben-Porath, Hostetler, Butcher, & Graham):

        Shyness / Self-Consciousness (Si1)   4             48
        Social Avoidance (Si2)               3             49
        Alienation--Self and Others (Si3)   10             65


Uniform T scores are used for Hs, D, Hy, Pd, Pa, Pt, Sc, Ma, and the Content
Scales; all other MMPI-2 scales use linear T scores.
```

FIGURE 6-2. Continued

```
        TM                                                         page 7
MMPI-2              TM
THE MINNESOTA REPORT:                 ID: 0037041      REPORT DATE: 23-AUG-89
ADULT CLINICAL SYSTEM
INTERPRETIVE REPORT


                          CRITICAL ITEMS

    The following critical items have been found to have possible significance in
    analyzing a client's problem situation.  Although these items may serve as a
    source of hypotheses for further investigation, caution should be taken in
    interpreting individual items because they may have been inadvertently
    checked.


Acute Anxiety State  (Koss-Butcher Critical Items)

     3. I wake up fresh and rested most mornings.  (F)
     5. I am easily awakened by noise.  (T)
    10. I am about as able to work as I ever was.  (F)
    28. I am bothered by an upset stomach several times a week.  (T)
   218. I have periods of such great restlessness that I cannot sit long in a
        chair.  (T)
   469. I sometimes feel that I am about to go to pieces.  (T)


Depressed Suicidal Ideation  (Koss-Butcher Critical Items)

    38. I have had periods of days, weeks, or months when I couldn't take care
        of things because I couldn't "get going."  (T)
   130. I certainly feel useless at times.  (T)
   411. At times I think I am no good at all.  (T)
   518. I have made lots of bad mistakes in my life.  (T)


Threatened Assault  (Koss-Butcher Critical Items)

    37. At times I feel like smashing things.  (T)


Situational Stress Due to Alcoholism  (Koss-Butcher Critical Items)

   264. I have used alcohol excessively.  (T)
   489. I have a drug or alcohol problem.  (T)
   518. I have made lots of bad mistakes in my life.  (T)


Mental Confusion  (Koss-Butcher Critical Items)

   299. I cannot keep my mind on one thing.  (T)
   325. I have more trouble concentrating than others seem to have.  (T)


Persecutory Ideas  (Koss-Butcher Critical Items)

   124. I often wonder what hidden reason another person may have for doing
        something nice for me.  (T)
   241. It is safer to trust nobody.  (T)
   251. I have often felt that strangers were looking at me critically.  (T)
   333. People say insulting and vulgar things about me.  (T)
```

FIGURE 6-2. Continued

```
          TM                                                        page 8
MMPI-2                    TM
THE MINNESOTA REPORT:                    ID: 0037041    REPORT DATE: 23-AUG-89
ADULT CLINICAL SYSTEM
INTERPRETIVE REPORT


Antisocial Attitude  (Lachar-Wrobel Critical Items)

   27. When people do me a wrong, I feel I should pay them back if I can, just
       for the principle of the thing.  (T)
   35. Sometimes when I was young I stole things.  (T)
   84. I was suspended from school one or more times for bad behavior.  (T)
  105. In school I was sometimes sent to the principal for bad behavior.  (T)
  227. I don't blame people for trying to grab everything they can get in this
       world.  (T)
  266. I have never been in trouble with the law.  (F)


Family Conflict  (Lachar-Wrobel Critical Items)

   21. At times I have very much wanted to leave home.  (T)


Somatic Symptoms  (Lachar-Wrobel Critical Items)

   28. I am bothered by an upset stomach several times a week.  (T)
   33. I seldom worry about my health.  (F)
   47. I am almost never bothered by pains over my heart or in my chest.  (F)
   53. Parts of my body often have feelings like burning, tingling, crawling,
       or like "going to sleep."  (T)
   57. I hardly ever feel pain in the back of my neck.  (F)
  142. I have never had a fit or convulsion.  (F)
  159. I have never had a fainting spell.  (F)
  224. I have few or no pains.  (F)
  229. I have had blank spells in which my activities were interrupted and I
       did not know what was going on around me.  (T)
  247. I have numbness in one or more places on my skin.  (T)
  255. I do not often notice my ears ringing or buzzing.  (F)
  295. I have never been paralyzed or had any unusual weakness of any of my
       muscles.  (F)


Sexual Concern and Deviation  (Lachar-Wrobel Critical Items)

   12. My sex life is satisfactory.  (F)


Anxiety and Tension  (Lachar-Wrobel Critical Items)

  218. I have periods of such great restlessness that I cannot sit long in a
       chair.  (T)
  261. I have very few fears compared to my friends.  (F)
  299. I cannot keep my mind on one thing.  (T)
  320. I have been afraid of things or people that I knew could not hurt
       me.  (T)
```

FIGURE 6-2. Continued

```
        TM                                                          page 9
   MMPI-2                    TM
   THE MINNESOTA REPORT:                ID: 0037041      REPORT DATE: 23-AUG-89
   ADULT CLINICAL SYSTEM
   INTERPRETIVE REPORT


   Sleep Disturbance   (Lachar-Wrobel Critical Items)

      5. I am easily awakened by noise.   (T)
    328. Sometimes some unimportant thought will run through my mind and bother
         me for days.   (T)


   Deviant Thinking and Experience   (Lachar-Wrobel Critical Items)

    122. At times my thoughts have raced ahead faster than I could speak
         them.   (T)
    298. Peculiar odors come to me at times.   (T)


   Depression and Worry   (Lachar-Wrobel Critical Items)

      3. I wake up fresh and rested most mornings.   (F)
     10. I am about as able to work as I ever was.   (F)
     73. I am certainly lacking in self-confidence.   (T)
    130. I certainly feel useless at times.   (T)
    339. I have sometimes felt that difficulties were piling up so high that I
         could not overcome them.   (T)
    411. At times I think I am no good at all.   (T)
    415. I worry quite a bit over possible misfortunes.   (T)


   Deviant Beliefs   (Lachar-Wrobel Critical Items)

    106. My speech is the same as always (not faster or slower, no slurring or
         hoarseness).   (F)
    333. People say insulting and vulgar things about me.   (T)
    466. Sometimes I am sure that other people can tell what I am thinking.   (T)


   Substance Abuse   (Lachar-Wrobel Critical Items)

    168. I have had periods in which I carried on activities without knowing
         later what I had been doing.   (T)
    264. I have used alcohol excessively.   (T)
```

FIGURE 6-2. Continued

TM
MMPI-2
TM
MINNESOTA MULTIPHASIC PERSONALITY INVENTORY-2

By Starke R. Hathaway and J. Charnley McKinley

TM
THE MINNESOTA REPORT:
ADULT CLINICAL SYSTEM
INTERPRETIVE REPORT

By James N. Butcher

```
       Client ID:  0015211
     Report Date:  23-AUG-89
            Age:  25
            Sex:  Male
         Setting:  Chronic Pain
       Education:  12
  Marital Status:  Never Married
```

FIGURE 6-3. Computer-Generated MMPI-2 Interpretive Report for Case Study #3

```
        TM                                                          page 1
MMPI-2                  TM
THE MINNESOTA REPORT:                   ID: 0015211     REPORT DATE: 23-AUG-89
ADULT CLINICAL SYSTEM
INTERPRETIVE REPORT


PROFILE VALIDITY

This is a valid MMPI-2 profile.  The client's responses to the MMPI-2
validity items suggest that he cooperated with the evaluation enough to
provide useful interpretive information.  The resulting clinical profile is
an adequate indication of his present personality functioning.


SYMPTOMATIC PATTERNS

The client presents a picture of multiple physical problems and a reduced
level of psychological functioning.  His physical problems may be vague, may
have appeared suddenly after a period of stress, and may not be traceable to
actual organic changes.  He may be manifesting fatigue, vague pain,
weakness, or unexplained periods of dizziness.

He may view himself as highly virtuous and show a "Pollyannish" attitude
toward life.  He may not appear greatly anxious or depressed over his
symptoms and may show "La belle indifference."  Apparently sociable and
rather exhibitionistic, he seems to manage conflict by excessive denial and
repression.

The client seems to have a rather limited range of interests and tends to
prefer stereotyped masculine activities over literary and artistic pursuits
or introspective experiences.  He tends to be somewhat competitive and needs
to see himself as masculine.  He probably prefers to view women in
subservient roles.  Interpersonally, he is likely to be intolerant and
insensitive, and others may find him rather crude, coarse, or narrow-minded.


In addition, the following description is suggested by the content of this
client's responses.  He views his physical health as failing and reports
numerous somatic concerns.  He feels that life is no longer worthwhile and
that he is losing control of his thought processes.  According to his
self-report, there is a strong possibility that he has seriously
contemplated suicide.  He complains about feeling quite uncomfortable and in
poor health.  The symptoms he reports reflect vague weakness, fatigue, and
difficulties in concentration.  In addition, he feels that others are
unsympathetic toward his perceived health problems.


INTERPERSONAL RELATIONS

He tends to be somewhat passive-dependent and demanding in interpersonal
relationships.  He may attempt to control others by complaining about
physical symptoms.

His social interests appear to be high and he seems to enjoy social
participation.  However, his interpersonal behavior may be problematic at
times in the sense that he may lose his temper in frustrating situations.
```

FIGURE 6-3. Continued

```
        TM                                                          page 2
MMPI-2                      TM
THE MINNESOTA REPORT:                ID: 0015211     REPORT DATE: 23-AUG-89
ADULT CLINICAL SYSTEM
INTERPRETIVE REPORT


The content of this client's MMPI-2 responses suggests the following
additional information concerning his interpersonal relations.  He feels
intensely angry, hostile, and resentful of others, and would like to get
back at them.  He is competitive and uncooperative, tending to be very
critical of others.


BEHAVIORAL STABILITY

The personality pattern characterized by this profile is long-standing and
quite stable.  The client is likely to have a hysteroid adjustment to life,
but under stress might experience periods of exacerbated symptom
development.  Some individuals with this profile develop a lifestyle of
"invalidism" in which they become incapacitated and dependent upon others.
His interpersonal style is not likely to change significantly if retested at
a later date.


DIAGNOSTIC CONSIDERATIONS

Individuals with this profile typically show a neurotic pattern of
adjustment and would probably receive a clinical diagnosis of Conversion
Disorder or Somatization Disorder.  They might also receive an Axis II
diagnosis of Dependent Personality.

There is some possibility that he is having difficulties of an addictive
nature.  He may be abusing or over-using addicting substances.  Further
evaluation of alcohol or drug usage is recommended.

His MMPI-2 profile most closely matches the "A" Type pattern found in
cluster analytic studies of chronic pain patient profiles.  The "A" Type
pattern is thought to characterize one of the most frustrating groups of
pain patients with which to work because of their initial defensiveness and
denial of psychological problems.

Patients with this pattern typically show low psychological mindedness and a
seeming lack of awareness of psychological mechanisms involved in their pain
behavior.  Individuals with this pattern are frequently diagnosed as having
conversion symptoms.


TREATMENT CONSIDERATIONS

Individuals with this MMPI-2 profile tend to be defensive toward
psychological interpretations of their physical symptoms.  They show
reluctance to engage in self-exploration and are generally not very open to
the idea that their own thinking may be influencing their problems.  He
shows little anxiety about his symptoms and is unmotivated to improve his
personal adjustment.
```

FIGURE 6-3. Continued

```
        TM                                                                page 3
MMPI-2                    TM
THE MINNESOTA REPORT:                ID: 0015211        REPORT DATE: 23-AUG-89
ADULT CLINICAL SYSTEM
INTERPRETIVE REPORT


He appears to be difficult to approach with long-term treatment goals or
insight-oriented approaches to psychotherapy.  However, if he is to make
significant, enduring gains in personality adjustment, a long-term treatment
commitment may be called for.  In the beginning of therapy, individuals with
this profile type may be too defensive to engage in productive
self-reflection.  They tend to lose interest in psychological treatment or
continue to fall back on somatic explanations for their problems,
particularly if treatment sessions are aimed at exploring emotional content.

In many cases, the somatic symptoms reflected in this profile pattern are
influenced or exacerbated by environmental stress.  His low level of
psychological functioning may be improved by stress inoculation therapy
aimed at reducing his situational stress and providing him with more
adaptive approaches to living.

Many individuals with this profile type persist in pursuing medical
treatments for problems that have no organic basis.  Some individuals may
actually seek radical treatments such as surgery even though the basis of
their condition is vague or uncertain.  This profile type is associated with
negative outcomes to surgical interventions.


---------------------------------------------------------------------------
NOTE:  This MMPI-2 interpretation can serve as a useful source of hypotheses
about clients.  This report is based on objectively derived scale indexes
and scale interpretations that have been developed in diverse groups of
patients.  The personality descriptions, inferences and recommendations
contained herein need to be verified by other sources of clinical
information since individual clients may not fully match the prototype.  The
information in this report should most appropriately be used by a trained,
qualified test interpreter.  The information contained in this report should
be considered confidential.
---------------------------------------------------------------------------
```

FIGURE 6-3. Continued

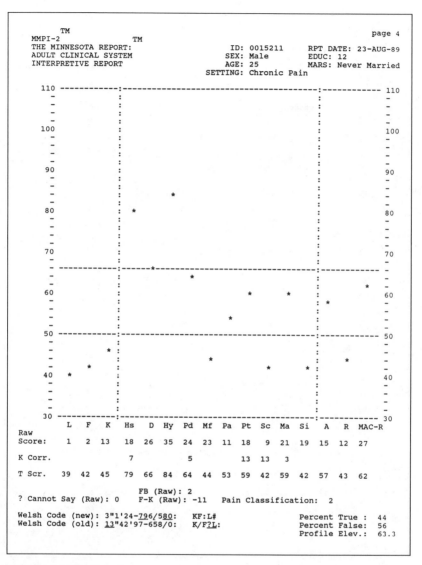

```
                TM                                                        page 4
        MMPI-2                     TM
        THE MINNESOTA REPORT:                   ID: 0015211    RPT DATE: 23-AUG-89
        ADULT CLINICAL SYSTEM                   SEX: Male      EDUC: 12
        INTERPRETIVE REPORT                     AGE: 25        MARS: Never Married
                                            SETTING: Chronic Pain
```

	L	F	K	Hs	D	Hy	Pd	Mf	Pa	Pt	Sc	Ma	Si	A	R	MAC-R
Raw Score:	1	2	13	18	26	35	24	23	11	18	9	21	19	15	12	27
K Corr.				7			5			13	13	3				
T Scr.	39	42	45	79	66	84	64	44	53	59	42	59	42	57	43	62

```
                                  FB (Raw): 2
        ? Cannot Say (Raw): 0     F-K (Raw): -11   Pain Classification:  2

        Welsh Code (new): 3"1'24-796/580:    KF:L#          Percent True :  44
        Welsh Code (old): 13"42'97-658/0:    K/F?L:         Percent False:  56
                                                            Profile Elev.:  63.3
```

FIGURE 6-3. Continued

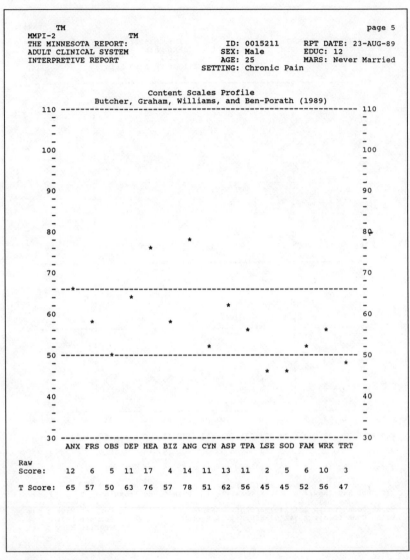

FIGURE 6-3. Continued

```
      TM                                                            page 6
MMPI-2                    TM
THE MINNESOTA REPORT:              ID: 0015211      REPORT DATE: 23-AUG-89
ADULT CLINICAL SYSTEM
INTERPRETIVE REPORT


                     SUPPLEMENTARY SCORE REPORT


                                      Raw Score       T Score

        Ego Strength (Es)                32              38
        Dominance (Do)                   17              51
        Social Responsibility (Re)       14              34
        Overcontrolled Hostility (O-H)   14              55
        PTSD - Keane (PK)                12              57
        PTSD - Schlenger (PS)            20              62
        True Response Inconsistency (TRIN)   9           50
        Variable Response Inconsistency (VRIN)  4        46


Depression Subscales (Harris-Lingoes):

        Subjective Depression (D1)       13              66
        Psychomotor Retardation (D2)      3              37
        Physical Malfunctioning (D3)      7              83
        Mental Dullness (D4)              3              53
        Brooding (D5)                     5              68


Hysteria Subscales (Harris-Lingoes):

        Denial of Social Anxiety (Hy1)    5              56
        Need for Affection (Hy2)          7              51
        Lassitude-Malaise (Hy3)          10              84
        Somatic Complaints (Hy4)          7              72
        Inhibition of Aggression (Hy5)    4              55


Psychopathic Deviate Subscales (Harris-Lingoes):

        Familial Discord (Pd1)            3              58
        Authority Problems (Pd2)          4              55
        Social Imperturbability (Pd3)     5              58
        Social Alienation (Pd4)           3              46
        Self-Alienation (Pd5)             7              67


Paranoia Subscales (Harris-Lingoes):

        Persecutory Ideas (Pa1)           2              52
        Poignancy (Pa2)                   4              62
        Naivete (Pa3)                     3              41
```

FIGURE 6-3. Continued

```
        TM                                                                page 7
MMPI-2                    TM
THE MINNESOTA REPORT:                      ID: 0015211        REPORT DATE: 23-AUG-89
ADULT CLINICAL SYSTEM
INTERPRETIVE REPORT


                                         Raw Score      T Score

Schizophrenia Subscales (Harris-Lingoes):

        Social Alienation (Sc1)                1             43
        Emotional Alienation (Sc2)             2             59
        Lack of Ego Mastery, Cognitive (Sc3)   0             42
        Lack of Ego Mastery, Conative (Sc4)    2             49
        Lack of Ego Mastery, Def. Inhib. (Sc5) 0             40
        Bizarre Sensory Experiences (Sc6)      4             60


Hypomania Subscales (Harris-Lingoes):

        Amorality (Ma1)                        3             58
        Psychomotor Acceleration (Ma2)         7             58
        Imperturbability (Ma3)                 5             59
        Ego Inflation (Ma4)                    4             56


Social Introversion Subscales (Ben-Porath, Hostetler, Butcher, & Graham):

        Shyness / Self-Consciousness (Si1)     3             45
        Social Avoidance (Si2)                 2             45
        Alienation--Self and Others (Si3)      6             53


Uniform T scores are used for Hs, D, Hy, Pd, Pa, Pt, Sc, Ma, and the Content
Scales; all other MMPI-2 scales use linear T scores.
```

FIGURE 6-3. Continued

```
          TM                                                      page 8
MMPI-2                  TM
THE MINNESOTA REPORT:                      ID: 0015211     REPORT DATE: 23-AUG-89
ADULT CLINICAL SYSTEM
INTERPRETIVE REPORT


                          CRITICAL ITEMS

   The following critical items have been found to have possible significance in
   analyzing a client's problem situation.  Although these items may serve as a
   source of hypotheses for further investigation, caution should be taken in
   interpreting individual items because they may have been inadvertently
   checked.


Acute Anxiety State  (Koss-Butcher Critical Items)

    3. I wake up fresh and rested most mornings.  (F)
    5. I am easily awakened by noise.  (T)
   10. I am about as able to work as I ever was.  (F)
   15. I work under a great deal of tension.  (T)
   28. I am bothered by an upset stomach several times a week.  (T)
   39. My sleep is fitful and disturbed.  (T)
   59. I am troubled by discomfort in the pit of my stomach every few days or
       oftener.  (T)
  140. Most nights I go to sleep without thoughts or ideas bothering me.  (F)
  172. I frequently notice my hand shakes when I try to do something.  (T)
  208. I hardly ever notice my heart pounding and I am seldom short of
       breath.  (F)
  301. I feel anxiety about something or someone almost all the time.  (T)
  444. I am a high-strung person.  (T)
  469. I sometimes feel that I am about to go to pieces.  (T)


Depressed Suicidal Ideation  (Koss-Butcher Critical Items)

    9. My daily life is full of things that keep me interested.  (F)
   71. These days I find it hard not to give up hope of amounting to
       something.  (T)
   95. I am happy most of the time.  (F)
  130. I certainly feel useless at times.  (T)
  146. I cry easily.  (T)
  215. I brood a great deal.  (T)
  273. Life is a strain for me much of the time.  (T)
  388. I very seldom have spells of the blues.  (F)
  518. I have made lots of bad mistakes in my life.  (T)


Threatened Assault  (Koss-Butcher Critical Items)

   37. At times I feel like smashing things.  (T)
  134. At times I feel like picking a fist fight with someone.  (T)
  213. I get mad easily and then get over it soon.  (T)
  389. I am often said to be hotheaded.  (T)
```

FIGURE 6-3. Continued

```
              TM                                                    page 9
MMPI-2                     TM
THE MINNESOTA REPORT:                    ID: 0015211      REPORT DATE: 23-AUG-89
ADULT CLINICAL SYSTEM
INTERPRETIVE REPORT


Situational Stress Due to Alcoholism  (Koss-Butcher Critical Items)

   264. I have used alcohol excessively.  (T)
   487. I have enjoyed using marijuana.  (T)
   502. I have some habits that are really harmful.  (T)
   518. I have made lots of bad mistakes in my life.  (T)


Persecutory Ideas  (Koss-Butcher Critical Items)

   241. It is safer to trust nobody.  (T)


Antisocial Attitude  (Lachar-Wrobel Critical Items)

    27. When people do me a wrong, I feel I should pay them back if I can, just
        for the principle of the thing.  (T)
    35. Sometimes when I was young I stole things.  (T)
   105. In school I was sometimes sent to the principal for bad behavior.  (T)
   227. I don't blame people for trying to grab everything they can get in this
        world.  (T)
   254. Most people make friends because friends are likely to be useful to
        them.  (T)
   266. I have never been in trouble with the law.  (F)
   324. I can easily make other people afraid of me, and sometimes do for the
        fun of it.  (T)


Family Conflict  (Lachar-Wrobel Critical Items)

    83. I have very few quarrels with members of my family.  (F)


Somatic Symptoms  (Lachar-Wrobel Critical Items)

    28. I am bothered by an upset stomach several times a week.  (T)
    33. I seldom worry about my health.  (F)
    53. Parts of my body often have feelings like burning, tingling, crawling,
        or like "going to sleep."  (T)
    57. I hardly ever feel pain in the back of my neck.  (F)
    59. I am troubled by discomfort in the pit of my stomach every few days or
        oftener.  (T)
   142. I have never had a fit or convulsion.  (F)
   159. I have never had a fainting spell.  (F)
   175. I feel weak all over much of the time.  (T)
   176. I have very few headaches.  (F)
   224. I have few or no pains.  (F)
   295. I have never been paralyzed or had any unusual weakness of any of my
        muscles.  (F)
   464. I feel tired a good deal of the time.  (T)
```

FIGURE 6-3. Continued

```
        TM                                                    page 10
MMPI-2                TM
THE MINNESOTA REPORT:                ID: 0015211      REPORT DATE: 23-AUG-89
ADULT CLINICAL SYSTEM
INTERPRETIVE REPORT


Anxiety and Tension  (Lachar-Wrobel Critical Items)

   15. I work under a great deal of tension.  (T)
  172. I frequently notice my hand shakes when I try to do something.  (T)
  261. I have very few fears compared to my friends.  (F)
  301. I feel anxiety about something or someone almost all the time.  (T)


Sleep Disturbance  (Lachar-Wrobel Critical Items)

    5. I am easily awakened by noise.  (T)
   39. My sleep is fitful and disturbed.  (T)
  140. Most nights I go to sleep without thoughts or ideas bothering me.  (F)


Deviant Thinking and Experience  (Lachar-Wrobel Critical Items)

  122. At times my thoughts have raced ahead faster than I could speak
       them.  (T)
  427. I have never seen a vision.  (F)


Depression and Worry  (Lachar-Wrobel Critical Items)

    3. I wake up fresh and rested most mornings.  (F)
   10. I am about as able to work as I ever was.  (F)
  130. I certainly feel useless at times.  (T)
  273. Life is a strain for me much of the time.  (T)
  415. I worry quite a bit over possible misfortunes.  (T)


Deviant Beliefs  (Lachar-Wrobel Critical Items)

  106. My speech is the same as always (not faster or slower, no slurring or
       hoarseness).  (F)
  466. Sometimes I am sure that other people can tell what I am thinking.  (T)


Substance Abuse  (Lachar-Wrobel Critical Items)

  264. I have used alcohol excessively.  (T)
  429. Except by doctor's orders I never take drugs or sleeping pills.  (F)


Problematic Anger  (Lachar-Wrobel Critical Items)

  134. At times I feel like picking a fist fight with someone.  (T)
  213. I get mad easily and then get over it soon.  (T)
  389. I am often said to be hotheaded.  (T)
```

FIGURE 6-3. Continued

```
                                 TM
                               MMPI-2
                                                       TM
             MINNESOTA MULTIPHASIC PERSONALITY INVENTORY-2

             By Starke R. Hathaway and J. Charnley McKinley


                                     TM
                      THE MINNESOTA REPORT:
                      ADULT CLINICAL SYSTEM
                      INTERPRETIVE REPORT

                      By James N. Butcher




                      Client ID:  0037038
                    Report Date:  23-AUG-89
                            Age:  53
                            Sex:  Female
                        Setting:  Chronic Pain
                      Education:  12
                 Marital Status:  Married




             MINNESOTA MULTIPHASIC PERSONALITY INVENTORY-2
          Copyright (c) by THE REGENTS OF THE UNIVERSITY OF MINNESOTA
             1942, 1943 (renewed 1970), 1989.  This Report 1989.
                           All Rights Reserved.
            Distributed Exclusively by NATIONAL COMPUTER SYSTEMS, INC.
              Under License from The University of Minnesota.

             "MMPI-2," "Minnesota Multiphasic Personality Inventory-2," and
      "The Minnesota Report" are trademarks owned by The University of Minnesota.
                      Printed in the United States of America.
```

FIGURE 6-4. Computer-Generated MMPI-2 Interpretive Report for Case Study #4

```
          TM                                                    page 1
MMPI-2                     TM
THE MINNESOTA REPORT:                ID: 0037038    REPORT DATE: 23-AUG-89
ADULT CLINICAL SYSTEM
INTERPRETIVE REPORT


PROFILE VALIDITY

This is a valid MMPI-2 profile.  The client has responded to the items in a
generally open and frank manner, neither denying problems nor claiming an
excessive number of unusual symptoms.  There is, however, some possibility
that she was overly critical in her self-appraisal, possibly presenting a
more negative picture than is warranted.  This may reflect low self-esteem,
or a need to gain attention for her problems.


SYMPTOMATIC PATTERNS

The client's MMPI-2 profile suggests that she is presently experiencing many
psychological problems.  Individuals with this profile tend to show a
pattern of chronic psychological maladjustment.  She is presently quite
depressed and anxious, extremely pessimistic, and disinterested in life.
She blames and belittles herself to the point that she cannot function in
routine daily activities.  She may experience vague physical complaints and
feel as if she cannot "get going."  She reports no significant sex-role
conflicts.

In addition, the following description is suggested by the content of this
client's responses.  She views her physical health as failing and reports
numerous somatic concerns.  She feels that life is no longer worthwhile and
that she is losing control of her thought processes.  According to her
self-report, there is a strong possibility that she has seriously
contemplated suicide.


INTERPERSONAL RELATIONS

She is socially withdrawn, fearful of others, does not make friends easily,
and lacks expressiveness and spontaneity in social situations.  She tends to
allow others to dominate her and fails to defend herself even when she has
been wronged.  She may become involved in relationships in which she is
mistreated or taken advantage of because she feels she "doesn't deserve
better."  Her marital situation is likely to be unrewarding and
impoverished.  Her marriage does not seem to provide her with sufficient
pleasure or happiness.

The content of this client's MMPI-2 responses suggests the following
additional information concerning her interpersonal relations.  Her social
relationships are likely to be viewed by others as problematic.  She may
visibly be uneasy around others, sits alone in group situations, and
dislikes engaging in group activities.


BEHAVIORAL STABILITY

Her depression may be partly situational and may diminish over time or with
treatment, or as stress dissipates.  Nevertheless, her profile also
indicates a stable pattern of behavior or a personality-trait pattern
reflecting social withdrawal.  Her many passive traits, including
dependency, low self-esteem, and social isolation, are likely to persist
even after the symptom pattern of depression and anxiety subsides.
```

FIGURE 6-4. Continued

```
       TM                                                            page 2
MMPI-2                    TM
THE MINNESOTA REPORT:            ID: 0037038       REPORT DATE: 23-AUG-89
ADULT CLINICAL SYSTEM
INTERPRETIVE REPORT


DIAGNOSTIC CONSIDERATIONS

A Dysthymic Disorder is the most likely clinical diagnosis.  She would
probably also be considered to have a Dependent Personality Disorder.


TREATMENT CONSIDERATIONS

Medical or pain patients with this MMPI-2 profile are usually experiencing a
great deal of emotional distress along with their physical symptoms.  Some
individuals with this profile require antidepressant medication to elevate
their mood.  This patient is probably feeling quite tense and may be
motivated to receive help for her depressive symptoms.

Individual psychotherapy, although possibly considered appropriate in her
case, may not be very easy to conduct.  Individuals with this MMPI-2 pattern
are very inhibited, have very low social skills, and have difficulty
relating well to others.  They are likely to have problems establishing a
therapeutic relationship.

Directive psychological treatment that requires less initial activity on the
part of the patient might have more chance of succeeding than
insight-oriented psychotherapy.  She might also benefit from some social
skills training.

If psychological treatment is being considered it may be profitable for the
therapist to explore the client's treatment motivation early in therapy.
The item content she endorsed includes some feelings and attitudes that
could be unproductive in psychological treatment and in implementing
self-change.  In any intervention or psychological evaluation program
involving occupational adjustment, her negative work attitudes could become
an important problem to overcome.  She holds a number of attitudes and
feelings that could interfere with work adjustment.


----------------------------------------------------------------------------
NOTE:  This MMPI-2 interpretation can serve as a useful source of hypotheses
about clients.  This report is based on objectively derived scale indexes
and scale interpretations that have been developed in diverse groups of
patients.  The personality descriptions, inferences and recommendations
contained herein need to be verified by other sources of clinical
information since individual clients may not fully match the prototype.  The
information in this report should most appropriately be used by a trained,
qualified test interpreter.  The information contained in this report should
be considered confidential.
----------------------------------------------------------------------------
```

FIGURE 6-4. Continued

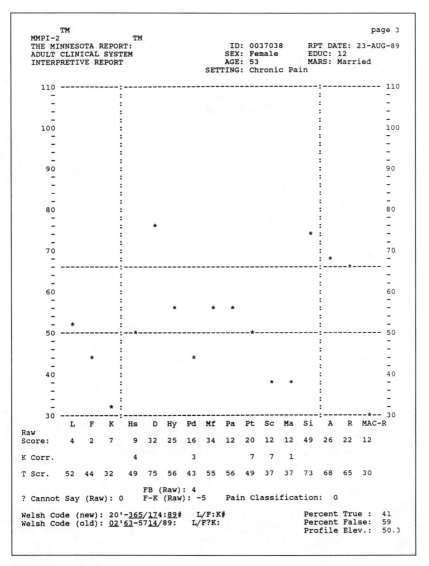

```
                TM                                                        page 3
MMPI-2                        TM
THE MINNESOTA REPORT:                      ID: 0037038     RPT DATE: 23-AUG-89
ADULT CLINICAL SYSTEM                      SEX: Female     EDUC: 12
INTERPRETIVE REPORT                        AGE: 53         MARS: Married
                                           SETTING: Chronic Pain
```

FIGURE 6-4. Continued

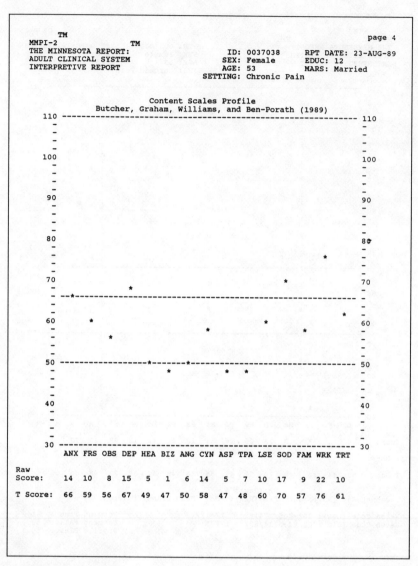

FIGURE 6-4. Continued

```
        TM                                                          page 5
MMPI-2                    TM
THE MINNESOTA REPORT:                  ID: 0037038      REPORT DATE: 23-AUG-89
ADULT CLINICAL SYSTEM
INTERPRETIVE REPORT


                          SUPPLEMENTARY SCORE REPORT


                                      Raw Score        T Score


        Ego Strength (Es)                 27              35
        Dominance (Do)                    15              46
        Social Responsibility (Re)        22              53
        Overcontrolled Hostility (O-H)    11              41
        PTSD - Keane (PK)                 18              64
        PTSD - Schlenger (PS)             23              62
        True Response Inconsistency (TRIN) 9              50
        Variable Response Inconsistency (VRIN) 11         74


Depression Subscales (Harris-Lingoes):

        Subjective Depression (D1)        18              75
        Psychomotor Retardation (D2)       7              57
        Physical Malfunctioning (D3)       6              70
        Mental Dullness (D4)               6              66
        Brooding (D5)                      6              68


Hysteria Subscales (Harris-Lingoes):

        Denial of Social Anxiety (Hy1)     1              35
        Need for Affection (Hy2)           4              38
        Lassitude-Malaise (Hy3)           11              83
        Somatic Complaints (Hy4)           3              49
        Inhibition of Aggression (Hy5)     3              46


Psychopathic Deviate Subscales (Harris-Lingoes):

        Familial Discord (Pd1)             2              50
        Authority Problems (Pd2)           1              40
        Social Imperturbability (Pd3)      1              36
        Social Alienation (Pd4)            6              60
        Self-Alienation (Pd5)              6              63


Paranoia Subscales (Harris-Lingoes):

        Persecutory Ideas (Pa1)            4              63
        Poignancy (Pa2)                    4              59
        Naivete (Pa3)                      3              41
```

FIGURE 6-4. Continued

```
       TM                                                              page 6
MMPI-2                TM
THE MINNESOTA REPORT:               ID: 0037038      REPORT DATE: 23-AUG-89
ADULT CLINICAL SYSTEM
INTERPRETIVE REPORT


                                          Raw Score      T Score

Schizophrenia Subscales (Harris-Lingoes):

        Social Alienation (Sc1)               6             61
        Emotional Alienation (Sc2)            1             49
        Lack of Ego Mastery, Cognitive (Sc3)  1             49
        Lack of Ego Mastery, Conative (Sc4)   3             54
        Lack of Ego Mastery, Def. Inhib. (Sc5) 1            46
        Bizarre Sensory Experiences (Sc6)     1             45


Hypomania Subscales (Harris-Lingoes):

        Amorality (Ma1)                       1             45
        Psychomotor Acceleration (Ma2)        4             45
        Imperturbability (Ma3)                0             30
        Ego Inflation (Ma4)                   6             68


Social Introversion Subscales (Ben-Porath, Hostetler, Butcher, & Graham):

        Shyness / Self-Consciousness (Si1)   13             71
        Social Avoidance (Si2)                5             60
        Alienation--Self and Others (Si3)    10             63


Uniform T scores are used for Hs, D, Hy, Pd, Pa, Pt, Sc, Ma, and the Content
Scales; all other MMPI-2 scales use linear T scores.
```

FIGURE 6-4. Continued

```
         TM                                                    page 7
MMPI-2                        TM
THE MINNESOTA REPORT:                ID: 0037038     REPORT DATE: 23-AUG-89
ADULT CLINICAL SYSTEM
INTERPRETIVE REPORT


                           CRITICAL ITEMS

The following critical items have been found to have possible significance in
analyzing a client's problem situation.  Although these items may serve as a
source of hypotheses for further investigation, caution should be taken in
interpreting individual items because they may have been inadvertently
checked.


Acute Anxiety State  (Koss-Butcher Critical Items)

    2. I have a good appetite.  (F)
    3. I wake up fresh and rested most mornings.  (F)
    5. I am easily awakened by noise.  (T)
   10. I am about as able to work as I ever was.  (F)
  140. Most nights I go to sleep without thoughts or ideas bothering me.  (F)
  223. I believe I am no more nervous than most others.  (F)
  444. I am a high-strung person.  (T)
  469. I sometimes feel that I am about to go to pieces.  (T)


Depressed Suicidal Ideation  (Koss-Butcher Critical Items)

   65. Most of the time I feel blue.  (T)
   71. These days I find it hard not to give up hope of amounting to
       something.  (T)
   75. I usually feel that life is worthwhile.  (F)
   95. I am happy most of the time.  (F)
  130. I certainly feel useless at times.  (T)
  146. I cry easily.  (T)
  233. I have difficulty in starting to do things.  (T)
  388. I very seldom have spells of the blues.  (F)
  411. At times I think I am no good at all.  (T)


Threatened Assault  (Koss-Butcher Critical Items)

   37. At times I feel like smashing things.  (T)


Situational Stress Due to Alcoholism  (Koss-Butcher Critical Items)

  125. I believe that my home life is as pleasant as that of most people I
       know.  (F)


Mental Confusion  (Koss-Butcher Critical Items)

   31. I find it hard to keep my mind on a task or job.  (T)
```

FIGURE 6-4. Continued

```
                  TM
    MMPI-2            TM                                          page 8
    THE MINNESOTA REPORT:               ID: 0037038     REPORT DATE: 23-AUG-89
    ADULT CLINICAL SYSTEM
    INTERPRETIVE REPORT


    Persecutory Ideas  (Koss-Butcher Critical Items)

      17. I am sure I get a raw deal from life.  (T)
      99. Someone has it in for me.  (T)
     124. I often wonder what hidden reason another person may have for doing
          something nice for me.  (T)
     145. I feel that I have often been punished without cause.  (T)
     251. I have often felt that strangers were looking at me critically.  (T)


    Family Conflict  (Lachar-Wrobel Critical Items)

     125. I believe that my home life is as pleasant as that of most people I
          know.  (F)


    Somatic Symptoms  (Lachar-Wrobel Critical Items)

     224. I have few or no pains.  (F)
     464. I feel tired a good deal of the time.  (T)


    Sexual Concern and Deviation  (Lachar-Wrobel Critical Items)

      62. I have often wished I were a girl. (Or if you are a girl) I have never
          been sorry that I am a girl.  (F)
     166. I am worried about sex.  (T)


    Anxiety and Tension  (Lachar-Wrobel Critical Items)

      17. I am sure I get a raw deal from life.  (T)
     223. I believe I am no more nervous than most others.  (F)
     261. I have very few fears compared to my friends.  (F)
     320. I have been afraid of things or people that I knew could not hurt
          me.  (T)
     405. I am usually calm and not easily upset.  (F)


    Sleep Disturbance  (Lachar-Wrobel Critical Items)

       5. I am easily awakened by noise.  (T)
     140. Most nights I go to sleep without thoughts or ideas bothering me.  (F)


    Deviant Thinking and Experience  (Lachar-Wrobel Critical Items)

     122. At times my thoughts have raced ahead faster than I could speak
          them.  (T)
     307. At times I hear so well it bothers me.  (T)
```

FIGURE 6-4. Continued

```
        TM                                                        page 9
MMPI-2                    TM
THE MINNESOTA REPORT:                   ID: 0037038      REPORT DATE: 23-AUG-89
ADULT CLINICAL SYSTEM
INTERPRETIVE REPORT


Depression and Worry  (Lachar-Wrobel Critical Items)

    2. I have a good appetite.  (F)
    3. I wake up fresh and rested most mornings.  (F)
   10. I am about as able to work as I ever was.  (F)
   65. Most of the time I feel blue.  (T)
   73. I am certainly lacking in self-confidence.  (T)
   75. I usually feel that life is worthwhile.  (F)
  130. I certainly feel useless at times.  (T)
  339. I have sometimes felt that difficulties were piling up so high that I
       could not overcome them.  (T)
  411. At times I think I am no good at all.  (T)
  415. I worry quite a bit over possible misfortunes.  (T)


Deviant Beliefs  (Lachar-Wrobel Critical Items)

   99. Someone has it in for me.  (T)
  466. Sometimes I am sure that other people can tell what I am thinking.˜  (T)
```

FIGURE 6-4. Continued

```
                              TM
                            MMPI-2
                                                          TM
               MINNESOTA MULTIPHASIC PERSONALITY INVENTORY-2

               By Starke R. Hathaway and J. Charnley McKinley


                                         TM
                         THE MINNESOTA REPORT:
                         ADULT CLINICAL SYSTEM
                         INTERPRETIVE REPORT

                         By James N. Butcher




                      Client ID:  0014026
                    Report Date:  23-AUG-89
                            Age:  43
                            Sex:  Female
                        Setting:  Chronic Pain
                      Education:  12
                 Marital Status:  Divorced




               MINNESOTA MULTIPHASIC PERSONALITY INVENTORY-2
          Copyright (c) by THE REGENTS OF THE UNIVERSITY OF MINNESOTA
             1942, 1943 (renewed 1970), 1989.  This Report 1989.
                           All Rights Reserved.
          Distributed Exclusively by NATIONAL COMPUTER SYSTEMS, INC.
               Under License from The University of Minnesota.

           "MMPI-2," "Minnesota Multiphasic Personality Inventory-2," and
       "The Minnesota Report" are trademarks owned by The University of Minnesota.
                     Printed in the United States of America.
```

FIGURE 6-5. Computer-Generated MMPI-2 Interpretive Report for Case Study #5

```
        TM                                                      page 1
MMPI-2                      TM
THE MINNESOTA REPORT:                ID: 0014026      REPORT DATE: 23-AUG-89
ADULT CLINICAL SYSTEM
INTERPRETIVE REPORT


PROFILE VALIDITY

This is a valid MMPI-2 profile.  The client has responded to the items in a
generally open and frank manner, neither denying problems nor claiming an
excessive number of unusual symptoms.  There is, however, some possibility
that she was overly critical in her self-appraisal, possibly presenting a
more negative picture than is warranted.  This may reflect low self-esteem,
or a need to gain attention for her problems.


SYMPTOMATIC PATTERNS

This individual is presenting with a somewhat mixed symptomatic pattern.
The client's MMPI-2 profile suggests that she currently has many
psychological problems.  Individuals with similar profiles tend to show a
pattern of chronic psychological maladjustment.  She appears to be
impulsive, immature, angry, and hostile, and she may have a history of
overly aggressive behavior.  Possibly complicating these many problems is a
poor work or achievement record.  Because she is hypersensitive to rejection
and has a low tolerance for frustration, she tends to lose control easily.
She may use denial and projection to avoid blame.

In addition, the following description is suggested by the content of this
client's responses.  She is preoccupied with feeling guilty and unworthy.
She feels that she deserves to be punished for wrongs she has committed.
She feels regretful and unhappy about life, and seems plagued by anxiety and
worry about the future.  She feels hopeless at times and feels that she is a
condemned person.  She views her physical health as failing and reports
numerous somatic concerns.  She feels that life is no longer worthwhile and
that she is losing control of her thought processes.  According to her
self-report, there is a strong possibility that she has seriously
contemplated suicide.  She has a self-acknowledged history of suicidal
ideation.  It is important to perform a suicide assessment and, if need be,
take appropriate precautions.  She has acknowledged having suicidal
thoughts recently.  Although she denies suicidal attempts in the past, given
her current mood an assessment of suicidal potential appears indicated.
She complains about feeling quite uncomfortable and in poor health.  The
symptoms she reports reflect vague weakness, fatigue, and difficulties in
concentration.  In addition, she feels that others are unsympathetic toward
her perceived health problems.  She has endorsed a number of items
reflecting a high degree of anger.  She appears to have a high potential for
explosive behavior at times.  She is rather high-strung and believes that
she feels things more, or more intensely, than others do.  She feels quite
lonely and misunderstood at times.


INTERPERSONAL RELATIONS

Her relationships tend to be rather superficial and she may be manipulative.
She may attempt to control others through intimidation.  Rocky interpersonal
relationships are the norm among individuals with this profile.  Marital
breakup is a relatively common problem.
```

FIGURE 6-5. Continued

```
          TM                                                      page 2
MMPI-2                     TM
THE MINNESOTA REPORT:                  ID: 0014026     REPORT DATE: 23-AUG-89
ADULT CLINICAL SYSTEM
INTERPRETIVE REPORT
```

The content of this client's MMPI-2 responses suggests the following
additional information concerning her interpersonal relations. She feels a
moderate degree of family conflict at this time, and reported some
troublesome family issues. She feels that her family life is not as
pleasant as that of other people she knows. She feels like leaving home to
escape a quarrelsome, critical situation, and to be free of family
domination. She feels intensely angry, hostile, and resentful of others,
and would like to get back at them. She is competitive and uncooperative,
tending to be very critical of others.

BEHAVIORAL STABILITY

This profile pattern tends to be generally stable over time and suggests
persistent personality problems in her clinical picture. Her interpersonal
style is not likely to change significantly if retested at a later date.

DIAGNOSTIC CONSIDERATIONS

Individuals with this profile are likely to be diagnosed as having a
Personality Disorder.

She has a number of personality characteristics that are associated with a
substance use or abuse disorder. The client's MacAndrew Alcoholism Scale -
Revised score, along with the personality characteristics reflected in the
profile, suggest that she resembles some individuals who develop addictive
disorders. A substance abuse evaluation is recommended to explore this
possibility.

TREATMENT CONSIDERATIONS

Her long-standing pain complaints may be related to her personality
problems. Possible secondary gain factors in her illness should be
carefully evaluated before any psychological treatment is begun.
Individuals with this MMPI-2 profile are usually seen as poor candidates for
psychotherapy. They do not ordinarily seek psychological treatment on their
own. When they are pressured into treatment, they tend to be only
marginally cooperative at best. They tend to use denial a great deal and to
have little psychological insight. They tend to be quite self-centered and
immature; they do not see a need for psychological therapy.

Individuals with this profile pattern are not amenable to changing their
behavior. They have anger control problems that are likely to interfere

FIGURE 6-5. Continued

```
        TM                                                            page 3
MMPI-2                  TM
THE MINNESOTA REPORT:                    ID: 0014026      REPORT DATE: 23-AUG-89
ADULT CLINICAL SYSTEM
INTERPRETIVE REPORT
```

with treatment. She is likely to terminate therapy early, possibly in
anger. The manipulative behavior that patients with this profile show is
likely to interfere with the development of trust in relationships, making
the treatment relationship stormy. Individuals with this profile may
develop substance abuse problems if treated with medication. Her item
content suggests some family conflicts which are giving her considerable
concern at this time. She feels unhappy about her life and resents having
an unpleasant home life. Psychological intervention with her could
profitably focus, in part, upon clarifying her feelings about her family.

```
-----------------------------------------------------------------------------
```

NOTE: This MMPI-2 interpretation can serve as a useful source of hypotheses
about clients. This report is based on objectively derived scale indexes
and scale interpretations that have been developed in diverse groups of
patients. The personality descriptions, inferences and recommendations
contained herein need to be verified by other sources of clinical
information since individual clients may not fully match the prototype. The
information in this report should most appropriately be used by a trained,
qualified test interpreter. The information contained in this report should
be considered confidential.

```
-----------------------------------------------------------------------------
```

FIGURE 6-5. Continued

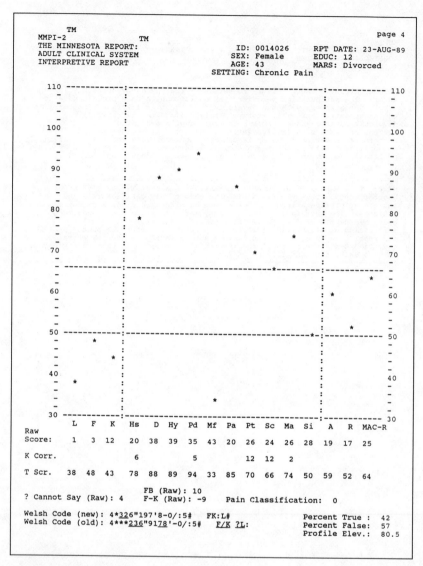

```
      TM
MMPI-2                TM                                              page 4
THE MINNESOTA REPORT:                        ID: 0014026      RPT DATE: 23-AUG-89
ADULT CLINICAL SYSTEM                        SEX: Female      EDUC: 12
INTERPRETIVE REPORT                          AGE: 43          MARS: Divorced
                                         SETTING: Chronic Pain

    110 -------------:--------------------------------------------:------------ 110
      -              :                                            :              -
      -              :                                            :              -
      -              :                                            :              -
    100              :                                            :            100
      -              :                 *                          :              -
      -              :                                            :              -
      -              :             *                              :              -
     90              :          *                                 :             90
      -              :                      *                     :              -
      -              :                                            :              -
     80              :   *                                        :             80
      -              :                                            :              -
      -              :                               *            :              -
     70              :                          *                 :             70
      - ------------:--------------------------------*-----------:------------   -
      -              :                                            :      *       -
     60              :                                            : *           60
      -              :                                            :              -
     50 -------------:--------------------------------------*-:------------      50
      -        *     :                                          *                -
      -              :   *                                                       -
     40              :                                                          40
      -    *         :                                                           -
      -              :                      *                                    -
     30 -------------:--------------------------------------------:------------  30
           L    F    K   Hs   D   Hy  Pd   Mf  Pa  Pt  Sc  Ma  Si   A    R  MAC-R
Raw
Score:     1    3   12   20  38  39  35   43  20  26  24  26  28  19   17   25

K Corr.                   6           5            12  12   2

T Scr.    38   48   43   78  88  89  94   33  85  70  66  74  50  59   52   64

                         FB (Raw): 10
? Cannot Say (Raw): 4    F-K (Raw): -9    Pain Classification:  0

Welsh Code (new): 4*326"197'8-0/:5#   FK:L#              Percent True :  42
Welsh Code (old): 4***236"9178'-0/:5#   F/K ?L:          Percent False:  57
                                                         Profile Elev.: 80.5
```

FIGURE 6-5. Continued

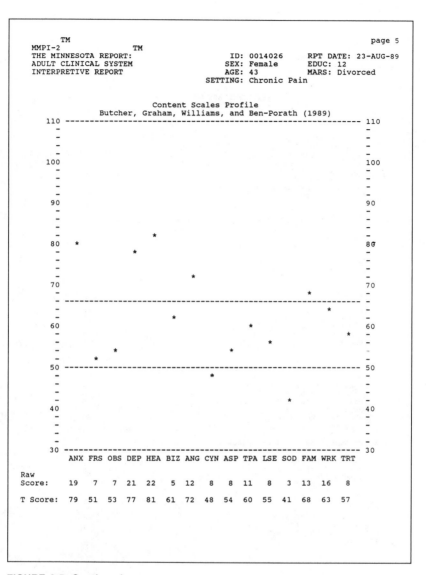

FIGURE 6-5. Continued

```
      TM                                                         page 6
MMPI-2                  TM
THE MINNESOTA REPORT:                ID: 0014026    REPORT DATE: 23-AUG-89
ADULT CLINICAL SYSTEM
INTERPRETIVE REPORT


                         SUPPLEMENTARY SCORE REPORT


                                        Raw Score     T Score

        Ego Strength (Es)                   25           31
        Dominance (Do)                      13           39
        Social Responsibility (Re)          13           30
        Overcontrolled Hostility (O-H)      13           48
        PTSD - Keane (PK)                   21           69
        PTSD - Schlenger (PS)               30           70
        True Response Inconsistency (TRIN)   9           50
        Variable Response Inconsistency (VRIN)  4        46


Depression Subscales (Harris-Lingoes):

        Subjective Depression (D1)          20           79
        Psychomotor Retardation (D2)         6           51
        Physical Malfunctioning (D3)         8           85
        Mental Dullness (D4)                 9           79
        Brooding (D5)                        7           73


Hysteria Subscales (Harris-Lingoes):

        Denial of Social Anxiety (Hy1)       5           56
        Need for Affection (Hy2)             8           55
        Lassitude-Malaise (Hy3)             14           95
        Somatic Complaints (Hy4)             6           61
        Inhibition of Aggression (Hy5)       4           54


Psychopathic Deviate Subscales (Harris-Lingoes):

        Familial Discord (Pd1)               6           74
        Authority Problems (Pd2)             7           85
        Social Imperturbability (Pd3)        4           54
        Social Alienation (Pd4)              8           71
        Self-Alienation (Pd5)                7           68


Paranoia Subscales (Harris-Lingoes):

        Persecutory Ideas (Pa1)              4           63
        Poignancy (Pa2)                      6           72
        Naivete (Pa3)                        7           60
```

FIGURE 6-5. Continued

```
      TM                                                        page 7
MMPI-2                    TM
THE MINNESOTA REPORT:                 ID: 0014026      REPORT DATE: 23-AUG-89
ADULT CLINICAL SYSTEM
INTERPRETIVE REPORT


                                         Raw Score       T Score

Schizophrenia Subscales (Harris-Lingoes):

        Social Alienation (Sc1)              5              57
        Emotional Alienation (Sc2)           3              67
        Lack of Ego Mastery, Cognitive (Sc3) 1              49
        Lack of Ego Mastery, Conative (Sc4)  6              70
        Lack of Ego Mastery, Def. Inhib. (Sc5) 5            72
        Bizarre Sensory Experiences (Sc6)    6              68


Hypomania Subscales (Harris-Lingoes):

        Amorality (Ma1)                      4              70
        Psychomotor Acceleration (Ma2)      10              75
        Imperturbability (Ma3)               3              50
        Ego Inflation (Ma4)                  3              49


Social Introversion Subscales (Ben-Porath, Hostetler, Butcher, & Graham):

        Shyness / Self-Consciousness (Si1)   1              38
        Social Avoidance (Si2)               1              42
        Alienation--Self and Others (Si3)    6              52


Uniform T scores are used for Hs, D, Hy, Pd, Pa, Pt, Sc, Ma, and the Content
Scales; all other MMPI-2 scales use linear T scores.
```

FIGURE 6-5. Continued

```
        TM                                                         page 8
MMPI-2                  TM
THE MINNESOTA REPORT:                   ID: 0014026     REPORT DATE: 23-AUG-89
ADULT CLINICAL SYSTEM
INTERPRETIVE REPORT


                             CRITICAL ITEMS

The following critical items have been found to have possible significance in
analyzing a client's problem situation. Although these items may serve as a
source of hypotheses for further investigation, caution should be taken in
interpreting individual items because they may have been inadvertently
checked.


Acute Anxiety State  (Koss-Butcher Critical Items)

     3. I wake up fresh and rested most mornings.  (F)
     5. I am easily awakened by noise.  (T)
    10. I am about as able to work as I ever was.  (F)
    15. I work under a great deal of tension.  (T)
    28. I am bothered by an upset stomach several times a week.  (T)
    39. My sleep is fitful and disturbed.  (T)
    59. I am troubled by discomfort in the pit of my stomach every few days or
        oftener.  (T)
   140. Most nights I go to sleep without thoughts or ideas bothering me.  (F)
   208. I hardly ever notice my heart pounding and I am seldom short of
        breath.  (F)
   218. I have periods of such great restlessness that I cannot sit long in a
        chair.  (T)
   223. I believe I am no more nervous than most others.  (F)
   301. I feel anxiety about something or someone almost all the time.  (T)
   444. I am a high-strung person.  (T)
   469. I sometimes feel that I am about to go to pieces.  (T)


Depressed Suicidal Ideation  (Koss-Butcher Critical Items)

     9. My daily life is full of things that keep me interested.  (F)
    38. I have had periods of days, weeks, or months when I couldn't take care
        of things because I couldn't "get going."  (T)
    65. Most of the time I feel blue.  (T)
    75. I usually feel that life is worthwhile.  (F)
    95. I am happy most of the time.  (F)
   130. I certainly feel useless at times.  (T)
   146. I cry easily.  (T)
   233. I have difficulty in starting to do things.  (T)
   273. Life is a strain for me much of the time.  (T)
   388. I very seldom have spells of the blues.  (F)
   454. The future seems hopeless to me.  (T)
   506. I have recently considered killing myself.  (T)
   518. I have made lots of bad mistakes in my life.  (T)
   520. Lately I have thought a lot about killing myself.  (T)
```

FIGURE 6-5. Continued

```
        TM                                                       page 9
MMPI-2                   TM
THE MINNESOTA REPORT:                ID: 0014026      REPORT DATE: 23-AUG-89
ADULT CLINICAL SYSTEM
INTERPRETIVE REPORT


Threatened Assault   (Koss-Butcher Critical Items)

   37. At times I feel like smashing things.   (T)
   85. At times I have a strong urge to do something harmful or shocking.   (T)
  213. I get mad easily and then get over it soon.   (T)
  389. I am often said to be hotheaded.   (T)


Situational Stress Due to Alcoholism  (Koss-Butcher Critical Items)

  125. I believe that my home life is as pleasant as that of most people I
       know.  (F)
  487. I have enjoyed using marijuana.   (T)
  489. I have a drug or alcohol problem.   (T)
  518. I have made lots of bad mistakes in my life.   (T)


Mental Confusion  (Koss-Butcher Critical Items)

   31. I find it hard to keep my mind on a task or job.   (T)


Persecutory Ideas  (Koss-Butcher Critical Items)

  251. I have often felt that strangers were looking at me critically.   (T)
  259. I am sure I am being talked about.   (T)
  333. People say insulting and vulgar things about me.   (T)


Antisocial Attitude  (Lachar-Wrobel Critical Items)

   35. Sometimes when I was young I stole things.   (T)
  105. In school I was sometimes sent to the principal for bad behavior.   (T)
  227. I don't blame people for trying to grab everything they can get in this
       world.   (T)
  266. I have never been in trouble with the law.   (F)


Family Conflict  (Lachar-Wrobel Critical Items)

   21. At times I have very much wanted to leave home.   (T)
   83. I have very few quarrels with members of my family.   (F)
  125. I believe that my home life is as pleasant as that of most people I
       know.  (F)


Somatic Symptoms  (Lachar-Wrobel Critical Items)

   28. I am bothered by an upset stomach several times a week.   (T)
   33. I seldom worry about my health.   (F)
```

FIGURE 6-5. Continued

```
       TM                                                        page 10
MMPI-2                    TM
THE MINNESOTA REPORT:                   ID: 0014026      REPORT DATE: 23-AUG-89
ADULT CLINICAL SYSTEM
INTERPRETIVE REPORT


   40. Much of the time my head seems to hurt all over.  (T)
   47. I am almost never bothered by pains over my heart or in my chest.  (F)
   57. I hardly ever feel pain in the back of my neck.  (F)
   59. I am troubled by discomfort in the pit of my stomach every few days or
       oftener.  (T)
  111. I have a great deal of stomach trouble.  (T)
  142. I have never had a fit or convulsion.  (F)
  175. I feel weak all over much of the time.  (T)
  176. I have very few headaches.  (F)
  182. I have had attacks in which I could not control my movements or speech
       but in which I knew what was going on around me.  (T)
  224. I have few or no pains.  (F)
  247. I have numbness in one or more places on my skin.  (T)
  295. I have never been paralyzed or had any unusual weakness of any of my
       muscles.  (F)
  464. I feel tired a good deal of the time.  (T)


Sexual Concern and Deviation  (Lachar-Wrobel Critical Items)

   12. My sex life is satisfactory.  (F)
   34. I have never been in trouble because of my sex behavior.  (F)


Anxiety and Tension  (Lachar-Wrobel Critical Items)

   15. I work under a great deal of tension.  (T)
  218. I have periods of such great restlessness that I cannot sit long in a
       chair.  (T)
  223. I believe I am no more nervous than most others.  (F)
  261. I have very few fears compared to my friends.  (F)
  301. I feel anxiety about something or someone almost all the time.  (T)
  405. I am usually calm and not easily upset.  (F)


Sleep Disturbance  (Lachar-Wrobel Critical Items)

    5. I am easily awakened by noise.  (T)
   39. My sleep is fitful and disturbed.  (T)
  140. Most nights I go to sleep without thoughts or ideas bothering me.  (F)


Deviant Thinking and Experience  (Lachar-Wrobel Critical Items)

  122. At times my thoughts have raced ahead faster than I could speak
       them.  (T)


Depression and Worry  (Lachar-Wrobel Critical Items)

    3. I wake up fresh and rested most mornings.  (F)
   10. I am about as able to work as I ever was.  (F)
   65. Most of the time I feel blue.  (T)
```

FIGURE 6-5. Continued

```
         TM                                                    page 11
MMPI-2                    TM
THE MINNESOTA REPORT:              ID: 0014026     REPORT DATE: 23-AUG-89
ADULT CLINICAL SYSTEM
INTERPRETIVE REPORT


  73. I am certainly lacking in self-confidence.   (T)
  75. I usually feel that life is worthwhile.   (F)
 130. I certainly feel useless at times.   (T)
 273. Life is a strain for me much of the time.   (T)
 339. I have sometimes felt that difficulties were piling up so high that I
      could not overcome them.   (T)
 415. I worry quite a bit over possible misfortunes.   (T)
 454. The future seems hopeless to me.   (T)


Deviant Beliefs   (Lachar-Wrobel Critical Items)

 106. My speech is the same as always (not faster or slower, no slurring or
      hoarseness).   (F)
 259. I am sure I am being talked about.   (T)
 333. People say insulting and vulgar things about me.   (T)
 466. Sometimes I am sure that other people can tell what I am thinking.   (T)


Substance Abuse   (Lachar-Wrobel Critical Items)

 429. Except by doctor's orders I never take drugs or sleeping pills.   (F)


Problematic Anger   (Lachar-Wrobel Critical Items)

  85. At times I have a strong urge to do something harmful or shocking.   (T)
 213. I get mad easily and then get over it soon.   (T)
 389. I am often said to be hotheaded.   (T)
```

FIGURE 6-5. Continued

```
      TM                                                           page 12
MMPI-2                 TM
THE MINNESOTA REPORT:                    ID: 0014026    REPORT DATE: 23-AUG-89
ADULT CLINICAL SYSTEM
INTERPRETIVE REPORT


                              OMITTED ITEMS


The following items were omitted by the client.  It may be helpful to
discuss these item omissions with this individual to determine the reason
for non-compliance with test instructions.

 185. I wish I were not so shy.
 199. I like science.
 278. I get all the sympathy I should.
 336. Someone has control over my mind.
```

FIGURE 6-5. Continued

```
                        TM
                     MMPI-2
                                             TM
      MINNESOTA MULTIPHASIC PERSONALITY INVENTORY-2

      By Starke R. Hathaway and J. Charnley McKinley


                               TM
               THE MINNESOTA REPORT:
               ADULT CLINICAL SYSTEM
               INTERPRETIVE REPORT

               By James N. Butcher




                 Client ID:   0013471
               Report Date:   23-AUG-89
                       Age:   41
                       Sex:   Male
                   Setting:   Chronic Pain
                 Education:   12
            Marital Status:   Married




          MINNESOTA MULTIPHASIC PERSONALITY INVENTORY-2
      Copyright (c) by THE REGENTS OF THE UNIVERSITY OF MINNESOTA
         1942, 1943 (renewed 1970), 1989.  This Report 1989.
                       All Rights Reserved.
      Distributed Exclusively by NATIONAL COMPUTER SYSTEMS, INC.
           Under License from The University of Minnesota.

        "MMPI-2," "Minnesota Multiphasic Personality Inventory-2," and
   "The Minnesota Report" are trademarks owned by The University of Minnesota.
                 Printed in the United States of America.
```

FIGURE 6-6. Computer-Generated MMPI-2 Interpretive Report for Case Study #6

```
        TM                                                          page 1
MMPI-2                    TM
THE MINNESOTA REPORT:                  ID: 0013471      REPORT DATE: 23-AUG-89
ADULT CLINICAL SYSTEM
INTERPRETIVE REPORT


PROFILE VALIDITY

This client has endorsed a number of psychological problems, suggesting that
he is experiencing a high degree of stress.  Although the MMPI-2 profile is
probably valid, it may reflect some exaggeration of symptoms.


SYMPTOMATIC PATTERNS

A severe psychological disorder is reflected in this profile.  The client
appears to be experiencing a florid psychotic process which includes
personality decompensation, social withdrawal, disordered affect, and
erratic, possibly assaultive, behavior.  He appears to be quite confused,
withdrawn, and preoccupied with occult or abstract ideas, and may feel that
others are against him because of his beliefs.  He may appear quite
apathetic, tends to spend a great deal of time in fantasy, and might suffer
from hallucinations, blunted or inappropriate affect, and hostile, irritable
behavior.  He appears confused and disoriented, and may behave in
unpredictable, highly aggressive ways.

The client seems to have a rather limited range of interests and tends to
prefer stereotyped masculine activities over literary and artistic pursuits
or introspective experiences.  He tends to be somewhat competitive and needs
to see himself as masculine.  He probably prefers to view women in
subservient roles.  Interpersonally, he is likely to be intolerant and
insensitive, and others may find him rather crude, coarse, or narrow-minded.


In addition, the following description is suggested by the content of this
client's responses.  The client's recent thinking is likely to be
characterized by obsessiveness and indecision.  He may feel somewhat
estranged from people, somewhat alienated and concerned over the actions of
others, and may tend to blame others for his negative frame of mind.  He
reports holding some antisocial beliefs and attitudes, admits to rule
violations, and acknowledges a history of antisocial behavior in the past.
He views the world as a threatening place, sees himself as having been
unjustly blamed for others' problems, and feels that he is getting a raw
deal out of life.  He is rather high-strung and believes that he feels
things more, or more intensely, than others do.  He feels quite lonely and
misunderstood at times.  He endorsed a number of extreme and bizarre
thoughts suggesting the presence of delusions and/or hallucinations.  He
apparently believes that he has special mystical powers or a special
"mission" in life which others do not understand or accept.  The client may
be having periods of clouded consciousness, irritability, and/or
uncontrollable emotionality.  The client reports bizarre or unusual sensory
experiences and confused thinking which should be evaluated carefully.
```

FIGURE 6-6. Continued

```
        TM                                                        page 2
MMPI-2              TM
THE MINNESOTA REPORT:              ID: 0013471      REPORT DATE: 23-AUG-89
ADULT CLINICAL SYSTEM
INTERPRETIVE REPORT
```

INTERPERSONAL RELATIONS

Disturbed interpersonal relationships are characteristic of individuals with
this profile type. The client feels socially inadequate and has very poor
social skills. He is rather introverted and is fearful and suspicious of
others. He may be blatantly negative in social interactions. He tends to
feel insecure in personal relationships, is hypersensitive to rejection, and
may become jealous at times. He tends to need a great deal of reassurance.
His mistrusting and jealous behaviors may place strain on his marriage.
Individuals with this profile are often petulant and testy with
relationships. He is likely to quarrel a great deal and continually bring
back "old" issues in his arguments. He may be experiencing marital discord
at this time.

The content of this client's MMPI-2 responses suggests the following
additional information concerning his interpersonal relations. He appears
to be an individual who holds rather cynical views about life. Any efforts
to initiate new behaviors may be colored by his negativism. He may view
relationships with others as threatening and harmful. He views his home
situation as unpleasant and lacking in love and understanding. He feels
like leaving home to escape a quarrelsome, critical situation, and to be
free of family domination.

BEHAVIORAL STABILITY

This MMPI-2 profile reflects chronic maladjustment, although he may
presently be experiencing an intensification of problems. Personality
decompensation and disorganization are likely. His interpersonal style is
not likely to change significantly if retested at a later date.

DIAGNOSTIC CONSIDERATIONS

The most likely diagnosis for individuals with this profile type is
Schizophrenia, possibly Paranoid type, or a Paranoid Disorder. The content
of his responses underscores the antisocial features in his history. These
factors should be taken into consideration in arriving at a clinical
diagnosis. His unusual thinking and bizarre ideas need to considered in any
diagnostic formulation.

TREATMENT CONSIDERATIONS

Individuals with this profile may be experiencing a great deal of
personality deterioration, which may require hospitalization if they are
considered dangerous to themselves or others. Psychotropic medication may
reduce their thinking disturbance and mood disorder. Outpatient treatment
may be complicated by their regressed or disorganized behavior. Day
treatment programs or other such structured settings may be helpful in
providing a stabilizing treatment environment.

FIGURE 6-6. Continued

```
         TM                                                    page 3
MMPI-2                TM
THE MINNESOTA REPORT:            ID: 0013471      REPORT DATE: 23-AUG-89
ADULT CLINICAL SYSTEM
INTERPRETIVE REPORT
```

Long-term adjustment is a problem. Frequent, brief "management" therapy contracts may be helpful in structuring their activities. Insight-oriented or uncovering therapies tend not to be helpful for individuals with this profile, and may actually exacerbate the problems. He is unlikely to be able to establish a trusting working relationship with a therapist.

The client endorsed item content which seems to indicate low potential for change. He may feel that his problems are not addressable through therapy and that he is not likely to benefit much from psychological treatment at this time. His apparently negative treatment attitudes may need to be explored early in therapy if treatment is to be initiated successfully. Examination of item content reveals a considerable number of problems with his home life. He feels extremely unhappy and alienated from his family. He related that he feels that his home life is unpleasant and feels pessimistic that the situation will improve. Any psychological intervention with him will need to focus upon his negative family feelings if treatment progress is to be made. In any intervention or psychological evaluation program involving occupational adjustment, his negative work attitudes could become an important problem to overcome. He holds a number of attitudes and feelings that could interfere with work adjustment.

NOTE: This MMPI-2 interpretation can serve as a useful source of hypotheses about clients. This report is based on objectively derived scale indexes and scale interpretations that have been developed in diverse groups of patients. The personality descriptions, inferences and recommendations contained herein need to be verified by other sources of clinical information since individual clients may not fully match the prototype. The information in this report should most appropriately be used by a trained, qualified test interpreter. The information contained in this report should be considered confidential.

FIGURE 6-6. Continued

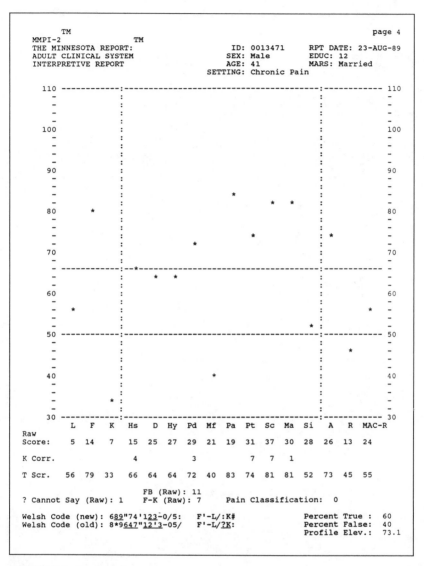

```
         TM                                                            page 4
MMPI-2                     TM
THE MINNESOTA REPORT:                   ID: 0013471      RPT DATE: 23-AUG-89
ADULT CLINICAL SYSTEM                   SEX: Male        EDUC: 12
INTERPRETIVE REPORT                     AGE: 41          MARS: Married
                                        SETTING: Chronic Pain

   110 ------------:-------------------------------------------:------------ 110
     -            :                                             :            -
     -            :                                             :            -
     -            :                                             :            -
     -            :                                             :            -
   100            :                                             :            100
     -            :                                             :            -
     -            :                                             :            -
     -            :                                             :            -
    90            :                                             :            90
     -            :                                             :            -
     -            :                            *                :            -
     -            :                                  *     *    :            -
    80      *     :                                             :            80
     -            :                                             :            -
     -            :                              *             *:            -
     -            :                  *                          :            -
    70            :                                             :            70
     -            :                                             :            -
     - -----------:-*----------------------------------------- :------------ -
     -            :    *     *                                  :            -
     -            :                                             :            -
    60            :                                             :            60
     -  *         :                                             *            -
     -            :                                             :            -
     -            :                                   *:        :            -
    50 -----------:-----------------------------------:---------:------------ 50
     -            :                                             :            -
     -            :                                        *    :            -
     -            :                                             :            -
    40            :               *                            :            40
     -            :                                             :            -
     -    *:                                                    :            -
     -            :                                             :            -
    30 -----------:---------------------------------:-----------:------------ 30
          L   F   K   Hs   D   Hy  Pd  Mf  Pa  Pt   Sc  Ma  Si   A   R  MAC-R
Raw
Score:    5  14   7   15  25  27  29  21  19  31   37  30  28   26  13  24

K Corr.           4           3               7   7   1

T Scr.   56  79  33  66  64  64  72  40  83  74   81  81  52   73  45  55

                         FB (Raw): 11
? Cannot Say (Raw): 1    F-K (Raw): 7      Pain Classification:  0

Welsh Code (new): 689"74'123-0/5:   F'-L/:K#        Percent True :   60
Welsh Code (old): 8*9647"12'3-05/   F'-L/?K:        Percent False:   40
                                                    Profile Elev.:  73.1
```

FIGURE 6-6. Continued

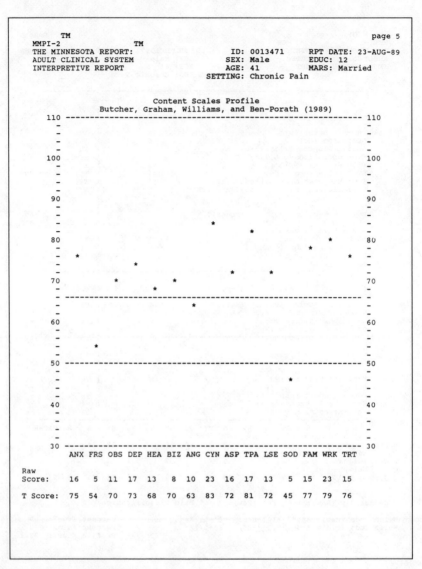

```
      TM                                                           page 5
MMPI-2                      TM
THE MINNESOTA REPORT:                   ID: 0013471      RPT DATE: 23-AUG-89
ADULT CLINICAL SYSTEM                  SEX: Male         EDUC: 12
INTERPRETIVE REPORT                    AGE: 41          MARS: Married
                                   SETTING: Chronic Pain


                        Content Scales Profile
               Butcher, Graham, Williams, and Ben-Porath (1989)
    110 -------------------------------------------------------------- 110
      -                                                                -
      -                                                                -
      -                                                                -
      -                                                                -
    100                                                               100
      -                                                                -
      -                                                                -
      -                                                                -
     90                                                                90
      -                                                                -
      -                                                                -
      -                                          *                     -
      -                                                                -
     80 -                            *                       *        80
      -           *                            *                  *    -
      -                                                    *          -
      -                  *                                       *    -
      -                                    *        *                 -
     70 -         *           *                                        70
      -                                                                -
      - ------------*------------------------------------------------- -
      -                                                                -
      -                            *                                   -
     60                                                                60
      -                                                                -
      -                                                                -
      -     *                                                          -
      -                                                                -
     50 -------------------------------------------------------------- 50
      -                                                                -
      -                                            *                   -
      -                                                                -
      -                                                                -
     40                                                                40
      -                                                                -
      -                                                                -
      -                                                                -
      -                                                                -
     30 -------------------------------------------------------------- 30
          ANX FRS OBS DEP HEA BIZ ANG CYN ASP TPA LSE SOD FAM WRK TRT

Raw
Score:   16   5  11  17  13   8  10  23  16  17  13   5  15  23  15

T Score: 75  54  70  73  68  70  63  83  72  81  72  45  77  79  76
```

FIGURE 6-6. Continued

```
        TM                                                  page 6
MMPI-2                    TM
THE MINNESOTA REPORT:              ID: 0013471    REPORT DATE: 23-AUG-89
ADULT CLINICAL SYSTEM
INTERPRETIVE REPORT


                        SUPPLEMENTARY SCORE REPORT


                                     Raw Score        T Score

        Ego Strength (Es)               26               30
        Dominance (Do)                   6               30
        Social Responsibility (Re)      11               30
        Overcontrolled Hostility (O-H)  14               55
        PTSD - Keane (PK)               26               80
        PTSD - Schlenger (PS)           37               83
        True Response Inconsistency (TRIN)  11           65T
        Variable Response Inconsistency (VRIN)  7        57


Depression Subscales (Harris-Lingoes):

        Subjective Depression (D1)      12               64
        Psychomotor Retardation (D2)     3               37
        Physical Malfunctioning (D3)     3               51
        Mental Dullness (D4)             7               72
        Brooding (D5)                    4               62


Hysteria Subscales (Harris-Lingoes):

        Denial of Social Anxiety (Hy1)   4               51
        Need for Affection (Hy2)         1               30
        Lassitude-Malaise (Hy3)         10               84
        Somatic Complaints (Hy4)         5               62
        Inhibition of Aggression (Hy5)   4               55


Psychopathic Deviate Subscales (Harris-Lingoes):

        Familial Discord (Pd1)           6               78
        Authority Problems (Pd2)         5               61
        Social Imperturbability (Pd3)    3               46
        Social Alienation (Pd4)         12               94
        Self-Alienation (Pd5)            5               58


Paranoia Subscales (Harris-Lingoes):

        Persecutory Ideas (Pa1)         10              100
        Poignancy (Pa2)                  6               76
        Naivete (Pa3)                    1               32
```

FIGURE 6-6. Continued

```
        TM                                                    page 7
MMPI-2                   TM
THE MINNESOTA REPORT:                 ID: 0013471    REPORT DATE: 23-AUG-89
ADULT CLINICAL SYSTEM
INTERPRETIVE REPORT


                                         Raw Score      T Score

Schizophrenia Subscales (Harris-Lingoes):

        Social Alienation (Sc1)              11            84
        Emotional Alienation (Sc2)            2            59
        Lack of Ego Mastery, Cognitive (Sc3)  7            84
        Lack of Ego Mastery, Conative (Sc4)   7            76
        Lack of Ego Mastery, Def. Inhib. (Sc5) 7           89
        Bizarre Sensory Experiences (Sc6)     8            80


Hypomania Subscales (Harris-Lingoes):

        Amorality (Ma1)                       3            58
        Psychomotor Acceleration (Ma2)       11            78
        Imperturbability (Ma3)                4            53
        Ego Inflation (Ma4)                   7            76


Social Introversion Subscales (Ben-Porath, Hostetler, Butcher, & Graham):

        Shyness / Self-Consciousness (Si1)    5            51
        Social Avoidance (Si2)                0            41
        Alienation--Self and Others (Si3)    14            77


Uniform T scores are used for Hs, D, Hy, Pd, Pa, Pt, Sc, Ma, and the Content
Scales; all other MMPI-2 scales use linear T scores.
```

FIGURE 6-6. Continued

```
        TM                                                          page 8
MMPI-2                   TM
THE MINNESOTA REPORT:                   ID: 0013471    REPORT DATE: 23-AUG-89
ADULT CLINICAL SYSTEM
INTERPRETIVE REPORT


                        CRITICAL ITEMS

The following critical items have been found to have possible significance in
analyzing a client's problem situation.  Although these items may serve as a
source of hypotheses for further investigation, caution should be taken in
interpreting individual items because they may have been inadvertently
checked.


Acute Anxiety State  (Koss-Butcher Critical Items)

    3. I wake up fresh and rested most mornings.  (F)
    5. I am easily awakened by noise.  (T)
   10. I am about as able to work as I ever was.  (F)
   15. I work under a great deal of tension.  (T)
   28. I am bothered by an upset stomach several times a week.  (T)
   39. My sleep is fitful and disturbed.  (T)
  140. Most nights I go to sleep without thoughts or ideas bothering me.  (F)
  172. I frequently notice my hand shakes when I try to do something.  (T)
  218. I have periods of such great restlessness that I cannot sit long in a
       chair.  (T)
  444. I am a high-strung person.  (T)
  463. Several times a week I feel as if something dreadful is about to
       happen.  (T)
  469. I sometimes feel that I am about to go to pieces.  (T)


Depressed Suicidal Ideation  (Koss-Butcher Critical Items)

   38. I have had periods of days, weeks, or months when I couldn't take care
       of things because I couldn't "get going."  (T)
   65. Most of the time I feel blue.  (T)
   71. These days I find it hard not to give up hope of amounting to
       something.  (T)
  130. I certainly feel useless at times.  (T)
  146. I cry easily.  (T)
  306. No one cares much what happens to you.  (T)
  411. At times I think I am no good at all.  (T)
  454. The future seems hopeless to me.  (T)
  485. I often feel that I'm not as good as other people.  (T)
  518. I have made lots of bad mistakes in my life.  (T)


Threatened Assault  (Koss-Butcher Critical Items)

   37. At times I feel like smashing things.  (T)
   85. At times I have a strong urge to do something harmful or shocking.  (T)
  213. I get mad easily and then get over it soon.  (T)
```

FIGURE 6-6. Continued

```
      TM                                                        page 9
MMPI-2                  TM
THE MINNESOTA REPORT:                   ID: 0013471     REPORT DATE: 23-AUG-89
ADULT CLINICAL SYSTEM
INTERPRETIVE REPORT


Situational Stress Due to Alcoholism  (Koss-Butcher Critical Items)

  125. I believe that my home life is as pleasant as that of most people I
       know.  (F)
  518. I have made lots of bad mistakes in my life.  (T)


Mental Confusion  (Koss-Butcher Critical Items)

   31. I find it hard to keep my mind on a task or job.  (T)
  299. I cannot keep my mind on one thing.  (T)
  311. I often feel as if things are not real.  (T)
  316. I have strange and peculiar thoughts.  (T)
  325. I have more trouble concentrating than others seem to have.  (T)


Persecutory Ideas  (Koss-Butcher Critical Items)

   17. I am sure I get a raw deal from life.  (T)
   42. If people had not had it in for me, I would have been much more
       successful.  (T)
   99. Someone has it in for me.  (T)
  124. I often wonder what hidden reason another person may have for doing
       something nice for me.  (T)
  138. I believe I am being plotted against.  (T)
  145. I feel that I have often been punished without cause.  (T)
  228. There are persons who are trying to steal my thoughts and ideas.  (T)
  241. It is safer to trust nobody.  (T)
  259. I am sure I am being talked about.  (T)


Antisocial Attitude  (Lachar-Wrobel Critical Items)

   27. When people do me a wrong, I feel I should pay them back if I can, just
       for the principle of the thing.  (T)
   35. Sometimes when I was young I stole things.  (T)
  105. In school I was sometimes sent to the principal for bad behavior.  (T)
  240. At times it has been impossible for me to keep from stealing or
       shoplifting something.  (T)
  254. Most people make friends because friends are likely to be useful to
       them.  (T)
  266. I have never been in trouble with the law.  (F)
  324. I can easily make other people afraid of me, and sometimes do for the
       fun of it.  (T)


Family Conflict  (Lachar-Wrobel Critical Items)

   21. At times I have very much wanted to leave home.  (T)
   83. I have very few quarrels with members of my family.  (F)
  125. I believe that my home life is as pleasant as that of most people I
       know.  (F)
```

FIGURE 6-6. Continued

```
        TM                                           page 10
MMPI-2                      TM
THE MINNESOTA REPORT:                ID: 0013471      REPORT DATE: 23-AUG-89
ADULT CLINICAL SYSTEM
INTERPRETIVE REPORT
```

Somatic Symptoms (Lachar-Wrobel Critical Items)

  28. I am bothered by an upset stomach several times a week. (T)
  33. I seldom worry about my health. (F)
  47. I am almost never bothered by pains over my heart or in my chest. (F)
  53. Parts of my body often have feelings like burning, tingling, crawling,
      or like "going to sleep." (T)
  57. I hardly ever feel pain in the back of my neck. (F)
 111. I have a great deal of stomach trouble. (T)
 182. I have had attacks in which I could not control my movements or speech
      but in which I knew what was going on around me. (T)
 224. I have few or no pains. (F)
 247. I have numbness in one or more places on my skin. (T)
 295. I have never been paralyzed or had any unusual weakness of any of my
      muscles. (F)
 464. I feel tired a good deal of the time. (T)

Sexual Concern and Deviation (Lachar-Wrobel Critical Items)

 166. I am worried about sex. (T)

Anxiety and Tension (Lachar-Wrobel Critical Items)

  15. I work under a great deal of tension. (T)
  17. I am sure I get a raw deal from life. (T)
 172. I frequently notice my hand shakes when I try to do something. (T)
 218. I have periods of such great restlessness that I cannot sit long in a
      chair. (T)
 299. I cannot keep my mind on one thing. (T)
 320. I have been afraid of things or people that I knew could not hurt
      me. (T)
 405. I am usually calm and not easily upset. (F)
 463. Several times a week I feel as if something dreadful is about to
      happen. (T)

Sleep Disturbance (Lachar-Wrobel Critical Items)

   5. I am easily awakened by noise. (T)
  30. I have nightmares every few nights. (T)
  39. My sleep is fitful and disturbed. (T)
 140. Most nights I go to sleep without thoughts or ideas bothering me. (F)
 328. Sometimes some unimportant thought will run through my mind and bother
      me for days. (T)
 471. I have often been frightened in the middle of the night. (T)
```

**FIGURE 6-6. Continued**
```

```
        TM                                                              page 11
MMPI-2                      TM
THE MINNESOTA REPORT:                     ID: 0013471      REPORT DATE: 23-AUG-89
ADULT CLINICAL SYSTEM
INTERPRETIVE REPORT


Deviant Thinking and Experience   (Lachar-Wrobel Critical Items)

   122. At times my thoughts have raced ahead faster than I could speak
        them.  (T)
   298. Peculiar odors come to me at times.  (T)
   316. I have strange and peculiar thoughts.  (T)


Depression and Worry   (Lachar-Wrobel Critical Items)

     3. I wake up fresh and rested most mornings.  (F)
    10. I am about as able to work as I ever was.  (F)
    65. Most of the time I feel blue.  (T)
   130. I certainly feel useless at times.  (T)
   150. Sometimes I feel as if I must injure either myself or someone
        else.  (T)
   165. My memory seems to be all right.  (F)
   339. I have sometimes felt that difficulties were piling up so high that I
        could not overcome them.  (T)
   411. At times I think I am no good at all.  (T)
   454. The future seems hopeless to me.  (T)


Deviant Beliefs   (Lachar-Wrobel Critical Items)

    42. If people had not had it in for me, I would have been much more
        successful.  (T)
    99. Someone has it in for me.  (T)
   106. My speech is the same as always (not faster or slower, no slurring or
        hoarseness).  (F)
   138. I believe I am being plotted against.  (T)
   228. There are persons who are trying to steal my thoughts and ideas.  (T)
   259. I am sure I am being talked about.  (T)
   466. Sometimes I am sure that other people can tell what I am thinking.  (T)


Problematic Anger   (Lachar-Wrobel Critical Items)

    85. At times I have a strong urge to do something harmful or shocking.  (T)
   213. I get mad easily and then get over it soon.  (T)
```

FIGURE 6-6. Continued

```
        TM                                                    page 12
MMPI-2                         TM
THE MINNESOTA REPORT:                ID: 0013471      REPORT DATE: 23-AUG-89
ADULT CLINICAL SYSTEM
INTERPRETIVE REPORT


                             OMITTED ITEMS

The following items were omitted by the client.  It may be helpful to
discuss these item omissions with this individual to determine the reason
for non-compliance with test instructions.

   20. I am very seldom troubled by constipation.
```

FIGURE 6-6. Continued

Chapter 7

Summary and Directions for Future Research

This book has addressed the use of the MMPI-2 with chronic pain patients—a clinical population that research and practice have shown differ from other medical patients and from psychiatric patients on a variety of dimensions. The chronic pain syndrome is an enormously frustrating and costly clinical problem in the United States as well as in many other industrialized countries. The past two decades have seen a rise in disability expenditures for the American labor force, with back injuries accounting for 20-30% of these claims. Viewing the chronic pain patient from an organic perspective alone has not proved sufficient to treat the lingering problems of a subset of patients suffering from pain. Instead, a multidimensional model of the chronic pain patient's disability has emerged, taking into account affective, cognitive, behavioral, and social components of the pain experience in addition to somatosensory aspects. Several models of chronic pain were reviewed in this volume. For any particular pain patient, it is likely that a combination of these factors is present and interacts to form a "chronic pain profile" unique to that individual.

New models of pain and new methods of treating chronic pain require detailed assessment of areas of a patient's functioning other than the traditional medical examination. Personality measurement is included in assessment batteries to help describe the individual's coping style, affective and psychiatric status, self-appraisal, and view of his or her environment. A number of personality factors related to the manifestation of chronic pain were explored such as excessive sensitivity to somatic cues and readiness to communicate needs through physical symptoms, somatic reactivity to stress, depressed mood, characterologic manipulativeness, dependency, and other personality styles. Clinicians and researchers working with chronic pain patients have noted the importance of viewing symptomatic behavior in the context of the patient's personality structure and the secondary gains accruing to that individual, if behavior change programs are going to be successful in ameliorating these persistent problems.

At this time, although many other assessment measures have been proposed, the Minnesota Multiphasic Personality Inventory is the most widely used standardized instrument with the chronic pain population. The MMPI has been found to be one of the most useful personality assessment techniques for appraising the personality variables influencing the maintenance of chronic pain and the degree of disability associated with pain problems.

Research using the MMPI has tended to focus on describing characteristics of the average chronic pain patient in relation to other clinical or nonclinical samples. This type of research has been relatively consistent in finding primary elevations on scales Hs and Hy, interpreted as somatic preoccupation with some associated denial of psychological distress. Researchers differ about the relative elevation of scale D compared to these two; some describe the average pain patient profile as a conversion V, suggesting conversion of psychological distress into physical complaints, and others describe a neurotic triad, which includes a significant degree of acknowledged depression and physical discomfort. Recent research has generally supported the contention that these average profiles are not necessarily indicative of functional pain because they are often found among patients with clear organic findings.

In the past few years researchers have begun to focus on another question: can subgroups of chronic pain patients that have distinctive treatment needs be identified? Several investigators have suggested grouping patients according to some common codetype groups (combinations of highest MMPI scales) that are expected to have differential correlates. These groups have included the conversion-V and neurotic-triad forms mentioned above, reactive depression and manipulative reaction groups, a normal-limits profile, and a borderline/psychotic or general-elevation group. Similar mean profile types have been identified through cluster analysis procedures. Research efforts have begun to support the prediction that at least some of these groups may have differential clinical or treatment outcome correlates, but much more work remains to be done.

Purpose of the MMPI-2 Chronic Pain Research Project

A large body of research and clinical literature has developed around the use of the MMPI with chronic pain patients. In 1989 a revised version of the MMPI, the MMPI-2, was published. This revised version includes new national norms, a new method of converting scale raw scores to T scores, item rewording, and some minor changes in scale length. It also incorporates newly developed content scales designed to expand the range of clinical content covered by the original MMPI.

The study described in this book was designed to address the comparability of the MMPI-2 to the original MMPI, as well as to provide some research data on the performance of the MMPI-2 among a large chronic pain population. The goal of this research was to provide clinicians and researchers with information on the applicability of previous MMPI chronic pain research to the new version of this test and to expand the body of information on clinical correlates of MMPI patterns to the MMPI-2 for this patient population.

Data for this study were collected at the Sister Kenny Chronic Pain Rehabilitation Program in Minneapolis, Minnesota. A sample of 268 men and 234 women, consecutive admissions to a three-week inpatient multidisciplinary pain program, were administered the MMPI-2 along with other questionnaires requesting life events and biographical information. Chart data were also abstracted for these patients. This sample was compared in several analyses to the national community normative sample used in restandardizing the MMPI and to a large group of hospitalized psychiatric patients.

Analyses reported in this book included description of the pain patient sample through frequency distributions and summary statistics on all non-MMPI measures collected, as well as by comparison on these measures with the normative and psychiatric samples. The group mean MMPI patterns of these groups were compared, as were scale scores and item endorsement frequencies. The original MMPI and the new MMPI-2 scores were contrasted for chronic pain patients by scoring their protocols by both methods, then looking at the similarities and differences in mean profiles and codetype distributions. Finally, correlates of MMPI-2 patterns among chronic pain patients were sought by comparing subgroups of patients on the biographical and clinical data collected. Subgroups were identified by three methods: 1) single scale elevations, 2) codetype groups, and 3) cluster analysis. Results and discussion of all analyses were presented in detail in Chapter 5.

Continuity of the MMPI-2 with the MMPI

Sample description from life events, biographical information, and chart review data supported the comparability of the Sister Kenny Institute chronic pain sample to those described in other studies of multidisciplinary pain programs. Pain patients tended to score as more distressed and dysfunctional than the normative sample on a wide variety of measures, including the MMPI. Compared to inpatient psychiatric patients, pain patients were more preoccupied with physical complaints, endorsed less psychopathology in general, but were just as depressed. Scoring the patients' MMPI profiles by old norms also supported the comparability of this sample to previous research samples: their average profile matched previous research in showing a neurotic-triad pattern (elevations on Hs, D, and Hy) with a secondary peak on Pt.

One of the goals of the MMPI Restandardization Committee was to maintain the continuity of the MMPI through the revision and the development of modern norms by keeping intact most of the items comprising the original validity and clinical scales and several supplementary scales such as the MAC scale. Consequently, it was hoped that these scales would operate in a similar manner with chronic pain patients even though the item context has changed and the comparison standard, i.e., the normative group, has been expanded in scope and updated. In this study, chronic pain patients were found to produce the same mean profile scale elevations (Hs, D, and Hy) on the MMPI-2 as they do on the original MMPI.

MMPI-2 profile codes were also found to identify several common codetype groups of pain patients consistent with those reported on the original MMPI. Similarly, chronic pain patients' MMPI-2 profiles can be grouped into cluster types very similar to those found in research with the original MMPI scales.

Despite these similarities, the clinician will need to alter clinical interpretation of profiles slightly in using the MMPI-2 norms. The MMPI-2 Restandardization Committee recommends the use of a T score of 65 and above for interpretation of "clinical scale elevation." The results of this study support this interpretive shift. A T-score elevation of 65 appears to optimally separate chronic pain patients from the MMPI-2 normative population on the scales most relevant to their clinical symptom picture, i.e., Hs, Hy, and the new content scale HEA (Health Concerns). Comparison of the Sister Kenny pain patients' mean profile revealed continuity in pattern from the MMPI to the MMPI-2, but the MMPI-2 profile was lower than the MMPI mean profile by an average of about 5 T-score points, suggesting interpretive strategies will need to use lower cutoffs to maintain continuity from one form to the other. In addition, the use of a T score of 65 or higher provides a high degree of codetype congruence between the MMPI-2 and the original MMPI, minimizing the degree of shift in codetype group categorizations that is more noticeable if a T score of 70 is used as the cutoff. Since some small shifts in relative scale elevations do occur from the MMPI to the MMPI-2, it was also recommended that the clinician or researcher not overinterpret small differences in configuration patterns, such as relative elevations of the neurotic-triad scales. If these recommendations are taken into account, data reported in this book indicate a high degree of comparability and continuity between the original MMPI and the MMPI-2 when used with chronic pain patients in a multidisciplinary inpatient setting.

Utility of the MMPI-2 in Chronic Pain Assessment

With an appropriate shift in the elevation level used for interpretation, this study strongly suggests that the MMPI-2 validity, clinical, and supplementary scales will provide the same type of personality and symptom information about the chronic pain patient as did the original MMPI scales. Correlate analyses revealed the MMPI-2 may be particularly useful among an inpatient chronic pain sample in discriminating patients according to their degree of depression. Other scales that seemed to have potential utility in identifying subgroups of patients with particular treatment problems included Sc, correlated with severe psychiatric problems, and Pd and Ma, associated with characterologic problems and acting-out behavior, including substance abuse. The MAC scale was also associated with behavioral problems including alcohol and drug abuse histories. The overall elevation of a client's profile was also an important indicator of degree of disability and associated life problems. More detailed correlate information and suggestions for interpretive strategies were discussed in Chapters 5 and 6.

In addition to the traditional MMPI scales, several new content scales have been developed for the MMPI-2. These scales contain more homogeneous item groups and are more easily interpretable in terms of this content than are the traditional, empirically developed clinical scales. Several of the MMPI-2 content scales appear to be relevant for the assessment of chronic pain patients. In particular, the HEA scale showed high discriminability between chronic pain patients and normals, and between chronic pain patients and chronically ill psychiatric patients. Several other scales that address specific personality or clinical problems such as Obsessiveness (OBS), Antisocial Practices (ASP), and Bizarre Ideation (BIZ) are likely to be important indexes to include in assessing chronic pain patients.

Two new general problem scales, WRK (Work Interference) and TRT (Negative Treatment Indicators) address problems or personal attitudes that could provide the clinician or researcher with suggestions on how the patient is likely to view or respond to rehabilitation efforts. Although this study did not allow for a full exploration of the utility of these scales, it did provide some suggestive data about their potential relevance for this population.

Future Research Directions

The results of this study support the continued use of the MMPI-2 for clinical assessment and research with chronic pain patients. As was discussed in detail in Chapter 5, we believe future research should concentrate on defining smaller, more deviant and non-overlapping codetype groups and using fewer, more well-defined clinical measures, including specific outcome measures, as potential correlates. In our view, the currently popular cluster analysis techniques provide little or no information not already available through codetype studies, as long as codetype rules take profile elevation into account. Cluster techniques have not resulted in the identification of new, unique pain patient groups differing substantially from those already suggested by clinicians using codetype groupings. Codetype systems are more easily replicable and result in more homogeneous profile groups than are obtained through cluster analyses. In addition, the results of such research will be more readily generalizable to clinical practice.

We suggest that future research with the MMPI-2 among chronic pain patients focus on delineating correlates of common codetypes and of the new content scales, and expand the current study to include pain patient groups at other stages of the assessment process. It will be vitally important to collect data on the new MMPI-2 items and scales in a general medical population to provide an appropriate comparison group in future chronic pain studies. Our prediction is that the MMPI-2 will prove of even greater utility in defining treatment-relevant groups of patients when used with a less highly selected population than the inpatient sample used in this study, and when used to make more clinically relevant decisions such as differentiating chronic pain patients from a general medical population rather than from the normative and psychiatric groups used here. We hope other researchers and clinicians will take up the challenge and expand this initial attempt at delineating the utility of the MMPI-2 in the assessment of patients suffering from chronic pain problems.

References

Abbott Northwestern Hospital (1984). *PACE: The program of aftercare, chronic pain rehabilitation program.* (Program pamphlet available through Sister Kenny Institute, 800 East 28th Street at Chicago Avenue, Minneapolis, MN 55407.)

Abse, D. W. (1974). Hysterical conversion and dissociative syndromes and the hysterical character. In S. Arieti (Ed.), *American handbook of psychiatry* (Vol. 3, 2nd ed., pp. 155-193). New York: Basic Books.

Adams, K. M., Heilbronn, M., & Blumer, D. P. (1987). A multimethod evaluation of the MMPI in a chronic pain patient sample. *Journal of Clinical Psychology, 42,* 878-886.

Adams, K. M., Heilbronn, M., Silk, S. D., Reider, E., & Blumer, D. P. (1981). Use of the MMPI with patients who report chronic back pain. *Psychological Reports, 48,* 855-866.

Ahern, D. K., & Follick, M. J. (1985). Distress in spouses of chronic pain patients. *International Journal of Family Therapy, 7,* 247-257.

Ahles, T. A., Yunus, M. B., Gaulier, B., Riey, S. D., & Masi, A. T. (1986). The use of contemporary MMPI norms in the study of chronic pain patients. *Pain, 24,* 159-163.

Anderson, D. B., & Pennebaker, J. W. (1980). Pain and pleasure: Alternative interpretations of identical stimulation. *European Journal of Social Psychology, 10,* 207-212.

Anderson, L. P., & Rehm, L. P. (1984). The relationship between strategies of coping and perception of pain in three chronic pain groups. *Journal of Clinical Psychology, 40,* 1170-1177.

Andersson, G. B. J. (1981). Epidemiologic aspects on low-back pain in industry. *Spine, 6,* 53-60.

Andersson, G. B. J., Pope, M. H., & Frymoyer, J. W. (1984). Epidemiology. In M. H. Pope, J. W. Frymoyer, & G. Andersson (Eds.), *Occupational low back pain* (pp. 101-114). New York: Praeger.

Armentrout, D. P., Moore, J. E., Parker, J. C., Hewett, J. E., & Feltz, C. (1982). Pain patient MMPI subgroups: The psychological dimensions of pain. *Journal of Behavioral Medicine, 5,* 201-211.

Aronoff, G. M. (1985). The role of the pain center in the treatment for intractable suffering and disability resulting from chronic pain. In G. M. Aronoff (Ed.), *Evaluation and treatment of chronic pain* (pp. 503-510). Baltimore: Urban & Schwarzenberg.

Aronoff, G. M., & Evans, W. O. (1982). The prediction of treatment outcome at a multidisciplinary pain center. *Pain, 14,* 67-73.

Aronoff, G. M., & Evans, W. O. (1985). Evaluation and treatment of chronic pain at the Boston Pain Center. In G. M. Aronoff (Ed.), *Evaluation and treatment of chronic pain* (pp. 495-502). Baltimore: Urban & Schwarzenberg.

Aronoff, G. M., Evans, W. O., & Enders, P. L. (1983). A review of follow-up studies of multi-disciplinary pain units. *Pain, 16,* 1-11.

Aronoff, G. M., & Rutrick, D. (1985). Psychodynamics and psychotherapy of the chronic pain syndrome. In G. M. Aronoff (Ed.), *Evaluation and treatment of chronic pain* (pp. 463-469). Baltimore: Urban & Schwarzenberg.

Atkinson, J. H., Ingram, R. E., Kremer, E. F., & Saccuzzo, D. P. (1986). MMPI subgroups and affective disorder in chronic pain patients. *Journal of Nervous and Mental Disease, 174,* 408-413.

Bandura, A. (1977a). Self-efficacy: Toward a unifying theory of behavioral change. *Psychological Review, 84,* 191–215.

Bandura, A. (1977b). *Social learning theory.* Englewood Cliffs, NJ: Prentice-Hall.

Barron, F. (1953). An ego strength scale which predicts response to psychotherapy. *Journal of Consulting Psychology, 17,* 327–333.

Barsky, A. J. (1986). Palliation and symptom relief. *Archives of Internal Medicine, 146,* 905–909.

Barsky, A. J., Wyshak, G., & Klerman, G. L. (1986). Hypochondriasis: An evaluation of the DSM-III criteria in medical outpatients. *Archives of General Psychiatry, 43,* 493–500.

Beals, R. K., & Hickman, N. W. (1972). Industrial injuries of the back and extremities: comprehensive evaluation—an aid in prognosis and management: A study of 180 patients. *Journal of Bone and Joint Surgery, 54,* 1593–1611.

Beck, A. T., Ward, C. H., Mendelson, M. M., Mock, J., & Erbaugh, J. (1961). An inventory for measuring depression. *Archives of General Psychiatry, 4,* 561–571.

Benedikt, R. A., & Kolb, L. C., (1986). Preliminary findings on chronic pain and post-traumatic stress disorder. *American Journal of Psychiatry, 143,* 908–910.

Ben-Porath, Y. S., & Butcher, J. N. (1988, March). *Exploratory analyses of rewritten MMPI items.* Paper presented at the 23rd Annual Symposium on Recent Developments in the Use of the MMPI, St. Petersburg, Florida.

Bergin, A. E. (1971). The evaluation of therapeutic outcomes. In A. E. Bergin & S. L. Garfield (Eds.), *Handbook of psychotherapy and behavior change: An empirical analysis.* New York: Wiley.

Bernstein, I. H., & Garbin, C. P. (1983). Hierarchical clustering of pain patients' MMPI profiles. *Journal of Personality Assessment, 47,* 171–172.

Beutler, L. E. (1979). Toward specific psychological therapies for specific conditions. *Journal of Consulting and Clinical Psychology, 47,* 882–897.

Blashfield, R. K. (1980). Propositions regarding the use of cluster analysis in clinical research. *Journal of Consulting and Clinical Psychology, 48,* 456–459.

Blazer, D. G. (1980–81). Narcissism and the development of chronic pain. *International Journal of Psychiatry in Medicine, 10,* 69–77.

Block, A. R., Kremer, E. F., & Gaylor, M. (1980). Behavioral treatment of chronic pain: The spouse as a discriminative cue for pain behavior. *Pain, 9,* 243–252.

Blumer, D., & Heilbronn, M. (1981). The pain-prone patient: A clinical and psychological profile. *Psychosomatics, 22,* 395–402.

Blumer, D., & Heilbronn, M. (1982). Chronic pain as a variant of depressive disease: The pain-prone disorder. *Journal of Nervous and Mental Disease, 170,* 381–406.

Blumer, D., & Heilbronn, M. (1984). "Chronic pain as a variant of depressive disease": A rejoinder. *Journal of Nervous and Mental Disease, 172,* 405–407.

Blumetti, A., & Modesti, L. (1976). Psychological predictors of success or failure of surgical intervention for intractable back pain. In J. J. Bonica & D. Albe-Fessard (Eds.), *Advances in pain research and therapy* (Vol. 1). New York: Raven.

Bokan, J. A., Ries, R. K., & Katon, W. J. (1981). Tertiary gain and chronic pain. *Pain, 10,* 331–335.

Bonica, J. J. (1980). Pain therapy research: past and current status and future needs. In L. K. Y. Ng and J. J. Bonica (Eds.), *Pain, discomfort and humanitarian care* (pp. 1–46). New York: Elsevier/North Holland.

Bouckoms, A. J., Litman, R. E., & Baer, L. (1985). Denial in the depressive and pain-prone disorders of chronic pain. In H. L. Fields, R. Dubner, & F. Cervero (Eds.), *Advances in pain research and therapy* (Vol. 9, pp. 879–887). New York: Raven.

Bradley, L. A. (1983). Relationships between the MMPI and the McGill Pain Questionnaire. In R. Melzack (Ed.), *Pain measurement and assessment* (pp. 129–136). New York: Raven.

Bradley, L. A., Prieto, E. J., Hopson, L., & Prokop, C. K. (1978). Comment on "personality organization as an aspect of back pain in a medical setting." *Journal of Personality Assessment,*

42, 573-578.

Bradley, L. A., Prokop, C. K., Gentry, W. D., Van der Heide, L. H., & Prieto, E. J. (1981). Assessment of chronic pain. In C. K. Prokop & L. A. Bradley (Eds.), *Medical psychology: Contributions to behavioral medicine* (pp. 91-117). New York: Academic Press.

Bradley, L. A., Prokop, C. K., Margolis, R., & Gentry, W. D. (1978). Multivariate analyses of the MMPI profiles of low back pain patients. *Journal of Behavioral Medicine, 1,* 253-272.

Bradley, L. A., & Van der Heide, L. H. (1984). Pain-related correlates of MMPI profile subgroups among back pain patients. *Health Psychology, 3,* 157-174.

Bradley, L. A., Van der Heide, L. H., Byrne, M., Troy, A., Prieto, E. J., & Marchisello, P. J. (1981). Pain-related correlates of MMPI profile subgroups among back pain patients. Paper presented at the Third World Congress on Pain, Edinburgh, Scotland.

Brandwin, M. A., & Kewman, D. G. (1982). MMPI indicators of treatment response to spinal epidural stimulation in patients with chronic pain and patients with movement disorders. *Psychological Reports, 51,* 1059-1064.

Brennan, A. F., Barrett, C. L., & Garretson, H. D. (1986-87). The prediction of chronic pain outcome by psychological variables. *International Journal of Psychiatry and Medicine, 16,* 373-387.

Butcher, J. N. (1972). *Objective personality assessment: Changing perspectives.* New York: Academic Press.

Butcher, J. N. (1989). *User's guide to the Minnesota Clinical Report for the MMPI-2* (revised edition). Minneapolis, MN: National Computer Systems.

Butcher, J. N. (1990). *The MMPI-2 in psychological treatment.* New York: Oxford University Press.

Butcher, J. N., Dahlstrom, W. G., Graham, J. R., Tellegen, A., & Kaemmer, B. (1989). *Manual for administration and scoring. MMPI-2.* Minneapolis, MN: University of Minnesota Press.

Butcher, J. N., Graham, J. R., Williams, C. L., & Ben-Porath, Y. S. (1989). *Development and use of the MMPI-2 content scales.* Minneapolis, MN: University of Minnesota Press.

Butcher, J. N., & Harlow, T. (1987). Personality assessment in personal injury cases. In A. Hess & I. Weiner (Eds.), *Handbook of forensic psychology* (pp. 128-154). New York: Wiley.

Butcher, J. N., & Owen, P. (1978). Objective personality inventories: Recent research and some contemporary issues. In B. Wolman (Ed.), *Handbook of clinical diagnosis.* New York: Plenum.

Butcher, J. N., & Tellegen, A. (1966). Objections to MMPI items. *Journal of Consulting Psychology, 30,* 527-534.

Butcher, J. N., & Tellegen, A. (1978). Common methodological problems in MMPI research. *Journal of Consulting and Clinical Psychology, 46,* 620-628.

Cairns, D., Mooney, V., & Crane, P. (1984). Spinal pain rehabilitation: Inpatient and outpatient treatment results and development of predictors for outcome. *Spine, 9,* 91-95.

Caldwell, A. B., & Chase, C. (1977). Diagnosis and treatment of personality factors in chronic low back pain. *Clinical Orthopaedics and Related Research, 129,* 141-149.

Calsyn, D. A., Louks, J., & Freeman, C. W. (1976). The use of the MMPI with chronic low back pain patients with a mixed diagnosis. *Journal of Clinical Psychology, 32,* 532-536.

Carron, H., DeGood, D. E., & Tait, R. (1985). A comparison of low back pain patients in the United States and New Zealand: Psychosocial and economic factors affecting severity of disability. *Pain, 21,* 77-89.

Catchlove, R. F., Cohen, D. R., Braha, R. E., & Demers-Desrosiers, L. A. (1985). Incidence and implications of alexithymia in chronic pain patients. *Journal of Nervous and Mental Disorders, 173,* 246-248.

Chapman, C. R. (1978). The perception of noxious events. In R. A. Sternbach (Ed.), *The psychology of pain* (pp. 169-202). New York: Raven.

Chapman, C. R., & Bonica, J. J. (1985). *Chronic pain.* Upjohn.

Chapman, S. L., & Brena, S. F. (1982). Learned helplessness and responses to nerve blocks in chronic low back pain patients. *Pain, 14,* 355–364.

Chapman, S. L., Brena, S. F., & Bradford, L. A. (1981). Treatment outcome in a chronic pain rehabilitation program. *Pain, 11,* 255–268.

Chodoff, P. (1974). The diagnosis of hysteria: An overview. *American Journal of Psychiatry, 131,* 1073–1078.

Chrzanowski, G. (1974). Neurasthenia and hypochondriasis. In S. Arieti (Ed.), *American handbook of psychiatry* (Vol. 3, 2nd ed., pp. 141–154). New York: Basic Books.

Clark, W. C., & Yang, J. C. (1983). Applications of sensory decision theory to problems in laboratory and clinical pain. In R. Melzack (Ed.), *Pain measurement and assessment* (pp. 15–25). New York: Raven.

Cohen, N. (1987). The response of chronic pain patients to the original and revised versions of the Minnesota Multiphasic Personality Inventory. Unpublished doctoral dissertation, University of Minnesota.

Colligan, R. C., Osborne, D., Swenson, W. M., & Offord, K. P. (1984). *The MMPI: A contemporary normative study.* New York: Praeger.

Costa, P. T., & McRae, R. R. (1985). Hypochondriasis, neuroticism, and aging: When are somatic complaints unfounded? *American Psychologist, 40,* 19–28.

Costello, R. M., Hulsey, T. L., Schoenfeld, L. S., & Ramamurthy, S. (1987). P-A-I-N: A four-cluster MMPI typology for chronic pain. *Pain, 30,* 199–209.

Cox, G. B., Chapman, C. R., & Black, R. G. (1978). The MMPI and chronic pain: The diagnosis of psychogenic pain. *Journal of Behavioral Medicine, 1,* 437–443.

Craig, K. D. (1978). Social modeling influences on pain. In R. A. Sternbach (Ed.), *The psychology of pain* (pp. 73–109). New York: Raven.

Craig, K. D. (1983). Modeling and social learning factors in chronic pain. In J. J. Bonica, U. Lindblom, & A. Iggo (Eds.), *Advances in pain research and therapy* (Vol. 5, pp. 813–827). New York: Raven.

Crook, J., Rideout, E., & Browne, G. (1984). The prevalence of pain complaints in a general population. *Pain, 18,* 299–314.

Crown, S. (1980). Psychosocial factors in low back pain. *Clinics in Rheumatic Diseases, 6,* 77–92.

Cypress, B. K. (1983). Characteristics of physician visits for back symptoms: A national perspective. *American Journal of Public Health, 73,* 389–395.

Dahlstrom, W. G., Welsh, G. S., & Dahlstrom, L. E. (1972). *An MMPI handbook (Vol. 1): Clinical interpretation* (rev. ed.). Minneapolis, MN: University of Minnesota Press.

Dahlstrom, W. G., Welsh, G. S., & Dahlstrom, L. E. (1975). *An MMPI handbook (Vol. 2): Research applications* (rev. ed.). Minneapolis, MN: University of Minnesota Press.

Deyo, R. A., Bass, J. E., Walsh, N. E., Shoenfeld, L. S., & Ramamurthy, S. (1988). Prognostic variability among chronic pain patients: Implications for study design, interpretation, and reporting. *Archives of Physical Medicine and Rehabilitation, 69,* 174–178.

Diehl, L. A. (1977). The relationship between demographic factors, MMPI scores and the social readjustment rating scale. *Dissertation Abstracts International, 38* (5-B), 2360.

Dieter, J. N., & Swerdlow, B. (1988). A replicative investigation of the reliability of the MMPI in the classification of chronic headaches. *Headache, 28,* 212–222.

Dolce, J. J. (1987). Self-efficacy and disability beliefs in behavioral treatment of pain. *Behaviour Research and Therapy, 25,* 289–299.

Dolce, J. J., Crocker, M. F., & Doleys, D. M. (1986). Prediction of outcome among chronic pain patients. *Behaviour Research and Therapy, 24,* 313–319.

Domino, J. V., & Haber, J. D. (1987). Prior physical and sexual abuse in women with chronic headache: Clinical correlates. *Headache, 27,* 310–314.

Duckworth, J. C., & Anderson, W. P. (1986). *MMPI interpretation manual for counselors and clinicians* (3rd ed.). Muncie, IN: Accelerated Development Inc.

Duncan, G. H., Gregg, J. M., & Ghia, J. N. (1978). The Pain Profile: A computerized system for assessment of chronic pain. *Pain, 5,* 275–284.

Dworkin, R. H., Handlin, D. S., Richlin, D. M., Brand, L., & Vannucci, C. (1985). Unraveling the effects of compensation, litigation, and employment on treatment response in chronic pain. *Pain, 23,* 49-59.

Dworkin, R. H., Richlin, D. M., Handlin, D. S., & Brand, L. (1986). Predicting treatment response in depressed and non-depressed chronic pain patients. *Pain, 24,* 343-353.

Edelbrock, C. (1979). Mixture model tests of hierarchical clustering algorithms: The problem of classifying everybody. *Multivariate Behavioral Research, 14,* 367-384.

Edwards, L. S. (1983). Workers' compensation insurance. *Orthopedic Clinics of North America, 14,* 661-668.

Edwards, P. W., Zeichner, A., Kuczmeirczyk, A. R., & Boczkowki, J. (1985). Familial pain models: The relationship between family history of pain and current pain experience. *Pain, 21,* 379-384.

Eisenberg, L. (1977). Disease and illness: Distinctions between professional and popular ideas of sickness. *Culture, Medicine and Psychiatry, 1,* 9-23.

Elkins, G. R., & Barrett, E. T. (1984). The MMPI in evaluation of functional vs. organic low back pain. *Journal of Personality Assessment, 48,* 259-264.

Ellertson, B., & Klove, H. (1987). MMPI patterns in chronic muscle pain, tension headaches, and migraine. *Cephalalgia, 7,* 65-71.

Engel, G. L. (1959). "Psychogenic" pain and the pain-prone patient. *American Journal of Medicine, 26,* 899-918.

Escobar, J. I., Burnam, M. A., Karno, M., Forsythe, A., & Golding, J. M. (1987). Somatization in the community. *Archives of General Psychiatry, 44,* 713-718.

Evans, W. O. (1985). A cognitive-behavioral approach to chronic pain. In G. M. Aronoff (Ed.), *Evaluation and treatment of chronic pain* (pp. 549-559). Baltimore: Urban & Schwarzenberg.

Feifel, H., Strack, S., & Nagy, V. T. (1988, August). *Coping profiles of medically ill patients.* Paper presented at the annual meeting of the American Psychological Association, Atlanta, Georgia.

Feinmann, C. (1985). Pain relief by antidepressants: Possible modes of action. *Pain, 23,* 1-8.

Fernandez, E. (1986). A classification system of cognitive coping strategies for pain. *Pain, 26,* 141-151.

Feuerstein, M., Papciak, A. S., & Hoon, P. E. (1987). Biobehavioral mechanisms of chronic low back pain. *Clinical Psychology Review, 7,* 243-273.

Feuerstein, M., Sult, S., & Houle, M. (1985). Environmental stressors and chronic low back pain: Life events, family and work environment. *Pain, 22,* 295-307.

Fishbain, D. A., Goldberg, M., Meagher, B. R., Steele, R., & Rosomoff, H. (1986). Male and female chronic pain patients categorized by DSM-III psychiatric diagnostic criteria. *Pain, 26,* 181-197.

Fleiss, J. L. (1971). Measuring nominal scale agreement among many raters. *Psychological Bulletin, 76,* 378-382.

Flor, H., & Turk, D. C. (1984). Etiological theories and treatment for chronic back pain. I. Somatic models and interventions. *Pain, 19,* 105-121.

Flor, H., Turk, D. C., & Birbaumer, N. (1985). Assessment of stress-related psychophysiological reactions in chronic back pain patients. *Journal of Consulting and Clinical Psychology, 53,* 354-364.

Follick, M. J., Smith, T. W., & Ahern, D. K. (1985). The sickness impact profile: A global measure of disability in chronic low back pain. *Pain, 21,* 67-76.

Ford, C. V. (1983). *The somatizing disorders: Illness as a way of life.* New York: Elsevier Biomedical Inc.

Ford, M. R. (1985). Interpersonal stress and style as predictors of biofeedback/relaxation training outcome. *Biofeedback and Self Regulation, 10,* 223-239.

Fordyce, W. E. (1976). *Behavioral methods for chronic pain and illness.* St. Louis: C. V. Mosby.

Fordyce, W. E. (1978). Learning processes in pain. In R.A. Sternbach (Ed.) *The psychology of pain* (pp. 49–72). New York: Raven.

Fordyce, W. E. (1979). Use of the MMPI in the assessment of chronic pain. *Clinical Notes on the MMPI, #3.* Nutley, NJ: Hoffman-LaRoche.

Fordyce, W. E. (1983). Behavioral conditioning concepts in chronic pain. In J. J. Bonica, U. Lindblom, & A. Iggo (Eds.), *Advances in pain research and therapy* (Vol. 5, pp. 781–788). New York: Raven.

Fordyce, W. E. (1984, February). Back pain, compensation, and public policy. In J. Rosen (Ed.), *Proceedings of the Vermont Conference on Primary Prevention of Psychopathology.*

Fordyce, W. E. (1988). Pain and suffering: A reappraisal. *American Psychologist, 43,* 276–283.

Fordyce, W. E., Brena, S. F., Holcomb, R. J., DeLateur, B. J., & Loeser, J. D. (1978). Relationship of patient semantic pain descriptions to physician diagnostic judgments, activity level measures and MMPI. *Pain, 5,* 293–303.

Fordyce, W. E., Brockway, J. A., Bergman, J. A., & Spengler, D. (1986). Acute back pain: A control-group comparison of behavioral vs. traditional management methods. *Journal of Behavioral Medicine, 9,* 127–140.

Fordyce, W. E., Lansky, D., Calsyn, D. A., Shelton, J. L., Stolov, W. C., & Rock, D. L. (1984). Pain measurement and pain behavior. *Pain, 18,* 199–203.

Fordyce, W. E., Roberts, A. H., & Sternbach, R. A. (1985). The behavioral management of chronic pain: A response to critics. *Pain, 22,* 113–125.

France, R. D., Krishnan, R. R. R., & Trainor, M. (1986). Chronic pain and depression. III. Family history study of depression and alcoholism in chronic low back pain patients. *Pain, 24,* 185–190.

Franz, C., Paul, R., Bautz, M., Choroba, G., & Hildebrandt, J. (1986). Psychosomatic aspects of chronic pain: A new way of description based on MMPI item analysis. *Pain, 26,* 33–43.

Freeman, C., Calsyn, D., & Louks, J. (1976). The use of the Minnesota Multiphasic Personality Inventory with low back pain patients. *Journal of Clinical Psychology, 32,* 294–298.

Frymoyer, J. W., Rosen, F. C., Clements, J., & Pope, M. H. (1985). Psychologic factors in low-back pain disability. *Clinical Orthopedics, 195,* 178–184.

Garron, D. C., & Leavitt, F. (1983a). Chronic low back pain and depression. *Journal of Clinical Psychology, 39,* 486–493.

Gatchel, R. J., Mayer, T. B., Capra, P., Diamond, P., & Barnett, J. (1986). Quantification of lumbar function part 6: The use of psychological measures in guiding physical functional restoration. *Spine, 11,* 36–42.

Gentry, W. D., & Bernal, G. A. A. (1977). Chronic pain. In R. B. Williams & W. D. Gentry (Eds.), *Behavioral approaches to medical treatment* (pp. 173–182). Cambridge, MA: Ballinger.

Gentry, W. D., Shows, W. D., & Thomas, M. (1974). Chronic low back pain: A psychological profile. *Psychosomatics, 151,* 174–177.

Getto, C. J., Heaton, R. K., & Lehman, R. A. W. (1983). PSPI: A standardized approach to the evaluation of psychosocial factors in chronic pain. In J. J. Bonica & D. Albe-Fessard (Eds.), *Advances in pain research and therapy* (Vol. 5, pp. 885–559). New York: Raven.

Gilberstadt, H., & Jancis, M. (1967). "Organic" vs. "functional" diagnoses from 1–3 MMPI profiles. *Journal of Clinical Psychology, 23,* 480–483.

Goldberg, P. J. (1985). The social worker, family systems, and the chronic pain family. In G. M. Aronoff (Ed.), *Evaluation and treatment of chronic pain* (pp. 571–588). Baltimore: Urban & Schwarzenberg.

Goldberg, R. T. (1982). The social and vocational rehabilitation of persons with chronic pain: A critical evaluation. *Rehabilitation Literature, 43,* 274–283.

Graham, J. R. (1987). *The MMPI: A practical guide (2nd ed.).* New York: Oxford University Press.

Graham, J. R. (1990). *The MMPI-2: A practical guide.* New York: Oxford University Press.

Graham, J. R., & Butcher, J. N. (1988, March). Differentiating schizophrenic and major affective disordered inpatients with the revised form of the MMPI. Paper presented at the *23rd Annual Symposium on Recent Developments in the Use of the MMPI*, St. Petersburg, Florida.

Graham, J.R., & Lilly, R. S. (1986, March). *Linear T-scores versus normalized T-scores: An empirical study.* Paper presented at the 21st Annual Symposium on Recent Developments in the Use of the MMPI, Clearwater Beach, Florida.

Green, P. E. (1978). *Analyzing multivariate data.* Hinsdale, IL: Dryden.

Green, S. B. (1982). Establishing behavioral correlates: The MMPI as a case study. *Applied Psychological Measurement, 6,* 219–224.

Greene, R. L. (1980). *The MMPI: An interpretive manual.* New York: Grune & Stratton.

Grove, W. M., & Andreasen, N. C. (1982). Simultaneous tests of many hypotheses in exploratory research. *Journal of Nervous and Mental Disease, 170,* 3–8.

Guck, T. P., Meilman, P. W., & Skultety, F. M. (1987). Pain assessment index: Evaluation following multidisciplinary pain treatment. *Journal of Pain and Symptom Management, 2,* 23–27.

Guck, T. P., Meilman, P. W., Skultety, F. M., & Dowd, E. T. (1986). Prediction of long-term outcome of multidisciplinary pain treatment. *Archives of Physical Medicine and Rehabilitation, 67,* 293–296.

Guck, T. P., Meilman, P. W., Skultety, F. M., & Poloni, L. D. (1988). Pain-patient Minnesota Multiphasic Personality Inventory (MMPI) subgroups: Evaluation of long-term treatment outcome. *Journal of Behavioral Medicine, 11,* 159–169.

Guck, T. P., Skultety, F. M., Meilman, P. W. & Dowd, E. T. (1985). Multidisciplinary pain center follow-up study: Evaluation with a no-treatment control group. *Pain, 21,* 295–306.

Gupta, M. A. (1986). Is chronic pain a variant of depressive illness? A critical review. *Canadian Journal of Psychiatry, 31,* 241–248.

Haber, J. D., & Roos, C. (1985). Effects of spouse abuse and/or sexual abuse in the development and maintenance of chronic pain in women. In H. L. Fields, R. Dubner, & F. Cervero (Eds.), *Advances in pain research and therapy* (Vol. 9, pp. 889–895). New York: Raven.

Hagedorn, S. D., Maruta, R., Swanson, D. W., & Colligan, R. C. (1982). Premorbid MMPI profiles of low back pain patients: Surgical successes vs. surgical failures. *Pain, Supp. 2,* 258.

Hamilton, M. (1960). A rating scale for depression. *Journal of Neurological and Neurosurgical Psychiatry, 23,* 53–62.

Hanvik, L. J. (1949). Some psychological dimensions of low back pain. Unpublished doctoral dissertation, University of Minnesota.

Hanvik, L. J. (1951). MMPI profiles in patients with low-back pain. *Journal of Consulting Psychology, 15,* 350–353.

Harkins, S. W., Kwentus, J., & Price, D. D. (1984). Pain and the elderly. In C. Benedetti, C. R. Chapman, & G. Moricca (Eds.), *Advances in pain research and therapy* (Vol. 7, pp. 103–121). New York: Raven.

Harris, G., & Rollman, G. B. (1985). Cognitive techniques for controlling pain: Generality and individual differences. In H. L. Fields, R. Dubner, & F. Cervero (Eds.), *Advances in pain research and therapy* (Vol. 9, pp. 847–851). New York: Raven.

Harris, J. G. (1982). The assessment of personality profiles. *Clinical Psychology Review, 2,* 27–47.

Harris, R. C., & Lingoes, J. C. (1955). Subscales for the MMPI: An aid to profile interpretation. Mimeographed materials, Department of Psychiatry, University of California.

Hart, R. L. (1984). Replicated multivariate clustering of personality profiles. *Journal of Clinical Psychology, 40,* 129–133.

Hathaway, S. R., & Briggs, P. F. (1957). Some normative data on new MMPI scales. *Journal of Clinical Psychology, 13,* 364–368.

Hathaway, S. R., & McKinley, J. C. (1940). A multiphasic personality schedule (Minnesota): I. Construction of the schedule. *Journal of Psychology, 10,* 249–254.

Hathaway, S. R., & McKinley, J. C. (1943). *The Minnesota Multiphasic Personality Schedule* (revised). Minneapolis, MN: University of Minnesota Press.

Haven, G. A., & Cole, K. M. (1972). Psychological correlates of low back pain syndrome and their relationship to the effectiveness of a low back pain program. *Newsletter for Research in Psychology, 14,* 31–33.

Heaton, R. K., Getto, C. J., Lehman, R. A., Fordyce, W. E., Brauer, E., & Groban, S. E. (1982). A standardized evaluation of psychosocial factors in chronic pain. *Pain, 12,* 165–174.

Hendler, H. (1984). Depression caused by chronic pain. *Journal of Clinical Psychiatry, 45,* 30–38.

Hendler, N., Mollett, A., Talo, S., & Levin, S. (1988). A comparison between the MMPI and the "Mensana Clinic Back Pain Test" for validating the complaint of chronic back pain. *Journal of Occupational Medicine, 30,* 98–102.

Henrichs, T. F. (1981). Using the MMPI in medical consultation. In J. Butcher, G. Dahlstrom, M. Gynther, & W. Schofield (Eds.), *Clinical Notes on the MMPI, #6.* Nutley, NJ: Hoffman-LaRoche.

Henrichs, T. F. (1987). MMPI profiles of chronic pain patients: Some methodological considerations that concern clusters and descriptors. *Journal of Clinical Psychology, 43,* 651–660.

Herron, L., Turner, J., & Weiner, P. (1986). A comparison of the Millon Clinical Multiaxial Inventory and the Minnesota Multiphasic Personality Inventory as predictors of successful treatment by lumbar laminectomy. *Clinical Orthopaedics and Related Research,* 232–238.

Holmes, T. H., & Rahe, R. H. (1967). The Social Readjustment Rating Scale. *Journal of Psychosomatic Research, 11,* 213–218.

Holzman, A. D., Rudy, T. E., Gerber, K. E., Turk, D. C., Sanders, S. H., Zimmerman, J., & Kerns, R. D. (1985). Chronic pain: A multiple-setting comparison of patient characterisitcs. *Journal of Behavioral Medicine, 8,* 411–422.

Hoon, P. W., Feuerstein, M., & Papciak, A. S. (1985). Evaluation of the chronic low back pain patient: Conceptual and clinical considerations. *Clinical Psychology Review, 5,* 377–401.

Hubbard, K. M. (1983). Patient response to pain treatment: Personality variables associated with the use of transcutaneous electrical nerve stimulation. *Dissertation Abstracts International, 43,* 2708.

Institute of Medicine Committee on Pain, Disability, and Chronic Illness Behavior (1987). *Pain and disability: clinical, behavioral, and public policy perspectives.* Washington, DC: National Academy Press.

International Association for the Study of Pain, Subcommittee on Classification (1986). Pain terms: A current list with definitions and notes on usage. *Pain,* Supp. 3, 215–221.

Jamison, K., Ferrer-Brechner, M., Brechner, V., & McCreary, C. (1976). Correlation of personality profile with pain syndrome. In J. J. Bonica & D. Albe-Fessard (Eds.), *Advances in pain research and therapy* (Vol. 1, pp. 317–321). New York: Raven.

Jessup, B. A. (1984). Biofeedback. In P. D. Wall & R. Melzack (Eds.), *Textbook of pain* (pp. 776–786). New York: Churchill-Livingstone.

Katon, W., Egan, K., & Miller, D. (1985). Chronic pain: Lifetime psychiatric diagnoses and family history. *American Journal of Psychiatry, 142,* 1156–1160.

Katon, W., Kleinman, A., & Rosen, G. (1982a). Depression and somatization: A review. Part I. *American Journal of Medicine, 72,* 127–135.

Katon, W., Kleinman, A., & Rosen, G. (1982b). Depression and somatization: A review. Part II. *American Journal of Medicine, 72,* 241–247.

Keefe, F. J. (1982). Behavioral assessment and treatment of chronic pain: Current status and future directions. *Journal of Consulting and Clinical Psychology, 50,* 896–911.

Keefe, F. J., Block, A. R., Williams, R. B., & Surwit, R. S. (1981). Behavioral treatment of chronic low back pain. *Pain, 11,* 221–231.

Keefe, F. J., & Dolan, E. (1986). Pain behavior and pain coping strategies in low back pain and myofascial pain dysfunction syndrome patients. *Pain, 24*, 49–86.

Keefe, F. J., Gil, K. M., & Rose, S. C. (1986). Behavioral approaches in the multidisciplinary management of chronic pain. *Clinical Psychology Review, 6*, 87–113.

Keller, L. S., Butcher, J. N., & Slutske, W. S. (1990). Objective personality assessment. In G. Goldstein & M. Hersen (Eds.), *Handbook of psychological assessment* (2nd ed.). New York: Pergamon.

Kelsey, J. L., White, A. A., Pastides, H., & Bisbee, G. E. (1979). The impact of musculoskeletal disorders on the population of the United States. *Journal of Bone and Joint Surgery, 61-A*, 959–964.

Kenyon, F. E. (1976). Hypochondriacal states. *British Journal of Psychiatry, 129*, 1–14.

Kerns, R. D., Turk, D. C., & Rudy, T. E. (1985). The West Haven-Yale Multidimensional Pain Inventory (WHYMPI). *Pain, 23*, 345–356.

Kiesler, D. J. (1966). Some myths of psychotherapy research and the search for a paradigm. *Psychological Bulletin, 65*, 110–136.

Klein, B. P., Jensen, R. C., & Sanderson, L. M. (1984). Assessment of workers' compensation claims for back strains/sprains. *Journal of Occupational Medicine, 26*, 443–448.

Kleinke, C. L., & Spangler, A. S. (1988). Predicting outcome of chronic back pain patients in a multidisciplinary pain clinic: Methodological issues and treatment implications. *Pain, 33*, 41–48.

Kramlinger, K. G., Swanson, D. W., & Maruta, T. (1983). Are patients with chronic pain depressed? *American Journal of Psychiatry, 140*, 747–749.

Kremer, E. F., Block, A., & Atkinson, J. H. (1983). Assessment of pain behavior: Factors that distort self-report. In R. Melzack (Ed.), *Pain measurement and assessment* (pp. 165–171). New York: Raven.

Kremer, E. F., Block, A., & Gaylor, M. S. (1981). Behavioral approaches to treatment of chronic pain: The inaccuracy of patient self-report measures. *Archives of Physical Medicine and Rehabilitation, 62*, 188–191.

Kremer, E. F., Sieber, W., & Atkinson, J. H. (1985). Spousal perpetuation of chronic pain behavior. *International Journal of Family Therapy, 7*, 258–270.

Krishnan, K. R. R., France, R. D., Pelton, S., McCann, U. D., Davidson, J., & Urban, B. J. (1985). Chronic pain and depression. II. Symptoms of anxiety in chronic low back pain patients and their relationship to subtypes of depression. *Pain, 22*, 289–294.

Kudrow, L., & Sutkus, B. J. (1979). MMPI pattern specificity in primary headache disorders. *Headache, 19*, 18–24.

Lachar, D. (1974). *The MMPI: Clinical assessment and automated interpretation*. Los Angeles: Western Psychological Services.

Lair, C. V., & Trapp, E. P. (1962). The differential diagnostic value of MMPI with somatically disturbed patients. *Journal of Clinical Psychology, 18*, 146–147.

Large, R. G. (1986). DSM-III diagnoses in chronic pain: Confusion or clarity? *Journal of Nervous and Mental Disease, 174*, 295–303.

Latimer, P. R. (1982). External contingency management for chronic pain: Critical review of the evidence. *American Journal of Psychiatry, 139*, 1308–1312.

Lawlis, G. F., & McCoy, C. E. (1983). Psychological evaluation: Patients with chronic pain. *Orthopedic Clinics of North America, 14*, 527–538.

Lazare, A. (1971). The hysterical character in psychoanalytic theory: Evolution and confusion. *Archives of General Psychiatry, 25*, 131–137.

Leavitt, F. (1985). The value of the MMPI conversion "V" in the assessment of psychogenic pain. *Journal of Psychosomatic Research, 29*, 125–131.

Leavitt, F., & Garron, D. C. (1982). Patterns of psychological disturbance and pain report in patients with low back pain. *Journal of Psychiatric Research, 26*, 301–307.

Leavitt, F., Garron, D. C., McNeill, T. W., & Whisler, W. W. (1982). Organic status, psychological disturbance, and pain report characteristics in low-back-pain patients on compensation. *Spine, 7*, 398-402.

Liebman, R., Honig, P., & Berger, H. (1976). An integrated program for psychogenic pain. *Family Processes, 15*, 307-406.

Lindsay, P. G., & Wykoff, M. (1981). The depression-pain syndrome and its response to antidepressants. *Psychosomatics, 22*, 571-577.

Linton, S. J. (1982). A critical review of behavioural treatments for chronic benign pain other than headache. *British Journal of Clinical Psychology, 21*, 321-337.

Linton, S. J. (1986). Behavioral remediation of chronic pain: A status report. *Pain, 24*, 125-141.

Lipton, J. A., & Marbach, J. J. (1984). Ethnicity and the pain experience. *Social Science in Medicine, 19*, 1279-1298.

Long, C. J. (1981). The relationship between surgical outcome and MMPI profiles in chronic pain patients. *Journal of Clinical Psychology, 37*, 744-749.

Louks, J. L., Freeman, C. W., & Calsyn, D. A. (1978). Personality organization as an aspect of back pain in a medical setting. *Journal of Personality Assessment, 42*, 152-158.

Love, A. W., & Peck, C. L. (1987). The MMPI and psychological factors in chronic low back pain: A review. *Pain, 28*, 1-28.

MacAndrew, C. (1965). The differentiation of male alcoholic out-patients from nonalcoholic psychiatric patients by means of the MMPI. *Quarterly Journal of Studies on Alcohol, 26*, 238-246.

Malec, J. F., Cayner, J. J., Harvey, R. F., & Timming, R. C. (1981). Pain management: Long-term follow-up of an inpatient program. *Archives of Physical Medicine and Rehabilitation, 62*, 369-372.

Marks, P. A., Seeman, W., & Haller, D. L. (1974). *The actuarial use of the MMPI with adolescents and adults.* Baltimore: Williams and Wilkins.

Maruta, T., Swanson, D. W., & Finlayson, R. E. (1979). Drug abuse and dependency in patients with chronic pain. *Mayo Clinic Proceedings, 54*, 241-244.

Maruta, T., Swanson, D. W., & Swenson, W. M. (1976). Pain as a psychiatric symptom: Comparison between low back pain and depression. *Psychosomatics, 17*, 123-127.

McArthur, D. L., Cohen, M. J., Gottlieb, H. J., Naliboff, B. D., & Schandler, S. L. (1987). Treating chronic low back pain. I. Admission to initial follow-up. *Pain, 29*, 1-22.

McCreary, C. (1985). Empirically derived MMPI profile clusters and characteristics of low back pain patients. *Journal of Consulting and Clinical Psychology, 53*, 558-560.

McCreary, C., & Colman, A. (1984). Medication usage, emotional disturbance and pain behavior in chronic low back pain patients. *Journal of Clinical Psychology, 40*, 15-19.

McCreary, C., Turner, J., & Dawson, E. (1977). Differences between functional and organic low back pain patients. *Pain, 4*, 73-78.

McCreary, C., Turner, J., & Dawson, E. (1979). The MMPI as a predictor of response to conservative treatment for low back pain. *Journal of Clinical Psychology, 35*, 278-284.

McCreary, C., Turner, J., & Dawson, E. (1980). Emotional disturbance and chronic low back pain. *Journal of Clinical Psychology, 36*, 709-715.

McGill, J., Lawlis, G. F., Selby, D., Mooney, V., & McCoy, C. E. (1983). The relationship of Minnesota Multiphasic Personality Inventory (MMPI) profile clusters to pain behaviors. *Journal of Behavioral Medicine, 6*, 77-92.

McGrath, R. E., & O'Malley, W. B. (1986). The assessment of denial and physical complaints: The validity of the Hy scale and associated MMPI signs. *Journal of Clinical Psychology, 42*, 754-760.

McNairy, S. L., Maruta, T., Ivnik, R. J., Swanson, D. W., & Ilstrup, D. M. (1984). Prescription medication dependence and neuropsychiatric function. *Pain, 18*, 169-177.

Mechanic, D. (1972). Social psychologic factors affecting the presentation of bodily complaints. *New England Journal of Medicine, 286*, 1132-1139.

Melzack, R. (1983). Concepts of pain measurement. In R. Melzack (Ed.), *Pain measurement and assessment* (pp. 1-5). New York: Raven.

Melzack, R., & Wall, P. D. (1965). Pain mechanisms: A new theory. *Science, 150,* 971–979.

Melzack, R., & Wall, P. D. (1983). *The challenge of pain.* New York: Basic Books.

Mendelson, G. (1982). Alexithymia and chronic pain: Prevalence, correlates and treatment results. *Psychotherapy and Psychosomatics, 37,* 154–164.

Mendelson, G. (1984). Compensation, pain complaints, and psychological disturbance. *Pain, 20,* 169–177.

Merskey, H. (1978). Pain and personality. In R. A. Sternbach (Ed.), *The psychology of pain* (pp. 111–127). New York: Raven.

Merskey, H. (1980). Some features of the history of the idea of pain. *Pain, 9,* 3–8.

Miller, E. (1987). Hysteria: Its nature and explanation. *British Journal of Clinical Psychology, 26,* 163–173.

Minuchin, S., Rosman, B. L., & Baker, L. (1978). *Psychosomatic families.* Cambridge, MA: Harvard University Press.

Mohamed, S. N., Weisz, G. M., & Waring, E. M. (1978). The relationship of chronic pain to depression, marital adjustment, and family dynamics. *Pain, 5,* 285–292.

Moore, J. E., Armentrout, D. P., Parker, J. C., & Kivlahan, D. R. (1986). Empirically derived pain-patient MMPI subgroups: Prediction of treatment outcome. *Journal of Behavioral Medicine, 9,* 51–63.

Moore, J. E., McFall, M. E., Kivlahan, D. R., & Capestany, F. (1988). Risk of misinterpretation of MMPI schizophrenia scale elevations in chronic pain patients. *Pain, 32,* 207–213.

Morey, L. C., Blashfield, R. K., & Skinner, H. A. (1983). A comparison of cluster analysis techniques within a sequential validation framework. *Multivariate Behavioral Research, 18,* 309–329.

Murray, J. B. (1982). Psychological aspects of low back pain: Summary. *Psychological Report, 50,* 343–351.

Muse, M. (1985). Stress-related, posttraumatic chronic pain syndrome. *Pain, 23,* 295–300.

Muse, M. (1986). Stress-related, posttraumatic chronic pain syndrome: Behavioral treatment approach. *Pain, 25,* 389–394.

Naliboff, B. D., Cohen, M. J., Swanson, B. A., Bonebakker, A. D., & McArthur, D. L. (1985). Comprehensive assessment of chronic low back pain patients and controls. *Pain, 23,* 121–134.

Naliboff, B. D., Cohen, M. J., & Yellen, A. N. (1982). Does the MMPI differentiate chronic illness from chronic pain? *Pain, 13,* 333–341.

Naliboff, B. D., Cohen, M. J., & Yellen, A. N. (1983). Frequency of MMPI profile types in three chronic illness populations. *Journal of Clinical Psychology, 39,* 843–847.

Norusis, M. J. (1985). *SPSS-X advanced statistics guide.* New York: McGraw-Hill.

O'Leary, A. (1985). Self-efficacy and health. *Behavior Research and Therapy, 23,* 437–451.

Oostdam, E. M., Duivenvoorden, H. J., & Pondaag, W. (1981). Predictive value of some psychological tests on the outcome of surgical intervention in low back pain patients. *Journal of Psychosomatic Research, 25,* 227–235.

Orne, M. T. (1983). Hypnotic methods for managing pain. In J. J. Bonica, U. Lindblom, & A. Iggo (Eds.), *Advances in pain research and therapy* (Vol. 5, pp. 847–856). New York: Raven.

Orne, M. T., & Dinges, D. F. (1984). Hypnosis. In P. D. Wall & R. Melzack (Eds.), *Textbook of pain* (pp. 806–816). New York: Churchill-Livingstone.

Osborne, D. (1985). The MMPI in medical practice. *Psychiatric Annals,* 534–541.

Page, R. D., & Schaub, L. H. (1978). EMG biofeedback applicability for differing personality types. *Journal of Clinical Psychology, 34,* 1014–1020.

Painter, J. R., Seres, J. L., & Newman, R. I. (1980). Assessing benefits of the pain center: Why some patients regress. *Pain, 8,* 101–113.

Parkison, S., & Fishburne, F. (1984). MMPI normative data for a male active duty Army population. Paper presented at the Department of Defense Psychology Symposium.

Patrick, J. (1988). Personality characteristics of work-ready workers' compensation clients. *Journal of Clinical Psychology, 44,* 1009–1012.

Payne, B., & Norfleet, M. A. (1986). Chronic pain and the family. *Pain, 26,* 1–22.

Penman, J. (1954). Pain as an old friend. *Lancet, 1,* 633–636.

Pennebaker, J. W. (1982). *The psychology of physical symptoms.* New York: Springer-Verlag.

Pennebaker, J. W., & Skelton, J. A. (1978). Psychological parameters of physical symptoms. *Personality and Social Psychology Bulletin, 4,* 524–530.

Philips, H. C. (1987). Avoidance behaviour and its role in sustaining chronic pain. *Behaviour Research and Therapy, 25,* 272–279.

Pichot, P., Perse, J., LeBeaux, M. O., Dureau, J. L., Perez, C. I., & Rychawaert, A. (1972). Le personalite des sujets presentant des douleurs dorsales fonchonelles valeur de l'inventaire multiphasique de personalite de Minnesota. *Revue de Psychologie Applique, 22,* 145–172.

Pilowsky, I. (1967). Dimensions of hypochondriasis. *British Journal of Psychiatry, 113,* 89–93.

Pilowsky, I. (1978). Psychodynamic aspects of the pain experience. In R. A. Sternbach (Ed.), *The psychology of pain* (pp. 203–217). New York: Raven.

Pilowsky, I., & Bassett, D. L. (1982). Pain and depression. *British Journal of Psychiatry, 141,* 30–36.

Pollack, D. R., & Grainey, T. F. (1984). A comparison of MMPI profiles for state and private disability insurance applicants. *Journal of Personality Assessment, 48,* 121–125.

Postone, N. (1986). Alexithymia in chronic pain patients. *General Hospital Psychiatry, 8,* 163–167.

Prokop, C. K. (1986). Hysteria scale elevations in low back pain patients: A risk factor for mis-diagnosis? *Journal of Consulting and Clinical Psychology, 46,* 425–427.

Prokop, C. K., Bradley, L. A., Margolis, R., & Gentry, W. K. (1980). Multivariate analysis of the MMPI profiles of patients with multiple pain complaints. *Journal of Personality Assessment, 44,* 246–252.

Rappaport, N. B., McAnulty, D. P., Waggoner, C. D., & Brantley, P. J. (1987). Cluster analysis of Minnesota Multiphasic Personality Inventory (MMPI) profiles in a chronic headache population. *Journal of Behavioral Medicine, 10,* 49–60.

Reich, J., Steward, M. S., Tupin, J. P., & Rosenblatt, R. M. (1985). Prediction of response to treatment in chronic pain patients. *Journal of Clinical Psychiatry, 46,* 425–427.

Reich, J., & Thompson, W. D. (1987). Comparison of psychiatric diagnoses in three populations. *Hillside Journal of Clinical Psychiatry, 9,* 36–46.

Reich, J., Tupin, J. P., & Abramowitz, S. I. (1983). Psychiatric diagnosis of chronic pain patients. *American Journal of Psychiatry, 140,* 1495–1498.

Reisbord, L. S., & Greenland, S. (1985). Factors associated with self-reported back-pain prevalence: A population-based study. *Journal of Chronic Diseases, 38,* 691–702.

Roberts, A. H., & Reinhardt, L. (1980). The behavioral management of chronic pain: Long-term follow-up with comparison groups. *Pain, 8,* 151–162.

Roberts, L. C. (1987). *The use of the MMPI in differential diagnosis of schizophrenia and depression.* Unpublished doctoral dissertation, University of Minnesota.

Romano, J. M., & Turner, J. A. (1985). Chronic pain and depression: Does the evidence support a relationship? *Psychological Bulletin, 97,* 18–34.

Rook, J. C., Pesch, R. N., & Keeler, E. C. (1981). Chronic pain and the questionable use of the Minnesota Multiphasic Personality Inventory. *Archives of Physical Medicine and Rehabilitation, 62,* 373–376.

Rosen, J. C., Frymoyer, J. W., & Clements, J. H. (1980). A further look at the validity of the MMPI with low back patients. *Journal of Clinical Psychology, 36,* 994–1000.

Rosen, J. C., Grubman, J. A., Bevins, T., & Frymoyer, J. W. (1987). Musculoskeletal status and disability of MMPI profile subgroups among patients with low back pain. *Health Psychology, 6,* 581–598.

Rosenstiel, A. K., & Keefe, F. J. (1983). The use of coping strategies in chronic low back pain patients: Relationship to patient characteristics and current adjustment. *Pain, 17,* 33–44.

Rosenthal, R. H., Ling, F. W., Rosenthal, T. L., & McNeeley, S. G. (1984). Chronic pelvic pain: Psychological features and laparoscopic findings. *Psychosomatics, 25,* 833–841.

Roy, R. (1984). "I have a headache tonight": Function of pain in marriage. *International Journal of Family Therapy, 6,* 165–176.

Roy, R. (1985). Family treatment for chronic pain: State of the art. *International Journal of Family Therapy, 7,* 297–309.

Roy, R., Thomas, M., & Matas, M. (1984). Chronic pain and depression: A review. *Comprehensive Psychiatry, 25,* 96–105.

Rylee, K. E. & Wu, N. N. (1984). Factors predicting the outcome of chronic pain management at an ambulatory pain clinic. *Pain,* Supp. 2, 437.

Schachter, S., & Singer, J. (1962). Cognitive, social and physiological determinants of emotional state. *Psychological Review, 69,* 379–399.

Schwartz, M. S., & Krupp, N. E. (1971). The MMPI "conversion V" among 50,000 medical patients: A study of incidence, criteria, and profile elevation. *Journal of Clinical Psychology, 27,* 89–95.

Shaffer, J. W., Nussbaum, K., & Little, J. M. (1972). MMPI profiles of disability insurance claimants. *American Journal of Psychiatry, 129,* 403–407.

Shipman, W. B., Greene, C. S., & Laskin, D. M. (1974). Correlation of placebo responses and personality characteristics in myofascial pain-dysfunction patients. *Journal of Psychosomatic Research, 18,* 475–483.

Sister Kenny Institute (undated). *Chronic pain rehabilitation.* (Program pamphlet available from Sister Kenny Institute, 800 East 28th Street at Chicago Avenue, Minneapolis, MN 55407.)

Sister Kenny Institute (1984). *Sister Kenny Institute.* (Program pamphlet available from Sister Kenny Institute, 800 East 28th Street at Chicago Avenue, Minneapolis, MN 55407.)

Smith, T. W., Follick, M. J., Ahern, D. K., & Adams, A. (1986). Cognitive distortion and disability in chronic low back pain. *Cognitive Therapy and Research, 10,* 201–210.

Smith, T. W., Snyder, C. R., & Perkins, S. C. (1983). The self-serving function of hypochondriacal complaints: Physical symptoms as self-handicapping strategies. *Journal of Personality and Social Psychology, 44,* 787–797.

Snibbe, J. R., Peterson, P. J., & Sosner, B. (1980). Study of psychological characteristics of a workers' compensation sample using the MMPI and Millon Clinical Multiaxial Inventory. *Psychological Reports, 47,* 959–966.

Snook, S. H., & Jensen, R. C. (1984). Cost. In M. H. Pope, J. W. Frymoyer, & G. Andersson (Eds.), *Occupational low back pain* (pp. 115–121). New York: Praeger.

Snyder, D. K. (in press). Assessing chronic pain with the Minnesota Multiphasic Personality Inventory (MMPI). In T. W. Miller (Ed.), *Chronic pain: Clinical issues in health care management.* International Universities Press.

Snyder, D. K., & Power, D. G. (1981). Empirical descriptors of unelevated MMPI profiles among chronic pain patients: A typological approach. *Journal of Clinical Psychology, 37,* 602–607.

Southwick, S. M., & White, A. A. (1983). The use of psychological tests in the evaluation of low-back pain. *Journal of Bone and Joint Surgery, 65,* 560–565.

Steinberg, G. G. (1982). Epidemiology of low back pain. In M. Stanton-Hicks & R. Boas (Eds.), *Chronic low back pain* (pp. 1–13). New York: Raven.

Sternbach, R. A. (1974a). *Pain patients: Traits and treatment.* New York: Academic Press.

Sternbach, R. A. (1974b). Psychological aspects of pain and the selection of patients. *Clinical Neurosurgery, 21,* 323–333.

Sternbach, R. A. (1974c). Varieties of pain games. In J. J. Bonica (Ed.), *Advances in Neurology* Vol. 4: *Pain.* New York: Raven.

Sternbach, R. A. (1984). Behaviour therapy. In P. D. Wall & R. Melzack (Eds.), *Textbook of pain* (pp. 800–805). New York: Churchill-Livingstone.

Sternbach, R. A., Dalessio, D. J., Kunzel, M., & Bowman, G. E. (1980). MMPI patterns in common headache disorders. *Headache, 311*–315.

Sternbach, R. A., & Rusk, T. N. (1973). Alternatives to the pain career. *Psychotherapy: Theory, Research and Practice, 10,* 321–324.

Sternbach, R. A., Wolf, S. R., Murphy, R. W., & Akeson, W. H. (1973). Traits of pain patients: The low-back "loser." *Psychosomatics, 14,* 226–229.

Stone, R. K., Jr., & Pepitone-Arreola-Rockwell, R. F. (1983). Diagnosis of organic and functional pain patients with the MMPI. *Psychological Report, 52,* 539–548.

Strang, J. P. (1985). The chronic disability syndrome. In G. M. Aronoff (Ed.), *Evaluation and treatment of chronic pain* (pp. 603–623). Baltimore: Urban & Schwarzenberg.

Strassberg, D. S., Reimherr, F., Ward, M., Russell, S., & Cole, A. (1981). The MMPI and chronic pain. *Journal of Consulting and Clinical Psychology, 49,* 220–226.

Swanson, D. W., Floreen, A. C., & Swenson, W. M. (1976). Program for managing chronic pain. II. Short-term results. *Mayo Clinic Proceedings, 51,* 409–411.

Swanson, D. W., Maruta, T., & Wolff, V. A. (1986). Ancient pain. *Pain, 25,* 383–387.

Swanson, D. W., Swenson, W. M., Maruta, T., & McPhee, M. C. (1976). Program for managing chronic pain. I. *Mayo Clinic Proceedings, 51,* 401–408.

Swenson, W. M., Pearson, J. S., & Osborne, D. (1973). *An MMPI source book: Basic item, scale, and pattern data on 50,000 medical patients.* Minneapolis, MN: University of Minnesota Press.

Szasz, T. S. (1968). The psychology of persistent pain: A portrait of l'homme douloureux. In A. Soulairac, J. Cahn, & J. Charpentier (Eds.), *Pain* (pp. 93–113). New York: Academic Press.

Tarsh, M. J., & Royston, C. (1985). A follow-up study of accident neurosis. *British Journal of Psychiatry, 146,* 18–25.

Tellegen, A. (1988a). The analysis of consistency in personality assessment. *Journal of Personality, 56,* 621–665.

Tellegen, A. (1988b). Derivation of uniform T scores for the restandardized MMPI. In R. D. Fowler (chair), Revision and restandardization of the MMPI: Rationale, normative sample, new norms, and initial validation. *Symposium conducted at the 96th Annual Convention of the American Psychological Association,* Atlanta, GA.

Towne, W. S., & Tsushima, W. T. (1978). The use of the Low Back and the Dorsal scales in the identification of functional low back pain patients. *Journal of Clinical Psychology, 34,* 88–91.

Trabin, T., Rader, C., & Cummings, C. (1987). A comparison of pain management outcomes for disability compensation and non-compensation patients. *Psychology and Health, 1,* 341–351.

Trief, P. M., Elliott, D. J., Stein, N., & Frederickson, B. E. (1987). Functional vs. organic pain: A meaningful distinction? *Journal of Clinical Psychology, 43,* 219–226.

Trief, P., & Stein, N. (1985). Pending litigation and rehabilitation outcome of chronic back pain. *Archives of Physical Medicine and Rehabilitation, 66,* 95–99.

Trief, P. M., & Yuan, H. A. (1983). The use of the MMPI in a chronic back pain rehabilitation program. *Journal of Clinical Psychology, 39,* 46–53.

Tryon, R. C., & Bailey, D. E. (1970). *Cluster analysis.* New York: McGraw-Hill.

Tsushima, W. T., & Towne, W. S. (1979). Clinical limitations of the Low Back Scale. *Journal of Clinical Psychology, 35,* 306–308.

Turk, D. C., & Flor, H. (1984). Etiological theories and treatments for chronic back pain. II. Psychological models and interventions. *Pain, 19,* 209–233.

Turk, D. C., & Kerns, R. D. (1983–84). Conceptual issues in the assessment of clinical pain. *International Journal of Psychiatry in Medicine, 13,* 57–68.

Turk, D. C., & Meichenbaum, D. (1984). A cognitive-behavioural approach to pain management. In P. D. Wall & R. Melzack (Eds.), *Textbook of pain* (pp. 787–794). New York: Churchill-Livingstone.

Turk, D. C., Meichenbaum, D. H., & Genest, M. (1983). *Pain and behavioral medicine: A cognitive-behavioral perspective.* New York: Guilford.

Turk, D. C., & Rudy, R. E. (1986). Assessment of cogntive factors in chronic pain: A worthwhile enterprise? *Journal of Consulting and Clinical Psychology, 54,* 760–768.

Turk, D. C., Rudy, T. E., & Flor, H. (1985). Why a family perspective for pain? *International Journal of Family Therapy, 7,* 223–234.

Turk, D. C., & Salovey, P. (1984). "Chronic pain as a variant of depressive disease": A critical reappraisal. *Journal of Nervous and Mental Disease, 172,* 398–404.

Turner, J. A. (1982). Comparison of group progressive-relaxation training and cognitive-behavioral group therapy for chronic low back pain. *Journal of Consulting and Clinical Psychology, 50,* 757–765.

Turner, J. A., Calsyn, D. A., Fordyce, W. E., & Ready, L. B. (1982). Drug utilization patterns in chronic pain patients. *Pain, 12,* 357–363.

Turner, J. A., & Chapman, C. R. (1982a). Psychological interventions for chronic pain: A critical review. I: Relaxation training and biofeedback. *Pain, 12,* 1–21.

Turner, J. A., & Chapman, C. R. (1982b). Psychological interventions for chronic pain: A critical review. II: Operant conditioning, hypnosis, and cognitive-behavioral therapy. *Pain, 12,* 23–46.

Turner, J. A., & Clancy, S. (1986). Strategies for coping with chronic low back pain: Relationship to pain and disability. *Pain, 24,* 355–364.

Turner, J. A., & Clancy, S. (1988). Comparison of operant behavioral and cognitive-behavioral group treatment for chronic low back pain. *Journal of Consulting and Clinical Psychology, 56,* 261–266.

Turner, J. A., Herron, L., & Weiner, P. (1986). Utility of the MMPI pain assessment index in predicting outcome after lumbar surgery. *Journal of Clinical Psychology, 42,* 764–769.

Turner, J. A., & Romano, J. M. (1984a). Evaluating psychologic interventions for chronic pain: Issues and recent developments. In C. Benedetti, C. R. Chapman, & G. Moricca (Eds.), *Advances in pain research and therapy* (Vol. 7, pp. 257–296). New York: Raven.

Turner, J. A. & Romano, J. M. (1984b). Review of prevalence of coexisting chronic pain and depression. In C. Benedetti, C. R. Chapman, & G. Moricca (Eds.), *Advances in pain research and therapy* (Vol. 7, pp. 123–129). New York: Raven.

Van Houdenhove, B. (1986). Prevalence and psychodynamic interpretation of premorbid hyperactivity in patients with chronic pain. *Psychotherapy and Psychosomatics, 45,* 195–200.

Violon, A., & Giurgea, D. (1984). Familial models for chronic pain. *Pain, 18,* 199–203.

Wall, P. D., & Melzack, R. (Eds., 1984). *Textbook of pain.* New York: Churchill-Livingstone.

Ward, J. H. (1963). Hierarchical grouping to optimize an objective function. *American Statistical Association Journal,* 236–244.

Waring, E. M. (1977). The role of the family in symptom selection and perpetuation of psychosomatic illness. *Psychotherapeutics and Psychosomatics, 28,* 253–259.

Waring, E. M., Weisz, G. M., & Bailey, S. I. (1976). Predictive factors in the treatment of low back pain by surgical intervention. In J. J. Bonica & D. Albe-Fessard (Eds.), *Advances in pain research and therapy* (Vol. 1, pp. 939–942). New York: Raven.

Watkins, R. G., O'Brien, J. P., Draugelis, R., & Jones, D. (1986). Comparisons of pre-operative and postoperative MMPI data in chronic back patients. *Spine, 11,* 385–390.

Watson, D. (1982). Neurotic tendencies among chronic pain patients: An MMPI item analysis. *Pain, 14,* 365–385.

Weisenberg, M. (1984). Cognitive aspects of pain. In P. D. Wall & R. Melzack (Eds.), *Textbook of pain* (pp. 162–172). New York: Churchill-Livingstone.

Weisenberg, M. (1987). Psychological intervention for the control of pain. *Behaviour Research and Therapy, 25,* 301–312.

Welsh, G. S. (1956). Factor dimensions A and R. In G. S. Welsh & W. G. Dahlstrom (Eds.), *Basic readings on the MMPI in psychology and medicine* (pp. 264–281). Minneapolis, MN: University of Minnesota Press.

Wilfling, F. J., Klonoff, H., & Kokan, P. (1973). Psychological, demographic, and orthopaedic factors associated with prediction of outcome of spinal fusion. *Clinical Orthopaedics, 90,* 153–160.

Williams, C. L., & Uchiyama, C. L. (in press). Assessment of life events during adolescence: The use of self-report inventories. *Adolescence.*

Wiltse, L. L., & Rocchio, P. D. (1975). Preoperative psychological tests as predictors of success of chemonucleolysis in the treatment of low back syndrome. *Journal of Bone and Joint Surgery, 57,* 478–483.

Yang, J. C., Wagner, J. M., & Clark, W. C. (1983). Psychological distress and mood in chronic pain and surgical patients: A sensory decision theory analysis. In J. J. Bonica, U. Lindblom, & A. Iggo (Eds.), *Advances in pain research and therapy* (Vol. 5, pp. 901–906). New York: Raven.

Zitman, F. G. (1983). Biofeedback and chronic pain. In J. J. Bonica, U. Lindblom, & A. Iggo (Eds.), *Advances in pain research and therapy* (Vol. 5, pp. 795–808). New York: Raven.

Appendix A
Distributions of Chart Review Data for Pain Patients

Chart Item		Men (N = 245)		Women (N = 218)	
Program status	Outpatient	48	(19.7%)	43	(19.7%)
	Inpatient	196	(80.3%)	175	(80.3%)
	Missing data	1	(0.0%)		0
Previous admissions to Sister Kenny	None	237	(96.7%)	215	(98.6%)
	One	8	(3.3%)	3	(1.4%)
Completion status	Completed program	231	(94.3%)	209	(95.9%)
	Left against staff advice	4	(1.6%)	2	(0.9%)
	Discharged early, psych or CD	4	(1.6%)		0
	Discharged early, medical		0	2	(0.9%)
	Discharged early, noncompliant	1	(0.4%)	1	(0.4%)
	Stayed for extra weeks	3	(1.2%)	2	(0.9%)
	No information	2	(0.8%)	2	(0.9%)
Aftercare status	Excused from Aftercare	6	(2.4%)	7	(3.2%)
	No/show for all Aftercare	9	(3.7%)	9	(4.1%)
	Completed up to chart review date but not yet 6 months follow-up	21	(8.6%)	10	(4.6%)
	Partially completed, but no/show for final evaluation	51	(20.8%)	53	(24.3%)
	Completed final PACE evaluation	129	(52.7%)	113	(51.8%)
	Dismissed early, noncompliant	8	(3.3%)	4	(1.8%)
	No information	21	(8.6%)	22	(10.1%)
Date of last follow-up information in chart	Less than six months	150	(61.2%)	139	(63.8%)
	Six months to less than one year	74	(30.2%)	61	(28.0%)
	One year to less than two years	20	(8.2%)	17	(7.8%)
	Two years to less than three years	1	(0.4%)	1	(0.5%)
		Mean = 5.8 mos.		Mean = 5.7 mos.	
		SD = 4.1 mos.		SD = 4.3 mos.	
Area of birth	United States	229	(93.5%)	208	(95.4%)
	Canada	2	(0.8%)		0
	Europe	3	(1.2%)	2	(0.9%)
	Mexico/South America	2	(0.8%)	2	(0.9%)
	Middle East	1	(0.4%)		0
	Africa	1	(0.4%)		0
	No information	7	(2.9%)	6	(2.8%)
Size of birth family (no. of siblings)	Mean		4.4		4.6
	S.D.		3.2		2.8
	Range		0-16		0-15
No. of children	Mean		2.4		2.3
	S.D.		2.1		2.0
	Range		0-15		0-10
Living situation at admission	Living alone	23	(9.4%)	29	(13.3%)
	With family including spouse/S.O.	183	(74.7%)	140	(64.2%)
	With children only (single parent)	8	(3.3%)	30	(13.8%)
	With parents or other relatives only	14	(5.7%)	7	(3.2%)
	With unrelated individual(s) only	11	(4.5%)	9	(4.1%)
	Nursing home or retirement home	4	(1.6%)	1	(0.5%)
	No information	2	(0.8%)	2	(0.9%)

Chart Item		Men (N = 245)		Women (N = 218)	
Current home	Minnesota	180	(73.5%)	145	(66.5%)
	Other Midwestern state	52	(21.2%)	63	(28.9%)
	Non-Midwest U.S.A.	12	(4.9%)	10	(4.6%)
	Canada	1	(0.4%)	0	
Pain complaints	Headache	90	(36.7%)	105	(42.9%)
(can be several)	Orofacial pain: TMJ, eye, ear	8	(3.3%)	21	(9.6%)
	Neck or shoulder pain	122	(49.8%)	117	(53.7%)
	Back pain	225	(91.8%)	193	(88.5%)
	Abdominal/pelvic pain	17	(6.9%)	22	(10.1%)
	Arm or leg pain	197	(80.4%)	169	(77.5%)
	Chest pain	12	(4.9%)	9	(4.1%)
	Hip pain	20	(81.6%)	16	(7.3%)
	Foot pain	6	(2.4%)	3	(1.4%)
	Hand pain	0		6	(2.8%)
	Testicular pain	4	(1.6%)	0	
	Total body pain	4	(1.6%)	8	(3.7%)
No. of pain	Mean		2.9		3.1
complaints (from	S.D.		1.1		1.3
list above)	Range		1-7		1-8
Primary pain	Back pain	179	(73.1%)	146	(66.9%)
complaint	Neck or shoulder pain	35	(14.3%)	41	(18.8%)
	Arm or leg pain	18	(7.3%)	12	(5.5%)
	Abdominal or pelvic pain	7	(2.9%)	4	(1.8%)
	Headache	3	(1.2%)	7	(3.2%)
	Foot pain	3	(1.2%)	2	(0.9%)
	Total body pain	0		2	(0.9%)
	Chest pain	0		1	(0.5%)
	Not specified	0		3	(1.4%)
Length of pain	Mean		4.2		5.1
problem (years)	S.D.		5.3		6.9
	Range		0-44		0-42
Pain onset	Sudden	201	(82.0%)	173	(79.4%)
	Gradual	43	(17.6%)	40	(18.3%)
	No information	1	(0.4%)	5	(2.3%)
Onset owing to	Yes	221	(90.2%)	179	(82.1%)
injury?	No	23	(9.4%)	36	(16.5%)
	No information	1	(0.4%)	3	(1.4%)
Was injury job-	Yes	194	(79.2%)	120	(55.0%)
related?	No or not applicable	50	(20.4%)	95	(43.6%)
	No information	1	(0.4%)	3	(1.4%)
Was injury related	Yes	54	(22.0%)	50	(22.9%)
to an auto	No or not applicable	191	(78.0%)	165	(75.7%)
accident?	No information	0		3	(1.4%)
No. of reinjuries	None	184	(75.1%)	154	(70.6%)
since original onset	One or two	54	(22.0%)	51	(23.4%)
	Three or more	4	(1.6%)	7	(3.2%)
	No information	3	(1.2%)	6	(2.8%)

Chart Item		Men (N = 245)		Women (N = 218)	
Did patient bring	Yes	51	(20.8%)	41	(18.8%)
lawsuit as result	No or not applicable	182	(74.3%)	166	(76.1%)
of injury?	No information	12	(4.9%)	11	(5.0%)
Course since onset	Gradually worsened	168	(68.6%)	153	(70.2%)
	Stayed the same	51	(20.8%)	48	(22.0%)
	Gradually improved	18	(7.3%)	13	(6.0%)
	No information	8	(3.3%)	4	(1.8%)
History of prior	Yes and somewhat incapacitating	49	(20.0%)	42	(19.3%)
pain problems?	Yes but no work/ADL incapacity	51	(20.8%)	49	(22.5%)
	No	131	(53.5%)	118	(54.1%)
	No information	14	(5.7%)	9	(4.1%)
No. of surgeries	None	138	(56.3%)	125	(57.3%)
	One or two	72	(29.4%)	68	(31.2%)
	Three to five	26	(10.6%)	19	(8.7%)
	Six or more	6	(2.4%)	5	(2.3%)
	No information	3	(1.2%)	1	(0.5%)
Other prior	Narcotic analgesics	159	(64.8%)	86	(39.4%)
treatments (can	Non-narcotic medications	221	(90.2%)	199	(91.3%)
be several)	Physical therapy	236	(96.3%)	209	(95.9%)
	Nerve blocks/trigger point injections	98	(40.0%)	98	(45.0%)
	Chymopapain injections	14	(5.7%)	10	(4.6%)
	TENS	139	(56.7%)	112	(51.4%)
	Acupuncture	27	(11.0%)	20	(9.2%)
	Relaxation/hypnosis/imagery	27	(11.0%)	28	(12.8%)
	Biofeedback	28	(11.4%)	29	(13.3%)
	Psychotherapy	59	(24.1%)	56	(25.7%)
	Chiropractor	93	(38.0%)	84	(38.5%)
	Medical hospitalization	117	(47.8%)	119	(54.6%)
	Operant pain program	20	(8.2%)	17	(7.8%)
	Supportive devices (braces, etc.)	113	(46.1%)	96	(44.0%)
No. of prior	Mean	7.1		7.0	
treatments (from	S.D.	2.3		2.1	
list above)	Range	1-13		2-13	
Employment status	Employed full-time	21	(8.6%)	13	(6.0%)
at admission	Employed part-time	19	(7.8%)	39	(17.9%)
	Not employed owing to pain disability	194	(79.2%)	145	(66.5%)
	Not employed owing to lack of jobs	6	(2.4%)	7	(3.2%)
	Retired	3	(1.2%)	7	(3.2%)
	Not employed out of choice	0		5	(2.3%)
	Retired owing to nonpain disability	1	(0.4%)	0	
	No information	1	(0.4%)	2	(0.9%)
Quit or changed	Yes	228	(93.1%)	187	(85.8%)
job or hours	No	16	(6.5%)	25	(11.5%)
owing to pain?	No information	1	(0.4%)	6	(2.8%)

Chart Item		Men (N = 245)		Women (N = 218)	
Years since last	Mean		1.9		1.8
worked	S.D.		2.2		2.6
	Range		0-17		0-20
Disability	Workers' Compensation	181	(73.9%)	111	(50.9%)
compensation	Private insurance	38	(15.5%)	33	(15.1%)
(can be more	Medical assistance	7	(2.9%)	15	(6.9%)
than one)	Social Security Disability Income	25	(10.2%)	18	(8.3%)
	Veterans' Disability Compensation	1	(0.4%)		0
Receiving any	Yes	227	(92.7%)	168	(77.1%)
disability	No or no information	18	(7.3%)	50	(22.9%)
compensation?					
Was litigation still	Yes	48	(19.6%)	39	(17.9%)
pending at	No	188	(76.7%)	173	(79.4%)
admission?	No information	9	(3.7%)	6	(2.8%)
Medical/psychiatric	Physical abuse	22	(9.0%)	67	(30.7%)
history	Sexual abuse	2	(0.8%)	21	(9.6%)
	Depression	144	(58.8%)	139	(63.8%)
	Psychosis	5	(2.0%)	7	(3.2%)
	Psychiatric hospitalization	17	(6.9%)	28	(12.8%)
	Alcohol abuse problem	101	(41.2%)	30	(13.8%)
	Alcohol abuse treatment	52	(21.2%)	16	(7.3%)
	Street drug use problem	24	(9.8%)	8	(3.7%)
	Street drug use treatment	5	(2.0%)	4	(1.8%)
	Prescription drug use problem	59	(24.1%)	45	(20.6%)
	Prescription drug use treatment	5	(2.0%)	12	(5.5%)
	Suicidal ideation	57	(23.3%)	56	(25.7%)
	Suicide attempt(s)	6	(2.4%)	15	(6.9%)
	Assaultiveness or property destruction	16	(6.5%)	3	(1.4%)
	Prison term	5	(2.0%)	1	(0.5%)
	Asthma	10	(4.1%)	15	(6.9%)
	Migraines	8	(3.3%)	39	(17.9%)
	Diabetes	7	(2.9%)	9	(4.1%)
	Hypertension	42	(17.1%)	29	(13.3%)
	Obesity	66	(26.9%)	84	(38.5%)
	Seizure disorder	5	(2.0%)	4	(1.8%)
	Ulcers/chronic g.i. distress	86	(35.1%)	83	(38.1%)
	Sexual dysfunction	35	(14.3%)	67	(30.7%)
Family models of	Mother with noncancer chronic pain	19	(7.8%)	34	(15.6%)
pain	Father with noncancer chronic pain	29	(11.8%)	27	(12.4%)
	Sibling with noncancer chronic pain	32	(13.1%)	31	(14.2%)
	Spouse with noncancer chronic pain	23	(9.4%)	20	(9.2%)
	Mother with cancer pain	16	(6.5%)	15	(6.9%)
	Father with cancer pain	20	(8.2%)	12	(5.5%)
	Sibling with cancer pain	12	(4.9%)	20	(9.2%)
	Spouse with cancer pain	2	(0.8%)	4	(1.8%)
Family models of	Mother	67	(27.3%)	94	(43.1%)
chronic illness or	Father	70	(28.6%)	74	(33.9%)
disability	Sibling(s)	50	(20.4%)	61	(28.0%)
	Spouse or ex-spouse	18	(7.3%)	24	(11.0%)

Chart Item		Men (N = 245)		Women (N = 218)	
Family history of substance abuse	Mother	11	(4.5%)	18	(8.3%)
	Father	66	(26.9%)	61	(28.0%)
	Sibling(s)	56	(22.9%)	114	(52.3%)
	Spouse or ex-spouse	14	(5.7%)	64	(29.4%)
Depression treatment during program	Depression not noted as issue	37	(15.1%)	21	(9.6%)
	Noted but not directly treated	61	(24.9%)	41	(18.8%)
	Specifically addressed, without meds.	38	(15.5%)	45	(20.6%)
	Treated with antidepressant meds.	106	(43.3%)	110	(50.4%)
	No information	3	(1.2%)	1	(0.5%)
Beck depression score at admission	Mean		16.1		18.8
	S.D.		8.8		9.6
	Range		0-53		0-49
Beck depression score at discharge	Mean		8.1		7.6
	S.D.		7.4		7.1
	Range		0-55		0-41
Depression treatment during follow-up	Depression not noted as issue	62	(25.3%)	47	(21.6%)
	Noted but not directly treated	56	(22.9%)	38	(17.4%)
	Specifically addressed, without meds.	12	(4.9%)	23	(10.6%)
	Treated with antidepressant meds.	97	(39.6%)	88	(40.4%)
	No follow-up or no information	18	(7.3%)	22	(10.1%)
At discharge, patient capable of return to previous job?	Yes	139	(56.7%)	152	(69.7%)
	No	94	(38.4%)	51	(23.4%)
	No information	12	(4.9%)	15	(6.9%)
Was returning to work a goal at discharge?	Yes	214	(87.3%)	179	(82.1%)
	No	24	(9.8%)	34	(15.6%)
	No information	7	(2.9%)	5	(2.3%)
Had patient met work goal at 6 month follow-up?	Completely	54	(22.0%)	72	(33.0%)
	Partially	44	(18.0%)	30	(13.8%)
	No	99	(40.4%)	64	(29.4%)
	No information or not applicable	48	(19.6%)	52	(23.9%)
Medication problems at admission	Muscle relaxant dependency/overuse	13	(5.3%)	18	(8.3%)
	Narcotic dependency/overuse	52	(21.2%)	54	(24.8%)
	Anxiolytic/sedative/hypnotic overuse	23	(9.4%)	27	(12.4%)
Rating of treatment compliance during program	Very poor	3	(1.2%)	1	(0.4%)
	Poor	11	(4.5%)	4	(1.8%)
	Fair	49	(20.0%)	32	(14.7%)
	Good	110	(44.9%)	113	(51.8%)
	Very good	68	(27.8%)	66	(30.3%)
	No information	4	(1.6%)	2	(0.9%)
Rating of treatment compliance during follow-up	Very poor	15	(6.1%)	6	(2.8%)
	Poor	31	(12.7%)	12	(5.5%)
	Fair	66	(26.9%)	62	(28.4%)
	Good	68	(27.8%)	77	(35.3%)
	Very good	32	(13.1%)	28	(12.8%)
	No information	33	(13.5%)	33	(15.1%)

Chart Item		Men (N = 245)		Women (N = 218)	
Rating of success	Very poor	10	(4.1%)	6	(2.8%)
in meeting	Poor	35	(14.3%)	11	(5.0%)
exercise goals as	Fair	65	(26.5%)	57	(26.1%)
of last follow-up	Good	81	(33.1%)	96	(44.0%)
	Very good	35	(14.3%)	25	(11.5%)
	No information	19	(7.8%)	23	(10.6%)
Rating of success	Very poor	10	(4.1%)	11	(5.0%)
in meeting	Poor	5	(2.0%)	7	(3.2%)
medication-reduc-	Fair	16	(6.5%)	8	(3.7%)
tion goals as of	Good	30	(12.2%)	24	(11.0%)
last follow-up	Very good	39	(15.9%)	31	(14.2%)
	Not a goal for patient	134	(54.7%)	126	(57.8%)
	No information	11	(4.5%)	11	(5.0%)
Rating of success	Very poor	30	(12.2%)	15	(6.9%)
in meeting	Poor	39	(15.9%)	31	(14.2%)
vocational or	Fair	56	(22.9%)	38	(17.4%)
educational goals	Good	38	(15.5%)	37	(17.0%)
as of last follow-up	Very good	33	(13.5%)	47	(21.6%)
	Not a goal for patient	18	(7.3%)	23	(10.6%)
	No information	31	(12.7%)	27	(12.4%)
Rating of success	Very poor	31	(12.7%)	30	(13.8%)
in meeting weight-	Poor	45	(18.4%)	42	(19.3%)
reduction goals as	Fair	23	(9.4%)	22	(10.1%)
of last follow-up	Good	13	(5.3%)	33	(15.1%)
	Very good	8	(3.3%)	8	(3.7%)
	Not a goal for patient	103	(42.0%)	66	(30.3%)
	No information	22	(9.0%)	17	(7.8%)
Rating of success	Very poor	5	(2.0%)	3	(1.4%)
in meeting	Poor	15	(6.1%)	9	(4.1%)
depression-treat-	Fair	61	(24.9%)	62	(28.4%)
ment goals as of	Good	67	(27.3%)	58	(26.6%)
last follow-up	Very good	5	(2.0%)	8	(3.7%)
	Not a goal for patient	64	(26.1%)	51	(23.3%)
	No information	28	(11.4%)	27	(12.4%)
Rating of	Not a factor	14	(5.7%)	7	(3.2%)
contribution of	Slight contribution	22	(9.0%)	15	(6.9%)
depression to	Moderately important	54	(22.0%)	40	(18.3%)
overall disability	Quite important	110	(44.9%)	109	(50.0%)
at admission	Majority of problem	42	(17.1%)	46	(21.1%)
	No information	3	(1.2%)	1	(0.5%)
Rating of	Not a factor	197	(80.4%)	166	(76.1%)
contribution of	Slight contribution	1	(0.4%)	2	(0.9%)
other psychiatric	Moderately important	9	(3.7%)	7	(3.2%)
disorder to overall	Quite important	8	(3.3%)	17	(7.8%)
disability at	Majority of problem	11	(4.5%)	8	(3.7%)
admission	No information	19	(7.8%)	18	(8.3%)

Chart Item		Men (N = 245)		Women (N = 218)	
Rating of	Not a factor	177	(72.2%)	201	(92.2%)
contribution of	Slight contribution	14	(5.7%)	6	(2.8%)
alcohol abuse to	Moderately important	29	(11.8%)	5	(2.3%)
overall disability	Quite important	14	(5.7%)	2	(0.9%)
at admission	Majority of problem	7	(2.9%)		0
	No information	4	(1.6%)	4	(1.8%)
Rating of	Not a factor	222	(90.6%)	213	(97.7%)
contribution of	Slight contribution	3	(1.2%)	2	(0.9%)
street drug abuse	Moderately important	5	(2.0%)		0
to overall disability	Quite important	6	(2.4%)		0
at admission	Majority of problem	2	(0.8%)		0
	No information	7	(2.9%)	3	(1.4%)
Rating of	Not a factor	173	(70.6%)	150	(68.8%)
contribution of	Slight contribution	8	(3.3%)	14	(6.4%)
narcotic	Moderately important	20	(8.2%)	19	(8.7%)
dependency to	Quite important	26	(10.6%)	20	(9.2%)
overall disability	Majority of problem	14	(5.7%)	13	(6.0%)
at admission	No information	4	(1.6%)	2	(0.9%)
Rating of	Not a factor	210	(85.7%)	187	(85.8%)
contribution of	Slight contribution	9	(3.7%)	5	(2.3%)
anxiolytic/sedative/	Moderately important	8	(3.3%)	7	(3.2%)
hypnotic drug	Quite important	8	(3.3%)	12	(5.5%)
dependency to	Majority of problem	6	(2.4%)	4	(1.8%)
overall disability	No information	4	(1.6%)	3	(1.4%)
at admission					
Rating of	Not a factor	108	(44.1%)	94	(43.1%)
contribution of	Slight contribution	34	(13.9%)	21	(9.6%)
family models or	Moderately important	39	(15.9%)	38	(17.4%)
reinforcement to	Quite important	34	(13.9%)	35	(16.1%)
overall disability	Majority of problem	10	(4.1%)	20	(9.2%)
at admission	No information	20	(8.2%)	10	(4.6%)
Rating of	Not a factor	173	(70.6%)	185	(84.9%)
contribution of lack	Slight contribution	20	(8.2%)	16	(7.3%)
of vocational	Moderately important	32	(13.1%)	11	(5.0%)
marketability to	Quite important	16	(6.5%)	5	(2.3%)
overall disability	Majority of problem	2	(0.8%)		0
at admission	No information	2	(0.8%)	1	(0.5%)
Rating of	Not a factor	211	(86.1%)	205	(94.0%)
contribution of	Slight contribution	17	(6.9%)	7	(3.2%)
intellectual	Moderately important	10	(4.1%)	5	(2.3%)
impairment to	Quite important	2	(0.8%)		0
overall disability	Majority of problem	1	(0.4%)		0
at admission	No information	4	(1.6%)	1	(0.5%)
Rating of	Not a factor	170	(69.4%)	167	(76.6%)
contribution of job	Slight contribution	12	(4.9%)	12	(5.5%)
dissatisfaction or	Moderately important	26	(10.6%)	17	(7.8%)
anger at employer	Quite important	17	(6.9%)	14	(6.4%)
to overall disability	Majority of problem	13	(5.3%)	4	(1.8%)
at admission	No information	7	(2.9%)	4	(1.8%)

Chart Item		Men (N = 245)		Women (N = 218)	
Rating of	Not a factor	150	(61.2%)	163	(74.8%)
contribution of	Slight contribution	24	(9.8%)	15	(6.9%)
financial	Moderately important	34	(13.9%)	20	(9.2%)
reinforcement of	Quite important	20	(8.2%)	11	(5.0%)
disability to overall	Majority of problem	7	(2.9%)	4	(1.8%)
disability at	No information	10	(4.1%)	5	(2.3%)
admission					
Rating of	Not a factor	180	(73.5%)	181	(83.0%)
contribution of	Slight contribution	24	(9.8%)	16	(7.3%)
conscious	Moderately important	21	(8.6%)	9	(4.1%)
malingering to	Quite important	6	(2.4%)	4	(1.8%)
overall disability	Majority of problem	1	(0.4%)	1	(0.5%)
at admission	No information	13	(5.3%)	7	(3.2%)
Rating of	Not a factor	35	(14.2%)	30	(13.8%)
contribution of	Slight contribution	24	(9.8%)	22	(10.1%)
physical	Moderately important	60	(24.5%)	44	(20.3%)
deconditioning or	Quite important	100	(40.8%)	91	(41.7%)
obesity to overall	Majority of problem	24	(9.8%)	30	(13.8%)
disability at	No information	2	(0.8%)	1	(0.5%)
admission					
Rating of	Not a factor	215	(87.8%)	196	(89.9%)
contribution of poor	Slight contribution	17	(6.9%)	12	(5.5%)
advice/education	Moderately important	9	(3.7%)	6	(2.8%)
from the medical	Quite important	1	(0.4%)	3	(1.4%)
system to overall	Majority of problem	0		0	
disability at	No information	3	(1.2%)	1	(0.5%)
admission					
Rating of	Not a factor	153	(62.4%)	77	(35.3%)
contribution of	Slight contribution	20	(8.2%)	13	(6.0%)
nonassertiveness or	Moderately important	31	(12.7%)	48	(22.0%)
"codependency" to	Quite important	25	(10.2%)	48	(22.0%)
overall disability at	Majority of problem	7	(2.9%)	24	(11.0%)
admission	No information	9	(3.7%)	8	(3.7%)
Rating of	Not a factor	0		0	
contribution of all	Slight contribution	5	(2.0%)	1	(0.5%)
"functional"	Moderately important	33	(13.5%)	21	(9.6%)
factors combined	Quite important	113	(46.2%)	115	(52.8%)
to patient's overall	Majority of problem	92	(37.6%)	80	(36.7%)
disability at	No information	2	(0.8%)	1	(0.5%)
admission					

Appendix B
Distributions of Biographical Information Form Data for Pain Patients

Bio. Form Item		Men (N = 257)		Women (N = 223)	
No. of times	Mean		1.1		1.2
married	S.D.		0.8		0.8
	Range		0-5		0-4
Employment	Presently employed	63	(24.5%)	45	(20.2%)
categories	Retired	5	(1.9%)	13	(5.8%)
(can be several)	Student	3	(1.2%)	9	(4.0%)
	Housewife		0	60	(26.9%)
	Self-employed	10	(3.9%)	9	(3.8%)
	Part-time employment	11	(4.3%)	20	(8.5%)
	On leave	19	(7.4%)	29	(13.0%)
	Disabled	156	(60.7%)	103	(46.2%)
	Have never held full-time job	6	(2.3%)	12	(5.4%)
Currently looking	Yes	48	(18.7%)	28	(12.6%)
for work?	No	183	(71.2%)	163	(73.1%)
	No answer	26	(10.1%)	32	(14.3%)
Non-employment	Disability pay	147	(57.2%)	97	(43.5%)
income	Welfare	7	(2.7%)	12	(5.4%)
(can be several)	Pension	7	(2.7%)	6	(2.7%)
	Unemployment compensation	3	(1.2%)	2	(0.9%)
Total family	Under $10,000	43	(16.7%)	63	(28.3%)
income	$10,000 to $14,999	52	(20.2%)	30	(13.5%)
	$15,000 to $24,999	63	(24.5%)	53	(23.8%)
	$25,000 to $34,999	40	(15.6%)	29	(13.0%)
	$35,000 to $44,999	24	(9.3%)	10	(4.5%)
	$45,000 to $64,999	9	(3.5%)	9	(4.0%)
	$65,000 and up		0	5	(2.2%)
	None of above or no answer	26	(10.1%)	24	(10.8%)
Native language	English	244	(94.9%)	212	(95.1%)
	Spanish	2	(0.8%)	1	(0.4%)
	Other	7	(2.7%)	7	(3.1%)
	No answer	4	(1.6%)	3	(1.3%)
Father's education	Mean		10.2		10.4
(years)	S.D.		3.2		3.5
	Range		2-20		1-20
Mother's education	Mean		11.1		10.5
(years)	S.D.		2.6		2.9
	Range		3-18		2-18
Father's occupation	Laborer	76	(29.6%)	67	(30.0%)
	Clerical worker	2	(0.8%)	1	(0.4%)
	Skilled craftsperson	40	(15.6%)	22	(9.9%)
	Manager	19	(7.4%)	16	(7.2%)
	Professional	28	(10.9%)	23	(10.3%)
	None of above or no answer	92	(35.8%)	94	(42.2%)
Mother's	Laborer	40	(15.6%)	47	(21.1%)
occupation	Clerical worker	20	(7.8%)	15	(6.7%)
	Skilled craftsperson	12	(4.7%)	7	(3.1%)

Bio. Form Item		Men (N = 257)		Women (N = 223)	
	Manager	12	(4.7%)	8	(3.6%)
	Professional	21	(8.2%)	23	(10.3%)
	None of above or no answer	152	(59.1%)	123	(55.2%)
Where have lived most of life	City	124	(48.2%)	90	(40.4%)
	Town	50	(19.5%)	58	(26.0%)
	Rural area	79	(30.7%)	69	(30.9%)
	No answer	4	(1.6%)	6	(2.7%)
Ever been given a ticket for speeding?	Yes	203	(79.0%)	99	(44.4%)
	No	49	(19.1%)	121	(54.3%)
	Not answered	5	(1.9%)	3	(1.3%)
Ever been arrested for other than a motor vehicle violation?	Yes	81	(31.5%)	11	(4.9%)
	No	171	(66.5%)	209	(93.7%)
	Not answered	5	(1.9%)	3	(1.3%)
Currently taking any meds. prescribed by a doctor?	Yes	153	(59.5%)	161	(72.2%)
	No	98	(38.1%)	56	(25.1%)
	Not answered	6	(2.3%)	6	(2.7%)
Ever been treated for emotional problems?	Yes	65	(25.3%)	81	(36.3%)
	No	187	(72.8%)	136	(61.0%)
	Not answered	5	(1.9%)	6	(2.7%)
Currently in psychological or psychiatric treatment?	Yes	37	(14.4%)	36	(16.1%)
	No	212	(82.5%)	183	(82.1%)
	Not answered	8	(3.1%)	4	(1.8%)
Ever been hospitalized for emotional problems?	Yes	20	(7.8%)	32	(14.3%)
	No	229	(89.1%)	185	(83.0%)
	Not answered	8	(3.1%)	6	(2.7%)
Ever been in treatment for drug or alcohol problems?	Yes	54	(21.0%)	18	(8.1%)
	No	195	(75.9%)	199	(89.2%)
	Not answered	8	(3.1%)	6	(2.7%)
Had an operation or major physical illness in the last year?	Yes	111	(43.2%)	102	(45.7%)
	No	138	(53.7%)	117	(52.5%)
	Not answered	8	(3.1%)	4	(1.8%)
Have a physical handicap?	Yes	173	(67.3%)	114	(51.1%)
	No	70	(27.2%)	94	(42.2%)
	Not answered	14	(5.4%)	15	(6.7%)
Last time went to a physician	Last week	71	(27.6%)	69	(30.9%)
	2-4 weeks ago	107	(41.6%)	90	(40.4%)
	2-6 months ago	64	(24.9%)	58	(26.0%)
	7-12 months ago	4	(1.6%)	3	(1.3%)
	2-3 years ago	2	(0.8%)	0	
	More than 3 years ago	1	(0.4%)	0	
	No response	8	(3.1%)	3	(1.3%)

Bio. Form Item		Men (N = 257)		Women (N = 223)	
Self-description of alcohol use (choose one)	Have never used alcohol	7	(2.7%)	29	(13.0%)
	Used to drink but do not now	68	(26.4%)	61	(27.4%)
	Drink socially but never to excess	92	(35.8%)	99	(44.4%)
	Sometimes drink to point of feeling "high"	31	(12.1%)	14	(6.3%)
	Usually drink moderately but will often drink more than should	17	(6.6%)	7	(3.1%)
	Often use alcohol to excess	2	(0.8%)	0	
	Have had serious problems	3	(1.2%)	0	
	Consider self an alcoholic	3	(1.2%)	0	
	Have been in alcohol treatment	28	(10.9%)	10	(4.5%)
	No response	6	(2.3%)	3	(1.3%)
Self-description of drug use	Have never used drugs such as marijuana, cocaine, etc.	152	(59.1%)	157	(70.4%)
	Have used such drugs but they are not a problem	66	(25.7%)	49	(22.0%)
	Have had a drug problem	23	(8.9%)	11	(4.9%)
	No response	16	(6.2%)	6	(2.7%)
Family history of treatment for chemical dependency or emotional problems	First-degree* relative, psych treatment	44	(17.1%)	65	(29.1%)
	Second-degree relative, psych treatment	43	(16.7%)	45	(20.2%)
	First-degree relative, CD treatment	72	(28.0%)	71	(31.8%)
	Second-degree relative, CD treatment	43	(16.7%)	37	(16.6%)

*First-degree relatives included parents, siblings, and children. Second-degree relatives included grandparents, aunts or uncles, and nieces or nephews.

Appendix C

Life Events Item-Endorsement Percentages for Pain Sample vs. Normative and Psychiatric Samples

Item	Men			Women		
	Pain N = 257	**Norms** N = 1138	**Psych** N = 166	**Pain** N = 222	**Norms** N = 1462	**Psych** N = 120
1) Death of spouse	0.4%	0.0%	0.0%	0.5%	0.5%	1.7%
2) Divorce	2.3	0.4	4.2	4.1	1.4	5.8
3) Marital separation	5.4	1.5*	8.4	4.1	2.0	11.7
4) Jail term	1.9	0.8	13.9*	0.0	0.3	4.2
5) Death of close family member	12.1	9.6	12.0	14.0	11.6	12.5
6) Personal injury or illness	47.6	13.3*	38.0	51.8	15.9*	40.0
7) Marriage	3.9	2.0	2.4	1.4	2.4	4.2
8) Fired from job	5.8	2.6	17.5*	4.5	1.6	15.8*
9) Got back together after marital separation	1.6	0.7	4.3	2.3	1.0	8.3
10) Retirement	1.6	2.1	1.2	3.2	1.2	0.0
11) Change in health of family member	18.3	12.4	21.7	29.7	18.3*	33.3
12) Pregnancy	1.6	1.1	1.2	0.9	5.8	9.2*
13) Sexual difficulties	42.1	7.8*	27.1	36.4	9.1*	30.0
14) Addition of new member to family	6.6	7.4	7.2	10.8	9.1	12.6
15) Business difficulties or loss	14.0	9.8	27.7*	16.2	7.5*	16.8
16) Change in financial status	49.8	25.6*	48.2	52.0	26.1*	59.2
17) Death of close friend	12.1	8.0	13.9	12.6	8.4	9.2
18) Change to different line of work	14.5	12.8	23.8	10.0	12.7	23.3
19) Change in number of arguments with family members	35.4	10.1*	33.1	33.3	15.2*	40.8
20) Assume high mortgage	3.9	4.4	0.0	5.4	4.6	5.8
21) Unable to pay mortgage or loan	16.7	4.2*	8.4	18.5	4.1*	16.0
22) Change in work responsibilities	30.1	26.1	28.5	26.6	25.4	29.2
23) Son or daughter leaving home	7.0	3.6	3.6	12.2	6.0*	15.8
24) Trouble with in-laws	12.5	3.3*	9.0	6.3	4.7	10.1
25) Outstanding personal achievement	10.4	15.9	21.7	90.5	14.8	16.7
26) Wife or husband begins or stops work	12.5	10.4	6.1	13.1	9.9	7.6
27) Begin or end school	5.5	11.0	15.7*	5.9	12.4	16.0
28) Change in living conditions	29.7	17.5*	60.8*	30.2	19.0*	61.7*
29) Change in personal habits	44.9	15.4*	46.4	42.5	21.4*	47.5
30) Trouble with boss	9.7	9.9	15.7	9.0	8.8	16.7
31) Change in work hours or conditions	26.5	26.3	35.2	29.1	29.2	34.2

*Significantly different from pain sample for same sex. A chi-square was considered significant at $p < = .0012$, equivalent to an overall alpha of $< = .05$ across 41 comparisons (Bonferroni criterion; Grove & Andreasen, 1982).

Item	Men			Women		
	Pain N = 257	**Norms** N = 1138	**Psych** N = 166	**Pain** N = 222	**Norms** N = 1462	**Psych** N = 120
32) Change in residence	14.0	15.1	54.2*	18.9	14.4	50.0*
33) Change in schools	1.6	3.7	6.0	0.9	3.3	8.3*
34) Change in recreation	44.4	15.9*	34.3	48.4	17.7*	37.5
35) Change in church activities	12.5	9.0	21.1	17.6	12.8	31.7
36) Change in social activities	45.5	16.6*	47.0	48.6	20.3*	40.0
37) Take out small loan	23.7	21.6	12.0	19.8	18.8	9.2
38) Change in sleeping habits	64.7	15.9*	62.4	63.8	20.8*	69.2
39) Change in number of family outings or holidays	34.0	12.3*	23.6	38.7	16.1*	30.8
40) Change in eating habits	46.9	18.9*	54.2	55.9	29.4*	65.8
41) Minor violations of the law	7.0	8.8	27.1*	3.6	3.6	16.7*

Appendix D

Chronic Pain Sample
Supplementary Scale
Statistics

Scale	Men (N = 268)					Women (N = 234)				
	Mean	SD	Median	Min	Max	Mean	SD	Median	Min	Max
Supplementary Scales										
Do	41.9	9.4	41	30	65	44.7	10.4	46	30	77
Re	42.7	9.3	42	30	73	48.2	9.5	50	30	71
Mt	63.5	12.8	64	37	91	62.6	11.2	62	38	87
O-H	50.3	10.1	48	30	76	49.7	10.2	52	30	77
Harris-Lingoes Subscales										
D1	65.6	14.6	64	37	108	64.2	13.4	63	37	96
D2	55.4	11.3	54	30	87	55.5	11.2	57	30	84
D3	71.3	11.5	75	43	100	70.1	11.4	70	41	100
D4	65.4	14.9	62	38	110	66.2	13.8	66	43	106
D5	59.4	13.2	57	40	96	59.1	12.2	58	37	89
Hy1	49.3	10.3	51	30	61	50.7	9.8	51	30	61
Hy2	49.8	9.9	51	30	71	52.5	10.4	55	30	71
Hy3	78.5	13.9	79	43	106	75.1	11.4	75	51	99
Hy4	70.3	16.3	67	43	115	67.6	14.2	65	41	101
Hy5	48.4	10.1	48	30	78	51.9	10.0	54	30	77
Pd1	53.4	11.4	51	38	84	52.8	11.6	50	38	92
Pd2	54.6	10.3	53	30	80	51.4	9.5	53	30	84
Pd3	49.8	10.5	51	30	63	50.5	9.9	52	30	64
Pd4	56.3	12.5	56	35	98	54.8	11.1	54	33	91
Pd5	59.0	12.7	58	34	91	57.9	11.9	58	34	87
Pa1	58.1	15.0	52	40	120	54.2	11.8	51	39	99
Pa2	54.3	11.8	55	34	82	52.6	11.0	53	34	84
Pa3	49.2	10.1	51	30	70	51.7	10.0	55	30	69
Sc1	52.7	12.9	51	39	105	51.4	10.5	50	38	84
Sc2	59.4	15.2	59	40	117	57.4	12.9	58	40	113
Sc3	56.3	14.5	54	42	103	57.9	14.2	55	43	104
Sc4	59.9	15.4	55	39	103	60.0	14.1	59	39	95
Sc5	55.0	11.9	54	40	117	53.4	10.2	53	40	97
Sc6	65.8	14.5	65	41	120	64.1	14.9	63	41	118
Ma1	51.0	10.4	50	35	81	48.4	9.3	45	37	87
Ma2	52.7	9.8	53	30	78	52.5	10.5	50	30	80
Ma3	48.3	10.1	47	30	77	49.3	10.5	50	30	75
Ma4	51.4	10.8	50	30	76	49.1	10.5	49	31	80
New Validity Scales										
FB	59.5	16.6	55	42	120	57.5	15.1	54	42	112
TRIN	50.9	10.9	50	30	86	49.6	10.8	50	30	80
VRIN	51.6	10.0	52	31	86	51.0	9.7	52	30	79

All values are linear T scores. See MMPI-2 manual (Butcher et al., 1989) for further discussion of these scales.

Appendix E

Comparison of Mean
Clinical and Content-
Scale MMPI-2
Profiles, Pain vs.
Psychiatric Samples

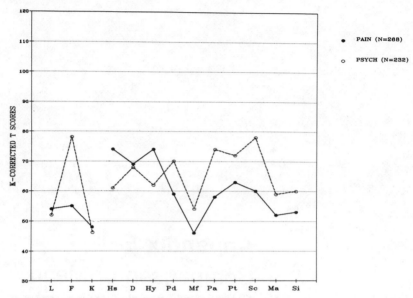

MMPI-2 Mean Profile, Pain vs. Psychiatric Sample Men

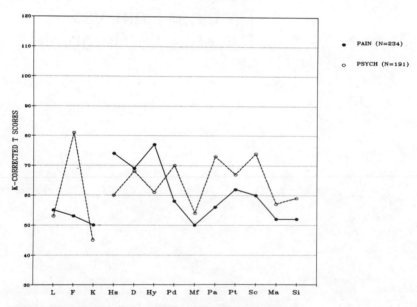

MMPI-2 Mean Profile, Pain vs. Psychiatric Sample Women

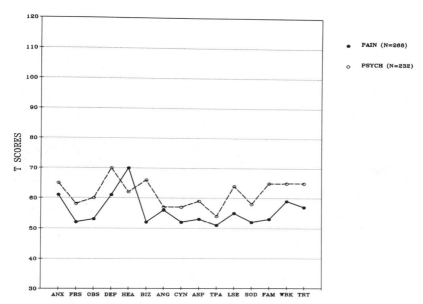

Content Scale Mean Profile, Pain vs. Psychiatric Sample Men

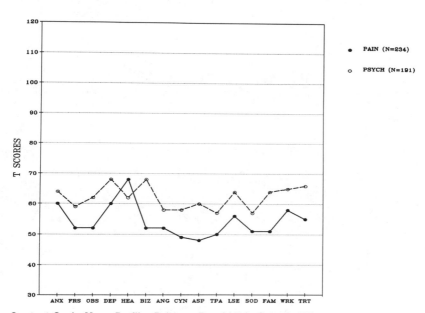

Content Scale Mean Profile, Pain vs. Psychiatric Sample Women

Appendix F
MMPI-2 Item-
Endorsement
Percentages for Men

Item No.	Normative Sample N	%T	Psychiatric Sample N	%T	Chronic Pain Sample N	%T
1.	1136	56.8	231	50.6	267	67.8
2.	1138	95.8*	232	83.6	267	82.0
3.	1137	68.5*	232	47.8*	268	16.0
4.	1136	20.4*	230	27.8*	267	8.6
5.	1137	41.4*	232	58.2	267	68.9
6.	1131	92.8	229	77.3*	268	92.9
7.	1138	48.9	232	40.9	268	42.5
8.	1137	87.0*	232	84.1*	268	65.7
9.	1137	85.6*	232	45.3	268	41.4
10.	1137	84.7*	232	60.3*	268	3.4
11.	1136	3.5*	232	18.5	268	14.2
12.	1135	73.3*	231	48.5	267	46.8
13.	1128	27.0	232	42.2	266	29.3
14.	1137	64.2	232	55.2	268	63.4
15.	1137	37.0	230	47.0	267	41.2
16.	1136	45.0	232	60.8	268	43.7
17.	1136	5.2*	229	39.7*	266	18.4
18.	1137	1.1*	232	14.2	268	7.8
19.	1126	37.9*	232	45.7*	268	21.3
20.	1137	87.5*	227	72.2	265	75.8
21.	1135	31.9	231	68.4*	267	38.2
22.	1138	8.8*	230	45.7*	268	21.3
23.	1135	5.6	232	35.8*	268	11.2
24.	1138	3.9	232	22.0*	268	3.4
25.	1138	41.6	232	44.8	268	28.7
26.	1136	47.2	232	52.6	267	47.6
27.	1136	26.7	231	41.6	268	31.0
28.	1137	8.1*	232	25.0	268	28.0
29.	1138	83.6	231	80.5	268	84.0
30.	1138	6.0*	232	33.2	268	19.0
31.	1138	13.3*	232	44.0	268	39.2
32.	1136	23.8	232	54.7*	266	27.8
33.	1138	62.9*	232	55.6*	268	27.6
34.	1136	80.7	232	72.4*	268	87.3
35.	1137	58.0	231	71.9	268	63.4
36.	1138	8.1	232	19.0	268	12.3
37.	1138	39.4	232	54.7	268	48.1
38.	1138	25.0*	231	67.1	268	50.7
39.	1137	11.4*	230	43.5*	267	65.5
40.	1138	3.3*	230	22.6	268	26.1
41.	1137	63.0*	231	65.4*	268	46.6
42.	1135	4.1	231	33.3*	268	6.0
43.	1135	79.0*	231	43.7	268	39.9
44.	1137	2.4*	232	24.6	268	19.0
45.	1138	86.9*	231	72.3*	268	14.9

*Significantly different from pain sample at $p < .0001$; equivalent to overall alpha of .05 for 567 comparisons.

Item No.	Normative Sample		Psychiatric Sample		Chronic Pain Sample	
	N	%T	N	%T	N	%T
46.	1137	18.8	232	41.4*	267	19.5
47.	1137	81.5*	232	63.4	268	66.4
48.	1137	11.7	231	39.0*	268	11.6
49.	1138	66.8	232	49.6	268	61.9
50.	1135	55.9	232	65.9	268	66.0
51.	1138	93.6	232	94.4	267	94.0
52.	1134	17.2*	231	60.6*	268	31.7
53.	1138	18.8*	232	46.6*	268	83.6
54.	1133	6.5	231	29.9*	267	9.4
55.	1137	43.6	231	51.5	268	39.6
56.	1131	31.5*	232	73.3	267	61.8
57.	1137	73.4*	232	67.2*	267	23.6
58.	1138	60.9	231	53.7	268	54.5
59.	1138	6.7*	232	29.7	268	22.4
60.	1138	2.5	231	21.2*	268	4.9
61.	1135	70.0	232	60.8	266	72.9
62.	1135	4.7	230	11.7	267	3.4
63.	1137	54.2	232	34.5	268	50.4
64.	1136	21.5	232	31.5	268	20.5
65.	1138	5.9*	231	49.4	268	31.3
66.	1135	4.6	232	12.5	268	6.0
67.	1135	51.3	232	56.0	267	39.0
68.	1138	27.8	232	31.0	268	34.7
69.	1137	62.0	232	63.4	268	71.6
70.	1134	18.7	230	40.4*	268	18.7
71.	1130	30.7*	232	59.9	268	57.5
72.	1136	4.3	231	16.9*	267	4.1
73.	1138	17.1*	232	57.3	268	41.4
74.	1138	11.9	232	23.7	268	13.1
75.	1138	94.8	231	68.8*	268	90.3
76.	1133	40.7	230	53.5	267	38.2
77.	1138	93.4	229	85.6	268	87.7
78.	1137	95.0	232	81.5	268	92.5
79.	1134	41.9	232	30.6	268	35.8
80.	1138	7.2	232	20.7	268	8.6
81.	1133	51.5	232	60.8	267	49.1
82.	1138	18.5	232	51.7*	267	27.7
83.	1136	78.8	231	58.9	268	70.9
84.	1138	17.3*	231	51.5	268	34.3
85.	1138	18.5	231	45.0*	268	20.9
86.	1135	45.2*	231	45.9	268	28.4
87.	1134	49.7	231	69.3	268	55.6
88.	1133	89.7	232	86.6	268	88.8
89.	1136	68.8	231	68.0	268	67.2
90.	1133	91.8	229	82.1	268	93.3
91.	1138	89.2*	230	72.6*	267	30.3
92.	1137	5.5	232	30.6*	267	12.4
93.	1138	86.5	231	83.5	268	92.2
94.	1138	4.8*	231	36.8*	268	13.1
95.	1136	89.4*	232	47.4	268	59.7

	Normative Sample		Psychiatric Sample		Chronic Pain Sample	
Item No.	N	%T	N	%T	N	%T
96.	1137	9.1	232	18.1	268	10.8
97.	1135	11.0*	228	31.1	267	21.7
98.	1137	36.9	232	51.7*	268	32.8
99.	1136	5.0	231	25.5*	268	9.0
100.	1137	27.6	232	38.4	268	25.0
101.	1138	3.4*	232	26.7	268	23.1
102.	1138	96.4	232	91.4	268	97.8
103.	1133	33.4	232	39.7	268	42.2
104.	1135	41.0	232	49.6	267	40.8
105.	1136	30.9*	232	62.5	268	51.9
106.	1136	81.9	230	68.3	268	78.4
107.	1138	66.6	232	56.9	268	57.8
108.	1138	90.6	232	86.6	268	96.6
109.	1138	94.3*	232	77.2	268	79.9
110.	1136	57.7	230	67.0	267	59.2
111.	1137	6.1*	232	15.1	267	18.7
112.	1137	57.7*	231	51.9	265	37.0
113.	1132	62.1	232	70.3	267	59.2
114.	1138	2.5	232	10.3	268	2.6
115.	1138	72.6	231	65.4	268	74.6
116.	1136	29.6*	232	44.4	268	44.8
117.	1138	82.9	232	65.1	268	73.5
118.	1138	63.4*	231	54.1	268	46.3
119.	1138	43.4	232	47.4	268	41.8
120.	1138	71.8	232	64.7	268	73.9
121.	1134	63.1	230	63.0	267	73.8
122.	1135	80.7	232	72.4	268	71.3
123.	1138	41.4	232	44.8	267	31.1
124.	1138	29.2	232	53.4*	268	34.7
125.	1138	89.2*	232	44.8*	268	78.4
126.	1134	96.6	231	90.5*	267	98.9
127.	1136	36.2	232	55.2	266	39.5
128.	1138	65.7	232	72.4	268	73.1
129.	1137	30.4	232	44.0*	268	22.8
130.	1138	34.3*	232	68.5	268	72.4
131.	1134	46.6	231	55.4	268	48.9
132.	1123	69.6	229	72.1	265	78.9
133.	1136	16.6	230	31.3	268	20.9
134.	1137	16.0	232	28.4	268	23.1
135.	1138	31.5	232	56.0	268	41.8
136.	1136	38.8	231	51.1	268	36.6
137.	1137	20.8*	231	32.9*	268	6.7
138.	1138	2.4	231	26.0*	268	7.1
139.	1135	93.4*	230	87.4	268	85.4
140.	1138	77.4*	232	48.7	268	36.9
141.	1138	94.3*	231	67.5*	268	43.3
142.	1138	92.8	232	68.5*	267	85.8
143.	1138	73.4*	231	56.3	267	46.4
144.	1138	1.3*	232	21.1*	268	5.6
145.	1136	9.1*	231	39.8*	268	19.8

Item No.	Normative Sample		Psychiatric Sample		Chronic Pain Sample	
	N	%T	N	%T	N	%T
146.	1138	12.9	232	30.2	268	20.5
147.	1137	15.4*	232	35.8	268	29.5
148.	1138	44.8*	232	28.9*	268	1.5
149.	1138	8.1*	232	26.7	268	22.8
150.	1136	6.1	231	34.6*	268	7.1
151.	1137	46.2	231	61.5*	268	38.4
152.	1136	70.6*	231	56.7*	268	25.7
153.	1135	49.8*	232	51.3*	268	32.1
154.	1137	42.3	230	46.5	268	47.0
155.	1138	30.4	232	37.9	268	27.6
156.	1138	6.5	231	27.7	268	13.4
157.	1148	40.8	231	41.1	268	42.5
158.	1130	52.0	231	60.6	268	52.2
159.	1137	73.0	231	56.3	268	67.9
160.	1138	78.5*	229	59.4	267	54.7
161.	1138	31.8	232	51.3	268	37.3
162.	1138	0.8	232	11.2*	268	0.7
163.	1137	70.8	231	71.9	268	64.6
164.	1136	90.8*	231	65.4	268	70.1
165.	1136	90.3*	232	67.2	268	75.7
166.	1136	15.1*	232	37.9	267	30.7
167.	1135	39.4	231	59.3	266	44.4
168.	1136	9.2	232	44.0*	268	14.6
169.	1136	43.4	232	52.6	268	52.2
170.	1138	7.1*	232	45.3*	268	16.0
171.	1135	42.3	232	38.4	268	48.1
172.	1138	9.2*	232	33.2	268	29.5
173.	1138	62.6*	232	53.9	267	40.1
174.	1138	89.5	231	81.8	268	85.8
175.	1137	4.2*	232	27.2	267	41.6
176.	1137	85.4*	232	69.8*	267	50.6
177.	1138	91.0*	232	75.4	267	73.4
178.	1136	24.3	232	38.8	268	32.5
179.	1136	92.9*	232	79.7*	268	49.6
180.	1138	4.6	229	43.2*	268	7.8
181.	1136	76.8	232	76.7	268	81.7
182.	1136	3.2*	232	28.9*	268	11.2
183.	1137	87.9	232	78.9	268	85.8
184.	1137	50.2	231	47.2	268	63.8
185.	1137	43.0	232	61.2*	268	42.2
186.	1138	94.1	232	83.6	268	94.0
187.	1137	25.9	232	34.1*	268	14.9
188.	1137	84.5	232	72.8	268	78.0
189.	1137	60.4	232	58.6	267	56.2
190.	1135	4.1	231	32.5*	268	6.0
191.	1138	35.3*	232	39.2*	268	18.3
192.	1137	97.6	230	85.2	268	95.9
193.	1138	7.2	232	16.4	268	9.0
194.	1138	50.2	231	42.9	268	51.1
195.	1137	8.5	231	46.3*	267	12.4

	Normative Sample		Psychiatric Sample		Chronic Pain Sample	
Item No.	N	%T	N	%T	N	%T
196.	1136	48.3*	230	66.1	268	66.4
197.	1137	51.2	231	48.9	268	58.2
198.	1138	1.7	231	21.6*	268	3.7
199.	1134	86.7*	232	76.3	268	70.9
200.	1136	45.0	231	39.8	268	36.2
201.	1137	23.7*	232	39.7*	268	61.2
202.	1136	19.1*	231	54.4*	268	31.3
203.	1138	80.2	231	71.0	268	79.1
204.	1137	81.4	232	84.9	268	74.3
205.	1137	48.5	230	55.2	268	45.1
206.	1137	78.0	231	69.3	268	80.2
207.	1137	31.9	232	43.5	268	35.1
208.	1135	70.0*	232	59.9	267	52.1
209.	1135	56.9	228	48.2	267	50.6
210.	1137	97.8	232	87.1	268	95.5
211.	1126	28.0	229	32.3	262	35.5
212.	1131	31.0	230	40.4	267	24.7
213.	1138	40.5	231	44.6	268	47.0
214.	1136	73.2	231	67.5	267	77.2
215.	1134	14.6	229	43.2*	265	24.9
216.	1137	2.6	231	14.3*	268	1.5
217.	1123	56.2	228	45.6	268	46.3
218.	1132	30.1*	231	59.7	268	72.4
219.	1134	51.3	231	70.6*	268	49.3
220.	1135	25.0	232	26.7	268	24.3
221.	1138	28.0	232	47.8*	268	29.5
222.	1133	89.2*	228	73.2	267	71.2
223.	1138	84.4*	231	55.0	268	68.3
224.	1137	81.8*	232	63.4*	267	3.4
225.	1137	33.7	231	60.6*	268	41.0
226.	1138	37.0	230	43.0	268	31.7
227.	1134	39.9*	230	60.4	268	57.8
228.	1135	3.8	227	14.5*	268	3.4
229.	1138	7.5	232	37.5*	268	15.3
230.	1137	73.5	232	59.1	268	66.4
231.	1137	30.8	232	25.4	268	34.0
232.	1137	70.3*	227	38.8	268	51.5
233.	1135	35.2	231	54.4	268	40.3
234.	1137	2.9*	231	26.4*	267	11.2
235.	1135	17.7*	230	44.3	268	41.4
236.	1136	30.8	232	42.7	268	31.3
237.	1136	77.6	232	60.3	268	75.0
238.	1137	25.9	232	32.3	267	35.2
239.	1136	42.0	232	33.6	268	41.8
240.	1138	6.6	232	19.0*	268	4.1
241.	1135	19.7	232	4.4*	267	26.2
242.	1137	34.7	232	39.7	268	36.9
243.	1137	32.4	232	57.3	268	41.4
244.	1135	67.0	232	51.3	267	57.3
245.	1135	31.6	232	37.5	268	36.9

Item No.	Normative Sample		Psychiatric Sample		Chronic Pain Sample	
	N	%T	N	%T	N	%T
246.	1135	3.3	232	19.0*	267	4.5
247.	1136	9.5*	232	21.1*	267	64.8
248.	1137	14.2	231	27.7	268	16.8
249.	1137	58.6	232	65.1	268	54.9
250.	1136	42.2	230	47.8	268	37.3
251.	1136	23.8	231	60.6*	268	33.6
252.	1138	1.4	232	12.5*	268	1.9
253.	1136	12.5	232	22.0	268	11.9
254.	1134	23.8	231	47.2	268	31.3
255.	1138	78.3*	232	72.0	268	60.4
256.	1138	31.8	231	50.6*	267	29.2
257.	1137	52.2	232	42.7	268	60.8
258.	1138	2.4*	231	20.3	268	14.2
259.	1136	18.4*	232	50.0	268	32.1
260.	1138	95.8	231	88.3	268	95.9
261.	1122	56.4*	231	40.7	268	41.8
262.	1138	78.3	232	63.4	268	73.5
263.	1136	72.5	230	55.2*	267	73.4
264.	1138	44.5	232	59.5	268	43.7
265.	1138	33.9	231	55.8*	268	35.4
266.	1137	59.1*	231	28.6	268	40.3
267.	1138	63.9	231	55.4	268	55.6
268.	1131	21.0	230	43.0*	267	18.7
269.	1132	27.6	230	47.4*	268	23.9
270.	1137	6.3	231	11.3	267	9.4
271.	1135	39.4	229	60.3	265	41.9
272.	1135	63.2	231	60.6	268	64.9
273.	1137	16.0*	232	56.0*	267	36.7
274.	1138	21.3	232	48.7*	268	25.7
275.	1138	53.2*	232	69.4	268	70.5
276.	1135	96.3	228	85.1*	267	96.6
277.	1137	17.5	231	57.6*	268	23.1
278.	1138	87.3	232	72.4	265	86.0
279.	1136	48.3	232	50.0	268	43.3
280.	1137	79.8	232	59.5*	268	81.3
281.	1138	5.4	230	21.3	267	9.4
282.	1136	4.8	231	16.9	268	7.5
283.	1136	37.9	228	55.3	266	49.2
284.	1137	53.8	232	60.3	268	48.9
285.	1135	40.7	231	63.2*	268	40.7
286.	1133	32.8	231	45.9	268	45.9
287.	1136	34.0*	232	32.8	267	18.4
288.	1136	10.6	231	49.4*	268	13.1
289.	1137	28.9	232	48.3	268	41.0
290.	1136	55.4*	232	62.1	267	70.8
291.	1137	3.6	232	16.4*	267	3.7
292.	1138	25.9	232	45.3	268	27.6
293.	1138	26.3	232	27.6	268	30.6
294.	1135	2.1	232	12.5	267	4.1
295.	1133	85.5*	229	70.7*	267	26.6

	Normative Sample		Psychiatric Sample		Chronic Pain Sample	
Item No.	N	%T	N	%T	N	%T
296.	1138	11.2*	232	39.7*	268	20.9
297.	1134	57.0	231	68.8	268	66.0
298.	1136	12.7	232	32.3	268	19.8
299.	1138	14.9*	232	47.0*	268	28.7
300.	1137	7.1	231	35.5*	268	8.6
301.	1138	14.8	230	52.6*	266	24.1
302.	1137	40.0	232	47.8	268	46.6
303.	1138	1.6	232	27.2*	267	4.9
304.	1137	48.3	232	61.2	268	58.2
305.	1138	29.3*	230	70.0	268	70.1
306.	1138	13.0	232	33.2*	268	12.3
307.	1137	8.9	232	28.4*	268	7.8
308.	1137	17.1	232	33.2	268	22.4
309.	1137	28.5	232	52.6	268	36.9
310.	1138	9.4	232	36.6*	268	11.2
311.	1138	8.3	230	36.5*	268	11.9
312.	1137	4.2	232	20.7*	267	6.7
313.	1136	19.5	232	28.4	268	16.4
314.	1138	88.4	232	68.5	268	82.8
315.	1138	48.2	229	63.8	268	50.4
316.	1137	14.9	232	44.0*	268	15.3
317.	1138	5.5*	231	25.1	268	15.3
318.	1138	94.6	230	77.8*	268	92.5
319.	1138	3.8	231	21.2*	268	4.5
320.	1138	13.9	231	39.8*	268	14.6
321.	1138	72.4	232	52.2	268	66.0
322.	1138	2.8	231	13.9*	268	2.2
323.	1137	4.8	231	17.3*	268	4.5
324.	1137	7.7	231	22.5*	267	9.0
325.	1138	18.9*	231	50.2	268	38.4
326.	1137	26.4	231	56.3*	268	31.7
327.	1138	9.5	231	29.0	268	14.2
328.	1138	23.4	230	46.1	268	32.1
329.	1138	1.6	230	28.3*	268	3.0
330.	1136	91.2*	232	75.9	266	69.9
331.	1137	30.7	232	61.2*	268	41.0
332.	1138	4.7	232	19.8*	268	5.2
333.	1138	6.2*	231	38.5*	268	14.6
334.	1138	2.5*	231	24.7	268	17.5
335.	1137	70.4	231	49.8	267	59.9
336.	1136	1.6	231	13.4*	268	2.2
337.	1138	42.1	232	60.3*	268	36.6
338.	1136	33.6	232	54.3	268	37.3
339.	1137	37.3*	231	71.9	268	57.5
340.	1138	38.2	232	47.0	268	45.9
341.	1138	64.8	232	62.9	268	66.4
342.	1136	51.7	232	40.9*	268	65.3
343.	1134	89.5	231	82.3	268	93.3
344.	1138	56.6	232	53.0	268	62.3
345.	1131	61.9	230	60.0	268	64.2

Item No.	Normative Sample		Psychiatric Sample		Chronic Pain Sample	
	N	%T	N	%T	N	%T
346.	1138	68.5	231	63.6	268	75.0
347.	1137	21.0	232	44.8*	268	25.0
348.	1137	23.4	231	42.0	268	26.9
349.	1138	8.0	230	25.7*	268	7.1
350.	1137	68.9	232	60.3	268	67.2
351.	1137	14.6	232	28.9*	268	11.9
352.	1136	72.5	232	70.7	268	73.5
353.	1136	72.6	232	61.6	268	66.0
354.	1138	81.6	232	71.6	268	80.6
355.	1138	1.2	232	21.6*	268	1.9
356.	1137	36.5*	230	49.1	268	56.3
357.	1136	49.1	230	67.4	265	59.6
358.	1138	20.4	232	39.7	268	28.7
359.	1137	60.2	230	58.3	268	58.6
360.	1137	85.5	232	72.0	268	83.6
361.	1138	4.3	231	33.3*	268	6.7
362.	1137	59.2	231	68.4	268	54.1
363.	1134	71.7	232	56.5	268	68.3
364.	1137	13.9	232	44.0*	268	18.7
365.	1138	76.0	230	71.7	268	81.7
366.	1137	15.3	232	40.5*	268	20.5
367.	1136	29.7	232	55.2	267	40.4
368.	1137	18.5	230	42.6*	267	19.9
369.	1134	33.5	230	53.9*	267	31.8
370.	1137	70.9	232	60.3	268	63.8
371.	1138	4.2	232	13.8*	268	2.6
372.	1137	68.9	232	62.1	267	59.6
373.	1133	51.8	232	50.9	268	38.8
374.	1138	42.9	232	57.8	268	47.4
375.	1136	30.8*	230	60.9	266	48.9
376.	1138	8.7*	231	38.5	268	29.9
377.	1137	25.1*	232	61.6	262	72.6
378.	1134	32.9	232	52.6	268	44.0
379.	1136	14.3	232	38.4*	268	19.8
380.	1137	15.7	232	31.5	268	17.2
381.	1136	8.9	230	28.3	268	13.8
382.	1137	22.7	232	47.0	268	33.2
383.	1137	89.8	229	58.1*	268	86.6
384.	1128	42.9*	229	45.0	267	27.3
385.	1136	69.0	230	62.6	268	61.9
386.	1138	39.0*	232	63.4	268	54.9
387.	1137	4.7	231	17.7*	268	4.5
388.	1136	75.0*	231	39.0	267	49.4
389.	1138	16.9*	231	33.8	268	38.1
390.	1133	36.4	231	61.0	268	44.0
391.	1137	35.2	232	52.6	268	39.2
392.	1138	17.0	232	28.4	268	23.5
393.	1136	29.4	232	35.3	268	27.2
394.	1138	18.9*	232	55.6	268	45.9
395.	1138	6.0	232	19.4*	268	4.9

	Normative Sample		Psychiatric Sample		Chronic Pain Sample	
Item No.	N	%T	N	%T	N	%T
396.	1136	39.5	229	53.3	267	50.2
397.	1137	10.0	232	18.1	268	15.7
398.	1136	50.3	232	48.3	268	54.5
399.	1138	11.5*	232	41.8	268	25.7
400.	1137	16.4	231	43.7	268	26.1
401.	1138	67.3	231	74.0	268	68.3
402.	1138	40.2	232	48.7	268	36.9
403.	1135	39.8	230	56.1	268	50.7
404.	1136	95.2	232	85.8	268	91.0
405.	1137	86.8*	231	63.6	268	70.1
406.	1132	45.9	229	48.9	268	47.0
407.	1134	10.7	230	24.3	268	15.7
408.	1134	26.9	232	57.3*	266	38.0
409.	1137	38.9*	231	60.6	268	54.1
410.	1136	39.7	232	40.5	268	38.1
411.	1138	19.5*	232	59.9*	268	34.0
412.	1137	15.8*	231	45.9	268	36.6
413.	1138	29.5	231	48.5	268	35.8
414.	1138	51.2	232	59.9	268	60.1
415.	1136	27.4*	232	60.3*	267	41.6
416.	1133	60.3*	232	40.9	268	42.2
417.	1137	32.5	232	44.8	268	44.8
418.	1134	45.1	231	60.6	268	53.7
419.	1137	52.6	232	54.7	268	47.0
420.	1138	46.1	232	59.5	268	56.7
421.	1137	20.1	231	47.2*	268	25.0
422.	1137	84.2	231	84.8	266	91.0
423.	1135	45.6	232	48.3	268	38.4
424.	1135	10.3	232	43.1*	267	13.5
425.	1136	36.3	230	48.7	267	46.4
426.	1136	44.0	232	46.6	268	38.1
427.	1137	83.0	232	61.2*	268	82.8
428.	1136	56.8	232	72.8	268	65.7
429.	1136	70.2	232	56.5*	267	79.0
430.	1136	37.6*	232	49.1*	268	70.5
431.	1137	8.5*	232	31.5	268	23.9
432.	1138	20.7	232	28.0*	268	11.6
433.	1134	55.1*	231	55.8	266	39.5
434.	1126	36.8*	232	46.6	268	50.7
435.	1135	7.0	232	16.8	268	6.3
436.	1131	36.5	230	42.6	268	31.3
437.	1136	63.1	232	62.5	267	67.0
438.	1137	31.2	231	41.1	268	42.9
439.	1136	42.6	230	50.4	266	41.7
440.	1135	74.4	232	70.7	268	72.4
441.	1137	10.9	232	29.3*	268	13.1
442.	1136	60.7	231	70.6	268	59.7
443.	1129	32.2	229	44.5	265	41.1
444.	1135	21.9*	232	50.0	268	42.2
445.	1133	38.7*	229	56.3	268	57.5

	Normative Sample		Psychiatric Sample		Chronic Pain Sample	
Item No.	N	%T	N	%T	N	%T
446.	1138	33.7	231	57.1*	267	25.8
447.	1138	10.6	230	18.7	268	13.1
448.	1136	18.4	232	39.2*	268	11.9
449.	1138	62.4	231	72.3	268	71.6
450.	1136	2.1	232	18.1*	268	4.5
451.	1133	12.1	232	25.4	267	15.0
452.	1137	68.6	230	65.2	268	77.6
453.	1137	65.0	232	58.6	268	69.8
454.	1136	4.8*	232	35.3*	268	16.8
455.	1134	83.3	231	68.4	268	83.2
456.	1137	57.6	232	65.9	268	55.2
457.	1137	14.6	232	35.8*	268	13.8
458.	1138	45.4	232	50.9	268	49.6
459.	1134	83.2	231	74.5	267	76.4
460.	1133	63.9	232	68.5	268	73.5
461.	1136	57.6	231	67.5	268	60.8
462.	1138	86.5	231	77.5	268	88.1
463.	1138	4.4	231	38.1*	268	10.4
464.	1138	24.5*	231	48.5	268	63.1
465.	1138	58.4	231	54.5	268	57.5
466.	1137	31.9	231	47.2	268	39.6
467.	1137	80.5*	232	68.5	268	61.9
468.	1137	2.8	231	18.2*	268	3.4
469.	1136	14.8*	230	58.7	268	44.0
470.	1129	32.2*	230	48.7	266	47.4
471.	1136	7.3	231	26.4*	268	9.0
472.	1135	32.1	232	44.4	268	42.9
473.	1127	50.6	232	61.2	265	52.8
474.	1135	89.6	230	73.9*	268	91.4
475.	1135	15.4*	232	43.1	268	28.7
476.	1136	3.8*	232	17.2	267	11.2
477.	1136	42.9	232	52.6	267	40.8
478.	1138	0.7	232	13.4*	268	0.7
479.	1136	43.4	232	58.2	267	40.8
480.	1138	27.7	232	60.8*	268	37.7
481.	1137	52.9	232	52.2	268	60.1
482.	1138	15.0	231	42.0*	267	21.0
483.	1134	11.2	231	31.6	267	20.2
484.	1138	3.8	231	25.1*	268	4.5
485.	1137	17.2*	232	52.2*	267	29.2
486.	1137	46.1	229	55.5	268	57.8
487.	1136	34.2*	230	44.3*	267	20.2
488.	1135	15.7	230	40.0	264	22.7
489.	1137	6.7*	232	37.5*	267	15.0
490.	1134	12.3	230	28.3	268	16.0
491.	1130	10.6	231	36.8*	267	18.7
492.	1132	78.6	230	77.4	266	77.4
493.	1136	85.3	232	75.0	267	84.6
494.	1135	82.1*	231	59.3	267	62.9
495.	1136	23.3	232	34.9	266	24.8

	Normative Sample		Psychiatric Sample		Chronic Pain Sample	
Item No.	N	%T	N	%T	N	%T
496.	1136	49.0*	232	33.6*	268	16.4
497.	1135	21.4*	232	40.1	268	39.9
498.	1135	13.1	231	31.2*	267	7.1
499.	1138	32.7*	231	43.7	268	50.0
500.	1126	8.2	231	27.3	268	15.3
501.	1137	92.3	231	81.0	267	87.6
502.	1138	27.8	232	54.3*	268	31.0
503.	1136	13.1	231	40.3*	268	11.6
504.	1135	38.0	232	44.0	268	30.2
505.	1134	10.7*	232	44.8*	267	26.6
506.	1136	4.2*	232	51.3*	268	19.4
507.	1138	30.8	232	48.3	268	38.8
508.	1138	20.7	232	26.7	268	17.2
509.	1137	25.0	232	50.9	268	34.7
510.	1138	33.5	232	34.1	268	34.3
511.	1138	19.6*	232	35.3*	267	7.5
512.	1138	14.8*	232	47.8*	267	29.2
513.	1138	17.3*	231	49.8	267	35.6
514.	1136	69.4	231	65.4	267	76.0
515.	1134	10.8	230	29.1*	268	10.1
516.	1137	3.3*	230	35.2*	268	10.8
517.	1136	3.7*	230	43.5*	268	11.2
518.	1137	27.3*	230	69.1*	267	46.8
519.	1134	25.7	230	48.3	268	32.1
520.	1138	1.8*	232	40.1*	267	10.1
521.	1138	72.6	232	53.0	268	68.7
522.	1133	49.8	232	40.1	267	42.7
523.	1137	63.8	232	58.6	267	64.0
524.	1135	1.5*	231	21.6*	268	6.7
525.	1137	6.8*	232	36.6	268	20.9
526.	1138	4.9*	231	40.7*	268	23.1
527.	1137	14.2	232	31.9*	268	7.1
528.	1132	7.2*	232	31.5	268	22.0
529.	1137	19.0	231	30.7	268	30.2
530.	1138	0.5	231	19.5*	268	2.2
531.	1132	17.0	231	29.0	268	22.8
532.	1134	28.9	232	55.6	266	41.7
533.	1136	36.9	232	44.4	268	49.3
534.	1137	64.4	231	31.6*	268	54.5
535.	1138	55.4	231	48.5	268	54.5
536.	1136	9.4*	232	33.6	268	20.1
537.	1137	39.1*	232	42.7	268	60.4
538.	1125	38.6	230	51.7	267	39.3
539.	1138	5.6*	232	42.7	268	25.4
540.	1137	7.5	232	30.2	268	15.3
541.	1138	72.2*	232	59.5	268	54.1
542.	1138	43.3*	231	62.3	268	57.5
543.	1138	16.5	232	37.5*	268	16.8
544.	1128	4.9	231	23.8*	268	93.3
545.	1138	36.5	232	36.2	268	31.3

Item No.	Normative Sample		Psychiatric Sample		Chronic Pain Sample	
	N	%T	N	%T	N	%T
546.	1137	12.5	232	39.2*	268	14.9
547.	1137	69.9	232	49.1	268	63.8
548.	1129	18.2*	231	42.0	267	29.6
549.	1137	13.4*	232	51.3	268	38.1
550.	1137	27.0	232	54.7*	268	32.5
551.	1137	12.6	232	36.6*	268	19.4
552.	1134	57.3	232	53.9	268	58.6
553.	1137	17.5	231	49.8*	268	17.2
554.	1137	8.6*	230	50.9*	268	23.1
555.	1138	2.4	232	15.5*	268	1.5
556.	1136	31.9*	232	55.2	267	50.9
557.	1129	53.5	231	66.7	268	65.7
558.	1138	14.3	231	35.9	268	24.3
559.	1130	15.4*	229	43.7	266	34.6
560.	1137	41.0*	232	27.6	268	26.5
561.	1135	92.4*	231	71.9	267	54.7
562.	1137	27.5	232	45.3	266	33.5
563.	1129	19.2	231	36.4	265	20.0
564.	1136	80.5*	229	58.5	268	67.9
565.	1137	11.1*	232	41.4	268	33.2
566.	1132	31.4	231	53.2	267	40.1
567.	1130	27.6	231	31.2	267	20.2

Appendix G
MMPI-2 Item-Endorsement Percentages for Women

Item No.	Normative Sample		Psychiatric Sample		Chronic Pain Sample	
	N	%T	N	%T	N	%T
1.	1456	10.0	191	17.8	234	17.5
2.	1461	95.9*	191	69.6	233	82.0
3.	1461	65.6*	191	44.0*	234	13.7
4.	1461	38.5*	191	33.0	233	19.3
5.	1462	54.0*	189	61.9	234	73.1
6.	1457	89.8	186	79.6	233	89.7
7.	1459	41.0	191	36.6	233	29.2
8.	1460	64.4*	191	65.4*	233	36.9
9.	1462	82.2*	189	54.0	234	44.0
10.	1462	86.5*	191	53.4*	233	2.6
11.	1461	5.3*	191	22.0	234	20.1
12.	1453	74.1*	186	51.6	231	52.4
13.	1455	34.5	190	47.9*	233	25.3
14.	1458	68.7	191	50.3	233	59.2
15.	1460	36.4	189	49.7	231	48.5
16.	1460	40.1	190	60.0*	234	31.6
17.	1461	6.0*	191	39.3*	233	15.5
18.	1461	3.8*	191	19.9	234	15.4
19.	1439	28.9*	189	34.4*	234	13.7
20.	1460	77.1*	190	65.8	234	63.7
21.	1457	41.2	190	72.6*	234	47.4
22.	1460	8.8*	189	45.5*	233	19.3
23.	1461	18.2	191	40.3	234	27.4
24.	1460	2.0	190	20.5*	232	2.2
25.	1461	44.4	191	49.2	234	38.9
26.	1461	39.7	190	52.6	233	38.6
27.	1461	13.6	190	27.4*	234	7.3
28.	1460	9.1*	191	28.3	234	37.2
29.	1460	81.9	191	78.5	234	77.4
30.	1461	6.0*	191	36.6*	233	18.0
31.	1461	12.5*	191	51.3	233	40.8
32.	1459	18.2	188	56.4*	232	17.7
33.	1460	64.0*	188	46.8	231	28.1
34.	1459	80.7	191	58.1*	232	83.6
35.	1462	36.9	191	57.6*	233	34.3
36.	1462	6.3	190	21.1	232	10.3
37.	1462	37.8	191	52.4	233	50.6
38.	1461	27.5*	191	63.9	233	59.2
39.	1461	13.8*	190	47.4*	231	67.5
40.	1462	7.0*	190	26.3	234	34.2
41.	1460	56.1	189	56.1	233	42.9
42.	1462	2.5	190	32.1*	232	2.6
43.	1455	77.6*	189	45.0	234	36.3
44.	1462	13.0*	191	37.2	234	28.6
45.	1462	86.5*	190	67.4*	234	15.4

*Significantly different from pain sample at $p < .0001$; equivalent to an overall alpha of .05 for 567 comparisons: Bonferroni criterion)

Item No.	Normative Sample		Psychiatric Sample		Chronic Pain Sample	
	N	%T	N	%T	N	%T
46.	1460	22.7	190	41.6*	232	21.6
47.	1460	84.5*	191	66.5	234	64.5
48.	1461	11.6	189	32.8*	233	8.6
49.	1460	75.2	191	54.5*	234	75.2
50.	1458	47.5	189	55.6	234	45.7
51.	1461	96.2	190	93.7	234	98.3
52.	1457	12.1	190	55.8*	233	17.6
53.	1459	25.4*	190	51.6*	234	79.1
54.	1453	4.8	190	23.2*	232	4.3
55.	1458	36.9	187	61.0*	233	36.1
56.	1454	34.0*	190	76.8	234	63.2
57.	1459	68.3*	190	68.9*	234	20.1
58.	1460	56.5	190	53.2	234	45.7
59.	1462	10.9*	189	33.9	234	27.8
60.	1461	2.7	189	24.9*	234	3.0
61.	1459	77.0	190	65.8	234	74.8
62.	1461	73.6	190	61.1	232	72.0
63.	1461	32.0	189	24.9	234	23.1
64.	1461	72.6	190	60.0	233	70.4
65.	1462	9.0*	190	45.3	233	30.9
66.	1462	2.1	191	45.3	234	1.3
67.	1461	72.1	189	78.3	232	68.1
68.	1462	13.7	189	30.7*	234	13.7
69.	1462	38.9	191	44.5	234	38.9
70.	1459	32.1	191	49.7	234	37.6
71.	1454	32.4*	190	70.0	234	55.1
72.	1460	4.5	191	20.9*	233	3.4
73.	1460	27.7*	191	59.7	233	46.8
74.	1462	33.6	191	49.7	233	44.6
75.	1460	95.2*	191	69.1*	233	86.3
76.	1448	33.5	189	50.8*	233	22.7
77.	1459	95.3	190	84.7	232	92.2
78.	1459	96.4	191	82.2*	234	95.3
79.	1459	29.1	191	29.3	234	24.8
80.	1462	26.7	191	44.0	233	37.8
81.	1461	44.3	190	53.2*	234	32.9
82.	1460	21.6	191	60.7*	234	28.2
83.	1462	78.4	190	60.5	232	70.7
84.	1462	7.0	191	34.0*	234	8.1
85.	1460	16.1	191	41.9*	233	15.9
86.	1459	39.4	190	38.9	234	31.2
87.	1452	53.5	188	69.1	234	55.6
88.	1449	83.4	188	69.1	230	77.4
89.	1460	77.6	190	81.1	233	82.8
90.	1456	91.9	188	81.4*	233	94.8
91.	1462	88.8*	191	68.1*	233	39.5
92.	1462	3.2*	191	27.2*	234	10.7
93.	1462	91.8	190	86.3*	234	97.4
94.	1462	5.4	191	46.1*	233	12.0
95.	1462	89.1*	191	48.7	232	56.9

	Normative Sample		Psychiatric Sample		Chronic Pain Sample	
Item No.	N	%T	N	%T	N	%T
96.	1456	4.8	190	16.3	234	5.1
97.	1460	10.9*	188	31.4	234	23.5
98.	1460	45.1	189	56.6	234	38.5
99.	1460	5.5	187	32.6*	232	8.2
100.	1460	49.7	191	50.8	233	54.5
101.	1461	7.0*	191	26.2	233	30.9
102.	1461	98.2	190	93.7	234	98.7
103.	1460	27.3	191	34.0	234	27.4
104.	1458	39.1	191	44.0	234	29.1
105.	1462	10.1	191	40.8*	234	13.7
106.	1461	84.7	191	67.5	233	70.4
107.	1462	66.8*	191	61.3	234	48.7
108.	1462	91.4	189	85.7	234	95.3
109.	1462	93.2*	189	69.3	234	79.5
110.	1454	50.3	190	61.6	232	41.6
111.	1462	8.9*	191	25.1	234	26.9
112.	1459	67.9*	186	54.8	232	50.0
113.	1452	70.5	190	76.3	234	61.1
114.	1462	1.2	189	10.6*	234	0.4
115.	1460	63.6	189	58.2	234	63.2
116.	1461	35.9	188	55.3	233	38.6
117.	1461	86.4	188	65.4	234	82.9
118.	1458	64.1	190	60.5	234	67.9
119.	1462	79.4	190	78.9	234	85.0
120.	1460	72.9	191	71.2	233	73.0
121.	1460	77.5*	188	60.1*	232	90.9
122.	1462	82.3	191	74.9	234	78.6
123.	1462	30.2	191	40.3*	234	17.1
124.	1462	24.9	191	60.2*	232	26.7
125.	1462	87.5*	191	44.5*	233	73.4
126.	1457	98.4	190	94.7	234	100.0
127.	1461	58.2	191	75.4	234	61.1
128.	1460	75.8	190	78.9	234	84.6
129.	1461	26.4	191	44.5*	234	19.7
130.	1461	38.1*	190	70.0	234	76.9
131.	1458	43.5	191	47.6	231	39.8
132.	1443	79.3	190	75.8	228	86.0
133.	1462	3.6	191	15.2	233	4.3
134.	1462	8.4	190	26.3	234	11.5
135.	1459	30.5	191	64.4*	234	33.3
136.	1461	35.6	191	53.9*	234	30.3
137.	1461	57.8	190	62.6	234	50.9
138.	1462	1.6	190	28.9*	232	2.6
139.	1461	87.5*	188	77.1	234	73.5
140.	1461	72.8*	191	47.1	234	33.8
141.	1460	90.9*	191	62.3*	234	32.1
142.	1462	93.5	191	69.6*	234	90.2
143.	1460	56.4*	191	46.6	234	33.3
144.	1462	0.5	191	23.6*	234	1.3
145.	1461	11.2	190	57.9*	234	15.8

	Normative Sample		Psychiatric Sample		Chronic Pain Sample	
Item No.	N	%T	N	%T	N	%T
146.	1462	46.4	191	58.6	233	59.7
147.	1459	14.5*	191	41.9	234	34.2
148.	1459	48.0*	190	27.4*	234	2.1
149.	1462	12.0*	191	27.2	234	34.2
150.	1461	5.3	189	37.0*	233	6.0
151.	1453	49.4	191	54.5	234	39.3
152.	1461	58.4*	190	41.6*	233	14.6
153.	1460	49.8*	191	56.0*	234	29.1
154.	1461	61.4	191	69.1	234	59.4
155.	1461	17.1	190	31.1	234	17.1
156.	1461	3.7	190	21.1*	234	5.1
157.	1457	31.2	189	29.6	233	27.0
158.	1453	63.2	188	64.4	234	62.8
159.	1461	55.0	190	44.2	234	44.0
160.	1460	86.2*	190	67.4	234	70.9
161.	1461	40.8	190	58.9*	232	37.9
162.	1462	0.3	191	11.0*	233	0.2
163.	1461	48.1	189	39.2	234	44.0
164.	1462	84.3*	190	61.6	234	64.1
165.	1461	90.4*	191	72.3	234	65.8
166.	1459	13.4	191	35.6	232	20.7
167.	1462	38.8	189	63.5*	234	32.5
168.	1461	8.5	191	37.7*	234	14.1
169.	1458	43.6	190	50.5	234	47.0
170.	1460	9.5*	191	46.1*	234	19.7
171.	1459	40.3	191	42.4	233	38.2
172.	1460	7.3*	191	36.1	234	29.5
173.	1461	69.6*	190	50.0	234	52.1
174.	1462	91.5	191	80.6	234	89.3
175.	1461	4.7*	191	35.6	234	42.7
176.	1460	74.5*	191	61.3*	233	38.2
177.	1461	89.7*	190	73.7	234	65.0
178.	1462	28.0	191	47.1	233	30.0
179.	1462	91.4*	191	70.7	233	51.9
180.	1461	3.4*	190	40.5*	234	9.8
181.	1459	76.0	191	75.9	234	73.5
182.	1460	3.8*	190	31.6*	234	10.7
183.	1461	90.8	191	78.5	234	84.6
184.	1458	53.8	191	47.1	234	61.1
185.	1460	46.5	191	66.5*	233	41.6
186.	1462	92.8	191	78.5	234	89.7
187.	1459	44.7	191	44.0	233	32.2
188.	1461	83.3	191	74.9	234	79.1
189.	1458	53.5	190	45.8	233	45.9
190.	1458	8.0	190	51.6*	234	9.0
191.	1461	38.4	191	41.4	233	25.8
192.	1460	97.3	189	89.4	234	95.3
193.	1462	8.6	190	17.9	234	5.6
194.	1461	44.0	191	42.9	234	52.1
195.	1462	9.5	190	40.5*	234	12.8

	Normative Sample		Psychiatric Sample		Chronic Pain Sample	
Item No.	N	%T	N	%T	N	%T
196.	1462	60.7*	190	72.6	234	78.6
197.	1459	17.2	191	22.5	234	14.5
198.	1462	1.5	191	27.2*	234	4.7
199.	1461	63.4	191	60.2	233	54.5
200.	1459	42.2	191	38.2	234	30.3
201.	1462	3.2*	191	16.8	234	12.4
202.	1462	18.9	191	55.5*	234	28.6
203.	1461	91.2	191	75.4*	234	90.6
204.	1462	89.5	191	83.2	234	88.0
205.	1462	66.2	191	58.6	234	58.5
206.	1462	75.0	191	63.4	234	73.9
207.	1460	34.5	191	43.5	234	29.9
208.	1459	72.1*	191	57.6	234	51.3
209.	1457	38.2*	190	32.1	232	21.1
210.	1461	98.1	191	87.4	234	97.0
211.	1433	26.6	187	39.0	229	24.9
212.	1452	23.8	190	42.1	233	26.6
213.	1461	42.4	191	53.4	234	41.9
214.	1462	62.7	190	56.8	234	62.0
215.	1454	17.5	189	43.4*	232	20.7
216.	1460	1.5	190	18.9*	234	1.3
217.	1440	54.0	189	41.3	232	53.9
218.	1459	23.7*	191	61.8	234	59.4
219.	1459	57.7	191	77.5*	232	55.6
220.	1457	10.6	190	17.4	234	9.4
221.	1461	26.6	191	49.2*	234	20.9
222.	1458	89.6	189	71.4	232	81.9
223.	1461	81.7*	191	48.7	234	61.5
224.	1462	81.3*	191	64.9*	233	0.4
225.	1461	27.9	191	70.7*	234	34.6
226.	1458	40.2	191	51.3	234	32.9
227.	1457	41.8	189	50.8	232	39.7
228.	1461	1.9	189	19.0*	233	0.9
229.	1462	4.7*	191	39.3*	234	12.0
230.	1461	72.6	189	76.7	234	76.5
231.	1460	17.5*	189	29.1	233	32.6
232.	1458	74.9	189	49.7	234	62.4
233.	1456	32.4	191	57.6	234	46.2
234.	1462	1.6	191	26.7*	233	3.9
235.	1459	10.1*	188	40.4	234	24.4
236.	1458	64.3	191	71.2	233	70.8
237.	1462	59.4	191	56.5	234	62.8
238.	1461	16.5	191	33.5	234	24.8
239.	1462	25.9	191	22.5	233	23.2
240.	1462	3.3	190	22.1*	234	2.1
241.	1462	14.4	191	41.4*	234	17.1
242.	1461	35.2	191	50.8*	234	29.1
243.	1462	34.7	190	61.6*	234	38.0
244.	1458	76.4	190	55.8	232	68.5
245.	1461	29.4	189	30.2	233	39.1

Item No.	Normative Sample		Psychiatric Sample		Chronic Pain Sample	
	N	%T	N	%T	N	%T
246.	1458	2.2	189	19.0*	232	4.7
247.	1461	8.7*	190	24.7*	233	61.4
248.	1458	10.5	189	20.6	234	9.0
249.	1461	55.2	191	53.9	234	49.6
250.	1461	23.6	191	30.9	233	15.0
251.	1462	24.6	191	57.6*	234	32.5
252.	1460	0.5*	191	9.4	234	3.8
253.	1461	11.7	191	30.9*	234	12.8
254.	1459	20.0	191	49.2*	233	15.0
255.	1462	83.6*	190	68.9	234	70.9
256.	1462	44.0	191	61.8*	234	33.3
257.	1461	17.3	191	29.8	234	15.4
258.	1462	2.6*	189	18.5	233	11.2
259.	1460	16.9	190	48.9*	233	23.2
260.	1461	92.9	191	85.3	234	92.7
261.	1442	52.0	190	30.5	231	39.0
262.	1461	72.3	190	58.4	234	62.8
263.	1457	82.0	190	65.3	233	81.1
264.	1462	22.9	191	42.4*	234	20.9
265.	1461	27.7	191	49.7*	234	29.5
266.	1460	83.9	191	52.4*	234	79.9
267.	1461	70.2	190	60.0	234	61.1
268.	1447	14.2	188	43.6*	232	17.2
269.	1450	19.6	191	43.5*	234	15.8
270.	1459	3.6	191	5.2	234	0.4
271.	1460	46.4	189	61.9*	232	40.1
272.	1460	11.0	188	16.5	234	8.1
273.	1461	17.9*	191	60.2	234	44.4
274.	1462	27.8	190	58.4*	234	34.6
275.	1461	59.4	191	77.0	234	70.9
276.	1457	96.0	189	90.5	234	96.2
277.	1462	19.0*	190	60.5*	234	35.9
278.	1457	83.8	191	66.5	232	82.8
279.	1461	48.4	191	62.3*	234	39.7
280.	1461	81.0	191	63.4*	234	81.6
281.	1459	3.6	191	14.1	234	5.6
282.	1462	6.0	191	16.2	234	6.4
283.	1461	39.6	191	58.1	234	50.0
284.	1458	49.7	191	49.7	233	39.5
285.	1462	49.0	191	72.8*	234	48.3
286.	1460	27.5	188	51.1*	234	27.4
287.	1461	13.8	189	20.6	234	6.8
288.	1458	13.6	190	48.4*	234	14.5
289.	1461	46.2	188	68.1	234	52.6
290.	1462	53.5*	191	63.9	234	71.4
291.	1462	3.6	190	11.6	234	4.3
292.	1462	35.0	191	57.1	234	41.9
293.	1461	25.2	191	26.7	234	29.5
294.	1461	4.9	188	10.1	234	7.3
295.	1459	83.6*	191	60.2*	232	23.7

	Normative Sample		Psychiatric Sample		Chronic Pain Sample	
Item No.	N	%T	N	%T	N	%T
296.	1462	13.2*	191	36.6	234	25.2
297.	1460	62.3	191	74.3	233	70.8
298.	1462	12.0	189	34.4*	234	11.5
299.	1462	14.8*	190	48.4	234	30.8
300.	1462	10.5	191	36.6*	234	8.5
301.	1462	20.2	190	50.5*	233	28.8
302.	1462	39.4	191	54.5	234	39.7
303.	1461	3.4	189	31.7*	234	7.7
304.	1461	54.1	190	63.2	234	51.3
305.	1458	36.2*	190	80.0	233	70.4
306.	1460	9.3	190	33.2*	234	9.8
307.	1462	11.1	191	34.0*	234	13.2
308.	1462	13.1	189	36.5	233	19.7
309.	1461	30.7	191	65.4*	233	30.9
310.	1461	11.3	190	32.1*	234	9.8
311.	1460	9.0	190	44.2*	234	9.0
312.	1462	6.0	190	20.5*	234	6.4
313.	1460	16.0	190	38.4*	234	14.1
314.	1457	92.2	190	63.2*	234	88.9
315.	1459	48.8	189	69.8*	232	42.7
316.	1461	10.0	186	41.9*	234	7.7
317.	1460	5.7	190	27.9	234	12.0
318.	1460	93.2	190	71.6*	234	90.6
319.	1460	7.0	189	19.6	234	6.4
320.	1459	16.9	191	37.7*	234	11.5
321.	1460	60.3	190	53.7	234	57.7
322.	1459	4.5	191	18.8*	234	2.6
323.	1460	4.9	191	19.4*	234	0.9
324.	1462	4.6	191	16.2*	234	2.6
325.	1461	17.0*	191	53.4	233	41.6
326.	1460	35.5	191	65.4*	234	39.7
327.	1461	7.9	191	32.5*	234	6.4
328.	1460	29.7	191	46.1	234	33.8
329.	1461	1.8	191	30.9*	234	5.6
330.	1462	94.1*	190	82.6	234	71.8
331.	1462	49.1*	191	68.6	234	64.5
332.	1462	3.8	191	22.0*	234	1.7
333.	1462	5.0	190	41.6*	234	9.8
334.	1462	2.6	190	29.5*	234	6.4
335.	1462	68.7	190	50.0	234	56.0
336.	1462	2.0	191	19.4*	233	2.6
337.	1460	42.5	191	66.5*	234	40.6
338.	1462	34.6	190	64.7*	234	36.3
339.	1462	43.2*	190	75.3	233	67.8
340.	1461	60.0	191	59.7	234	69.7
341.	1462	67.2	190	70.0	234	72.2
342.	1460	55.1	191	49.7	234	63.7
343.	1459	91.6	191	90.6	234	95.7
344.	1461	42.5*	191	42.4	234	57.3
345.	1458	52.5	190	59.5	232	53.4

Item No.	Normative Sample		Psychiatric Sample		Chronic Pain Sample	
	N	%T	N	%T	N	%T
346.	1460	64.5	191	65.4	234	60.7
347.	1462	22.3	191	46.6*	234	21.8
348.	1461	20.7	189	48.1*	234	20.1
349.	1461	8.4	188	20.2*	234	3.8
350.	1452	52.7	191	51.3	234	52.6
351.	1462	41.7	189	51.9	234	46.6
352.	1459	70.9	191	69.1	233	67.4
353.	1461	82.5	190	74.2	232	78.9
354.	1461	82.3	191	70.7	234	79.9
355.	1461	1.0	191	22.0*	234	0.4
356.	1462	32.8*	191	49.7	234	50.9
357.	1451	46.5	190	71.1	230	54.8
358.	1458	16.6	189	38.6*	234	19.2
359.	1459	59.2	190	56.3	234	59.0
360.	1460	81.9	191	62.3*	232	81.9
361.	1462	2.1	190	34.2*	234	5.6
362.	1461	59.4	191	67.0	234	50.0
363.	1456	76.5	190	65.8	233	68.7
364.	1454	26.2	191	54.5*	233	27.9
365.	1460	73.7	191	70.7	233	71.7
366.	1460	11.0	190	42.6*	234	14.5
367.	1455	28.4	191	46.6	234	30.8
368.	1459	25.2	191	52.9*	231	26.8
369.	1460	44.8	190	53.7	233	46.4
370.	1461	78.0	191	69.6	234	75.2
371.	1462	10.3	189	20.1	234	7.3
372.	1459	66.7	191	57.6	234	67.1
373.	1460	38.6	189	49.7*	234	28.2
374.	1461	37.7	191	62.8*	234	33.8
375.	1460	31.0	191	63.9*	234	41.9
376.	1462	13.3*	191	40.8	234	24.4
377.	1460	30.3*	190	67.9	232	78.0
378.	1459	38.8	191	55.0	233	43.8
379.	1462	13.5	191	33.5	234	19.2
380.	1462	15.5	191	27.7	234	20.9
381.	1460	8.7	190	25.3*	234	7.3
382.	1461	24.2	191	58.1*	234	28.2
383.	1462	91.3	191	60.7*	234	85.0
384.	1459	86.9	191	85.9	233	91.4
385.	1459	40.4	191	35.1	234	41.9
386.	1458	47.1	191	68.1	234	52.1
387.	1459	3.4	191	16.8*	234	3.0
388.	1462	64.3*	191	35.1	234	35.5
389.	1460	15.3	190	37.9	234	24.8
390.	1457	48.5	191	70.2*	234	49.6
391.	1461	33.7	191	57.1*	234	31.6
392.	1462	34.0	191	41.9	234	36.8
393.	1462	23.7	189	27.5	234	23.1
394.	1461	22.7*	191	63.4*	232	36.6
395.	1462	16.5	191	35.6	234	24.4

	Normative Sample		Psychiatric Sample		Chronic Pain Sample	
Item No.	N	%T	N	%T	N	%T
396.	1456	45.4	189	63.0	232	54.3
397.	1461	24.4	191	38.7	234	36.3
398.	1461	50.4	190	64.2	234	52.1
399.	1460	12.9	191	47.1*	234	23.1
400.	1461	17.3*	189	45.5	234	33.8
401.	1462	50.9	191	55.0	233	51.9
402.	1462	51.4	191	55.5	234	44.0
403.	1460	37.7	190	68.9*	234	37.6
404.	1461	94.1*	191	77.5	234	84.6
405.	1458	77.0*	190	57.4	233	61.4
406.	1457	29.4	188	36.2	232	25.4
407.	1456	7.0	190	29.5*	234	8.1
408.	1460	32.1	191	60.7*	233	39.1
409.	1460	54.0	191	68.1	234	52.6
410.	1457	38.1*	191	35.1	234	22.6
411.	1462	24.6*	190	62.1*	234	40.6
412.	1462	10.2*	191	36.6	234	20.1
413.	1460	35.0	191	57.1	234	41.0
414.	1461	40.0	190	52.6	233	43.8
415.	1461	29.1	191	57.6*	234	34.2
416.	1458	44.8	190	35.8	234	32.5
417.	1461	10.7	191	25.1	234	17.5
418.	1455	41.5	189	49.7	233	36.9
419.	1460	44.8	188	48.4	234	32.9
420.	1460	41.4	191	71.7	234	53.8
421.	1459	27.0	190	55.3*	234	32.1
422.	1461	77.7	191	82.2	234	89.3
423.	1456	37.6	188	48.4*	234	28.2
424.	1459	14.3	191	36.6	234	23.1
425.	1456	35.0*	191	52.4	233	49.8
426.	1462	95.2	191	89.5	233	94.0
427.	1462	82.4	191	56.0*	232	75.4
428.	1458	57.9	190	71.6	234	59.4
429.	1461	75.0	191	65.4	234	82.4
430.	1455	48.5*	191	66.5	234	73.9
431.	1460	3.4	189	23.3*	233	5.2
432.	1459	14.0	191	23.6*	233	8.2
433.	1455	50.9*	189	54.5	232	34.9
434.	1454	29.6*	190	44.2	233	52.8
435.	1458	17.4	190	37.4	232	20.3
436.	1452	29.4	191	53.9*	231	24.7
437.	1460	61.6	190	65.8	234	55.6
438.	1454	54.8	190	63.2	233	56.2
439.	1459	39.0	188	50.5	234	41.5
440.	1459	64.6	191	63.9	233	69.1
441.	1455	21.5	188	41.0	233	24.9
442.	1462	67.6	190	76.3	234	68.8
443.	1455	26.7	189	44.4	233	32.6
444.	1461	28.2	188	55.9	233	41.2
445.	1456	35.1	190	45.8	234	47.9

	Normative Sample		Psychiatric Sample		Chronic Pain Sample	
Item No.	N	%T	N	%T	N	%T
446.	1462	37.9	191	59.2*	233	38.6
447.	1458	14.4	188	36.2	234	20.9
448.	1460	18.4	191	41.9*	234	14.5
449.	1462	72.7	191	77.0	234	84.2
450.	1461	2.5	191	22.5*	234	4.3
451.	1459	15.0	191	29.3*	234	12.0
452.	1459	65.0	191	59.7	234	59.4
453.	1459	40.8	191	33.0	234	41.9
454.	1459	4.0*	191	34.6*	234	16.2
455.	1455	82.9	191	61.8*	233	80.3
456.	1462	79.3*	191	73.8	234	65.8
457.	1462	21.8	190	44.7	234	27.4
458.	1460	59.0	190	56.3	234	57.3
459.	1460	79.9	190	62.1	234	75.2
460.	1454	55.2*	190	65.3	232	73.3
461.	1462	56.8	191	72.8	234	56.4
462.	1457	51.5	191	46.1	234	50.0
463.	1461	5.5	191	40.8*	234	10.7
464.	1462	33.9*	191	56.0	234	74.8
465.	1455	24.6	190	26.3	233	24.0
466.	1459	33.7	190	57.4*	234	36.3
467.	1458	56.2	190	54.7	234	49.6
468.	1457	8.1	190	24.7	234	12.0
469.	1456	31.0*	190	66.8	234	65.0
470.	1452	36.4	189	58.2	231	43.7
471.	1456	18.4	190	51.6*	234	26.5
472.	1456	33.9	190	50.5	234	44.9
473.	1452	72.0	190	66.8	233	67.4
474.	1455	40.4	190	43.7	233	43.3
475.	1458	19.2*	190	52.1	234	39.3
476.	1460	7.1*	190	26.3	234	23.1
477.	1460	10.1	189	28.6*	234	11.5
478.	1461	1.4	190	7.4	234	0.4
479.	1456	38.0	191	66.0*	234	36.8
480.	1460	31.0	190	62.6*	234	40.2
481.	1459	47.2	191	54.5	232	52.6
482.	1459	21.2	191	52.9*	233	22.7
483.	1457	10.4*	190	30.5	229	21.4
484.	1460	2.3	191	24.6*	234	4.3
485.	1462	22.8*	191	60.7*	234	35.5
486.	1460	49.3	190	62.6	232	53.4
487.	1455	24.5*	189	38.6*	232	11.6
488.	1461	12.7	191	46.6*	232	16.4
489.	1462	3.5	191	28.8*	234	6.8
490.	1458	9.5	191	33.5*	231	10.0
491.	1455	20.3	184	49.5*	234	26.5
492.	1453	78.5	185	80.0	234	84.6
493.	1458	91.4	191	89.0	234	95.3
494.	1459	82.5*	188	67.6	233	64.4
495.	1459	21.0	190	37.9	233	23.6

Item No.	Normative Sample		Psychiatric Sample		Chronic Pain Sample	
	N	%T	N	%T	N	%T
496.	1461	44.3*	191	27.7	234	12.4
497.	1461	26.8	191	52.9	234	35.9
498.	1459	24.2*	191	41.4*	233	10.7
499.	1461	32.5*	191	56.0	234	56.0
500.	1446	12.4	190	31.6	233	15.0
501.	1459	96.2*	189	80.4	232	89.2
502.	1460	20.5	191	49.2	234	32.1
503.	1458	16.5	190	46.8*	234	17.9
504.	1460	38.4	190	45.3	232	27.2
505.	1459	14.6*	188	43.6	233	27.5
506.	1462	3.8*	189	49.2*	231	13.0
507.	1461	26.0	190	51.6*	234	29.9
508.	1461	23.4	190	27.4	234	23.9
509.	1462	42.5	189	69.3*	234	44.4
510.	1462	21.1	189	31.7	234	20.1
511.	1460	9.1	190	19.5*	234	3.0
512.	1462	23.5	189	49.7	234	33.8
513.	1461	22.7*	189	54.0	232	38.8
514.	1458	74.1	191	76.4	234	79.5
515.	1451	11.0	190	22.1	234	9.8
516.	1461	3.2*	190	35.8*	233	12.0
517.	1459	2.3*	188	40.4*	232	11.6
518.	1459	20.9*	190	71.1*	233	36.5
519.	1459	35.7*	190	57.9	233	54.5
520.	1461	1.9*	191	36.6*	231	10.8
521.	1461	62.2	191	48.7	234	51.7
522.	1459	49.1	190	38.4	232	48.3
523.	1459	46.9	190	62.1	234	50.9
524.	1461	4.5	190	24.2*	231	7.4
525.	1458	12.7*	191	44.5	234	28.2
526.	1460	3.7*	191	51.8*	234	26.5
527.	1460	7.9	191	18.3*	234	3.4
528.	1453	6.3*	190	27.4	233	17.2
529.	1460	24.8	191	39.3	234	32.5
530.	1460	1.1	191	21.5*	234	0.9
531.	1449	13.7	190	37.9	233	21.0
532.	1462	68.2	190	71.1	234	79.1
533.	1460	40.0	190	46.8	234	51.7
534.	1457	62.7*	190	32.1	234	46.6
535.	1456	60.9	189	51.9	232	58.2
536.	1462	25.2*	191	39.8	234	41.0
537.	1461	23.8	191	31.9	233	36.1
538.	1449	40.0	188	55.9*	233	29.6
539.	1459	7.0*	191	41.4*	233	21.5
540.	1460	3.5	190	15.8	232	4.3
541.	1462	77.8	190	58.9	232	69.8
542.	1462	56.2	190	63.7	234	66.7
543.	1458	21.1	191	49.7*	234	23.5
544.	1454	2.2	190	22.6*	231	3.0
545.	1460	44.0	191	47.6	234	40.6

Item No.	Normative Sample		Psychiatric Sample		Chronic Pain Sample	
	N	%T	N	%T	N	%T
546.	1457	14.3	191	38.7*	233	14.2
547.	1461	68.7	191	60.2	234	68.4
548.	1451	7.4	188	32.4*	232	5.6
549.	1462	10.9*	189	56.1*	234	35.0
550.	1461	16.4	191	49.7*	234	20.9
551.	1461	17.4	190	37.4	234	23.5
552.	1456	72.2	191	62.8	234	67.5
553.	1459	14.8	190	53.7*	234	17.9
554.	1461	14.2*	191	54.5*	232	31.9
555.	1461	3.7	191	19.4*	234	4.7
556.	1461	36.8*	190	62.1	234	58.1
557.	1458	36.8*	189	60.8	234	51.7
558.	1461	14.9*	191	36.1	234	26.9
559.	1444	10.9*	186	36.6	228	25.0
560.	1446	38.9	189	27.0	231	33.3
561.	1460	86.0*	190	66.3*	234	34.6
562.	1461	36.5	191	51.8	234	46.6
563.	1455	19.5	188	36.7*	233	18.0
564.	1458	72.2*	190	54.2	232	58.2
565.	1458	10.8*	191	42.4	234	32.9
566.	1453	27.9*	190	58.4	231	45.0
567.	1451	31.5	189	39.2	234	23.9

Appendix H

Item-Endorsement Percentage Differences for Pain (N = 268) vs. Normative (N = 1138) Sample Men

(Left margin = difference in item-endorsement percentages between pain and normative samples. Item numbers in body of table are from the MMPI-2 form.)

99 - 100	
97 - 98	
95 - 96	
93 - 94	
91 - 92	
89 - 90	
87 - 88	
85 - 86	
83 - 84	
81 - 82	10
79 - 80	224
77 - 78	
75 - 76	
73 - 74	
71 - 72	45
69 - 70	
67 - 68	
65 - 66	53
63 - 64	
61 - 62	
59 - 60	91 295
57 - 58	
55 - 56	39 247
53 - 54	3
51 - 52	141
49 - 50	57
47 - 48	377
45 - 46	9 152
43 - 44	148 179
41 - 42	218 305
39 - 40	43 140
37 - 38	130 175 201 464 561
35 - 36	33
33 - 34	176 430 496
31 - 32	
29 - 30	56 95 469
27 - 28	5 71 143 394
25 - 26	12 31 38 65 388 549
23 - 24	40 73 160 173 235
21 - 22	8 105 112 164 172 273 330 339 376 389 412 537 565
19 - 20	28 101 266 325 356 444 445 467 494 497 513 518 539 556 559
17 - 18	19 44 84 86 118 153 177 191 196 208 222 227 232 255 275 375 405 416 499 526 541
15 - 16	41 47 52 59 116 147 149 166 199 223 287 290 334 384 386 409 415 431 433 470 505 506 528 542

13 - 14	2 17 25 30 109 111 137 165 184 259 261 286 299 342 373 399 411 434 475 487 512 525 532 554 560 564
11 - 12	1 4 20 22 67 97 121 125 145 187 202 258 283 289 357 378 403 408 417 420 438 454 472 485 486 511 529 533 536 548 557
9 - 10	11 37 50 69 82 103 107 117 122 123 132 135 169 170 178 200 215 217 238 243 244 251 257 296 297 301 304 317 328 331 333 335 358 367 372 382 396 400 414 418 425 428 429 432 443 449 452 460 480 483 509 534 558 566
7 - 8	18 68 83 94 128 129 134 139 142 146 151 182 188 197 204 211 225 229 230 234 254 267 298 302 309 340 353 370 385 390 392 422 423 446 459 466 476 481 488 489 491 500 504 507 514 516 517 520 522 527 540 567
5 - 6	7 21 23 34 35 49 58 75 77 79 87 92 93 108 124 138 144 154 156 159 161 163 167 168 171 181 209 212 213 226 233 241 245 250 274 277 279 284 293 308 314 321 326 337 344 346 362 364 365 366 379 381 397 398 407 413 419 421 426 436 448 453 458 463 482 498 519 524 531 545 547 550 551 562
3 - 4	15 27 32 36 55 61 63 76 81 98 99 100 106 113 127 133 174 180 189 195 205 207 214 231 237 240 248 249 256 262 269 270 271 281 282 303 311 312 313 327 338 343 347 348 351 361 363 374 383 391 402 404 424 437 450 451 456 461 490 501 502 508 521
1 - 2	13 14 16 24 26 42 46 54 60 62 64 66 74 78 80 85 88 89 90 96 102 110 115 119 120 126 131 136 150 155 157 183 185 190 192 193 194 198 203 206 210 216 219 220 221 228 242 246 252 253 264 265 268 272 276 278 280 288 292 294 300 306 307 310 315 318 319 320 322 324 329 341 345 349 350 352 354 355 359 360 368 369 371 380 393 395 401 406 410 435 439 440 441 442 447 457 462 471 473 474 477 479 484 492 495 503 515 530 544 546 552 553 563
0	6 29 48 51 70 72 104 114 158 162 186 236 239 260 263 285 291 316 323 332 336 387 427 455 465 468 478 493 510 523 535 538 543 555

Appendix I

Item-Endorsement Percentage Differences for Pain (N = 234) vs. Normative (N = 1462) Sample Women

(Left margin = difference in item-endorsement percentages between pain and normative samples. Item numbers in body of text correspond to the MMPI-2 form.)

99 - 100	
97 - 98	
95 - 96	
93 - 94	
91 - 92	
89 - 90	
87 - 88	
85 - 86	
83 - 84	10
81 - 82	224
79 - 80	
77 - 78	
75 - 76	
73 - 74	
71 - 72	45
69 - 70	
67 - 68	
65 - 66	
63 - 64	
61 - 62	
59 - 60	141 295
57 - 58	
55 - 56	
53 - 54	39 53
51 - 52	3 247 561
49 - 50	91
47 - 48	57 377
45 - 46	148
43 - 44	152
41 - 42	43 464
39 - 40	130 140 179
37 - 38	9 175 176
35 - 36	33 218
33 - 34	305 469
31 - 32	38 95 496
29 - 30	56
27 - 28	8 28 31 40 388
25 - 26	177 273 325 339 430
23 - 24	71 101 143 165 172 434 499 526 549
21 - 22	12 65 149 153 208 330 556 565
19 - 20	4 5 47 73 147 164 223 475 494 519
17 - 18	59 107 111 112 173 196 209 277 290 356 400 460 554 566
15 - 16	11 19 44 106 125 160 231 299 331 405 410 411 425 433 476 513 518 525 534 536 539 557
13 - 14	2 15 20 37 41 97 109 121 123 139 146 187 232 233 235 255 261 335 344 394 420 444 445 456 485 487 498 505 559 564

11 - 12	7 18 30 58 74 76 80 81 159 191 200 256 275 296 373 375 376 397 416 419 422 449 454 472 483 502 504 528 532 533 537 542 558
9 - 10	13 14 17 22 23 63 75 104 113 128 151 170 201 202 245 250 262 267 283 284 297 301 340 342 362 389 396 399 404 412 423 424 471 480 497 506 512 516 517 520 521 538 562
7 - 8	1 16 27 83 86 92 94 110 132 137 166 180 182 184 189 194 199 205 222 225 226 229 236 238 244 251 258 274 279 287 289 292 308 357 363 395 402 408 417 427 429 447 470 491 501 529 531 541 551 567
5 - 6	21 25 29 52 70 82 88 89 93 98 100 119 129 136 145 167 168 183 185 207 221 242 249 254 259 271 293 303 315 317 320 333 341 351 378 379 380 383 386 413 415 418 421 432 437 443 452 457 459 463 467 473 481 492 511 514 527 550 560
3 - 4	34 35 36 48 64 67 77 79 90 105 108 116 117 118 122 127 131 134 142 157 161 163 169 174 186 188 193 195 198 212 215 230 237 239 241 243 246 252 266 268 269 270 272 304 314 323 326 328 329 334 343 346 349 352 353 361 366 367 370 371 374 382 384 392 406 414 435 436 439 440 441 448 451 455 468 474 486 488 489 493 495 500 507 523 535 543 545 552 553
1 - 2	26 46 50 51 54 55 61 62 66 72 78 84 87 99 102 114 115 124 126 135 138 150 154 156 171 178 181 190 192 197 204 206 210 211 214 216 219 220 227 228 234 240 248 253 257 263 264 265 278 280 281 285 286 288 294 300 302 306 307 310 313 316 318 319 321 322 324 327 332 336 337 338 348 354 355 358 364 365 368 369 381 385 390 391 393 398 401 407 409 426 428 431 438 442 446 450 453 458 461 462 465 466 477 478 479 482 484 503 508 509 510 515 522 524 544 547 548 555 563
0	6 24 32 42 49 60 68 69 85 96 103 120 133 144 155 158 162 203 213 217 260 276 282 291 298 309 311 312 345 347 350 359 360 372 387 403 490 530 540 546

Appendix J

Item-Endorsement Percentage Differences for Pain (N = 268) vs. Psychiatric (N = 232) Sample Men

(Left margin = difference in item-endorsement percentages between pain and psychiatric samples. Item numbers in body of table correspond to the MMPI-2 form.)

99 - 100	
97 - 98	
95 - 96	
93 - 94	
91 - 92	
89 - 90	
87 - 88	
85 - 86	
83 - 84	
81 - 82	
79 - 80	
77 - 78	
75 - 76	
73 - 74	
71 - 72	
69 - 70	
67 - 68	
65 - 66	
63 - 64	
61 - 62	
59 - 60	224
57 - 58	10 45
55 - 56	
53 - 54	
51 - 52	
49 - 50	
47 - 48	
45 - 46	
43 - 44	57 91 247 295
41 - 42	
39 - 40	
37 - 38	53
35 - 36	180 277 288
33 - 34	125 195 517 553
31 - 32	3 152 446 506
29 - 30	21 52 168 170 179 301 316 383 424 520
27 - 28	32 33 42 48 148 150 190 251 300 448 463 503 511 554
25 - 26	19 22 23 137 141 310 311 320 329 361 364 411 527
23 - 24	82 85 94 151 229 268 269 274 326 333 337 342 368 480 485 487 489 498 502 516 534 546
21 - 22	17 39 46 54 70 75 129 191 201 202 219 256 265 280 285 303 306 369 421 427 429 430 457 482 518 543 550

19 - 20	4 24 92 98 138 145 153 176 185 187 225 273 296 307 331 347 349 355 366 408 484 512 515
17 - 18	1 8 16 41 65 67 84 86 99 124 142 182 184 198 215 221 241 257 259 263 271 292 299 338 351 379 384 390 400 415 454 471 474 479 488 491 496 505 526 530 537 539 544 551 561
15 - 16	6 25 34 38 60 63 73 76 112 127 144 156 167 175 212 233 234 237 240 243 254 264 287 309 318 319 327 332 348 367 380 399 432 433 441 455 468 469 509 519 521 524 525 540 547 563
13 - 14	13 30 72 87 95 100 123 135 136 161 173 223 232 246 278 312 314 315 321 324 328 339 362 381 382 387 391 395 413 450 452 464 475 504 513 532 536 538 549 555 566
11 - 12	5 27 49 55 56 61 64 74 78 80 81 83 90 105 113 121 140 159 192 204 206 216 218 226 228 236 248 250 252 255 262 266 276 281 284 291 298 308 313 322 323 325 336 343 346 358 360 363 371 373 374 375 377 402 435 436 442 453 456 477 478 483 490 500 514 548 558 562 567
9 - 10	35 62 69 97 104 106 108 115 117 120 133 143 146 155 158 162 165 171 186 197 205 207 210 214 231 249 253 282 290 294 317 335 344 354 365 376 378 388 394 412 423 426 451 462 493 495 507 508 528 559 564
7 - 8	14 36 37 59 66 93 96 102 110 114 118 126 132 163 166 183 193 194 203 208 230 239 260 279 289 334 350 356 357 386 393 398 407 409 418 419 428 431 439 444 461 466 467 473 481 501 565
5 - 6	11 15 18 26 31 44 79 119 131 134 147 164 178 181 188 199 244 258 283 330 401 403 404 405 422 447 460 476 499 523 531 533 535 541 545 552
3 - 4	9 20 28 29 40 43 47 68 101 109 111 130 149 160 172 174 189 200 209 211 220 235 238 242 272 293 297 304 341 345 352 353 370 389 392 396 410 420 425 434 437 443 465 494 522 542 556
1 - 2	2 7 12 58 71 77 88 89 103 107 116 122 128 139 157 169 177 213 222 227 245 261 267 270 275 302 340 359 372 385 397 406 416 438 440 445 458 459 470 472 486 529 557 560
0	50 51 154 196 217 286 305 414 417 449 492 497 510

Appendix K

Item-Endorsement Percentage Differences for Pain (N = 234) vs. Psychiatric (N = 191) Sample Women

(Left margin = difference in item-endorsement percentages between pain and psychiatric samples. Item numbers in body of table correspond to the MMPI-2 form.)

99 - 100	
97 - 98	
95 - 96	
93 - 94	
91 - 92	
89 - 90	
87 - 88	
85 - 86	
83 - 84	
81 - 82	
79 - 80	
77 - 78	
75 - 76	
73 - 74	
71 - 72	
69 - 70	
67 - 68	
65 - 66	224
63 - 64	
61 - 62	
59 - 60	
57 - 58	
55 - 56	
53 - 54	
51 - 52	45
49 - 50	10 57
47 - 48	
45 - 46	
43 - 44	190
41 - 42	145
39 - 40	
37 - 38	32 52
35 - 36	225 247 295 311 506 553
33 - 34	82 94 124 254 288 309 316 518
31 - 32	121 135 150 167 180 333 403 488 561
29 - 30	3 42 141 256 338 374 382 436 463 479 482 498 503 550
27 - 28	8 16 22 53 76 91 105 125 152 153 195 202 221 229 266 268 269 300 315 327 348 361 364 366 448 487 517
25 - 26	21 34 55 84 85 99 129 138 148 170 185 251 259 277 285 314 320 326 329 337 347 368 391 394 471 485 509 520 526 538 543 546 548
23 - 24	13 17 35 48 123 136 144 168 176 234 241 243 274 286 303 306 313 334 383 399 415 421 480 490 491 516 554
21 - 22	39 60 161 182 198 215 219 242 264 271 279 298 301 307 310 355 373 375 407 408 411 466 484 489 507 530 549

19 - 20	19 24 27 30 33 46 49 54 81 110 142 179 240 265 280 318 332 358 360 390 423 427 433 446 450 454 464 539 544 563
17 - 18	68 72 75 98 117 178 216 226 228 253 299 308 323 362 376 381 412 420 429 431 435 451 455 457 461 477 497 500 502 504 511 524 525 531
15 - 16	71 92 104 113 116 151 156 166 191 203 212 235 250 257 263 273 278 289 292 302 312 317 322 336 344 349 357 367 379 386 409 413 419 432 441 444 447 496 505 512 513 527 534 567
13 - 14	4 23 26 41 56 65 73 78 87 90 127 134 140 143 155 184 207 211 217 223 244 246 287 319 324 342 371 387 389 418 424 428 459 468 470 475 495 551 555 566
11 - 12	2 5 36 62 70 93 96 107 109 114 133 137 162 186 187 193 206 209 213 222 227 232 233 248 296 304 325 328 330 378 395 398 400 402 406 410 443 510 515 523 540 541 559
9 - 10	6 9 14 25 28 31 43 50 61 64 67 83 108 132 154 177 194 210 238 245 272 282 284 305 340 354 372 377 396 414 434 437 439 453 483 486 501 522 528 557 558 565
7 - 8	7 40 44 58 66 77 86 88 95 97 103 118 130 131 147 149 174 175 197 200 208 220 258 260 261 281 283 290 291 339 345 369 380 385 404 417 422 430 438 442 449 456 460 478 532 545 547
5 - 6	18 38 59 69 74 80 101 102 112 115 119 126 128 163 165 172 183 192 196 199 201 204 214 237 252 262 270 275 276 335 343 351 353 370 384 392 393 440 467 472 492 493 529 533 535 552 560 562
3 - 4	51 79 100 122 139 157 160 169 171 188 218 231 249 293 294 297 321 331 346 359 363 397 401 405 416 426 462 476 494 508 514 519 521 537 542 556 564
1 - 2	11 15 20 29 37 47 63 89 106 111 120 146 158 164 173 181 255 267 341 350 352 356 365 388 425 445 452 458 465 469 474 481 536
0	1 12 159 189 205 230 236 239 473 499

Appendix L

Correlates of Top
Quartiles of Validity,
Clinical, Content, and
Supplementary Scales
for Chronic Pain Men

(Items are positively associated with upper quartile of scale unless followed by (-) notation.)

SCALE L

Biographical Information Form

Ever arrested for other than motor vehicle violation (-)
Ever treated for emotional problems (-)

Life Events Form

Total life events (-)
Change in eating habits (-)

Chart Review Form

History of suicidal ideation (-)

SCALE F

Biographical Information Form

Last time went to physician (more recent)
History of arrest for other than motor vehicle violation
Currently in psychological or psychiatric treatment

Life Events Form

Total life events
Sexual difficulties
Change in number of arguments with family members

Chart Review Form

Beck Depression Inventory score at admission
Beck Depression Inventory score at discharge
Depression was a focus of treatment during program
Depression was a focus of treatment during follow-up
History of suicidal ideation

SCALE K

Life Events Form

Total life events (-)
Change in number of arguments with family members (-)
Change in social activities (-)
Take out small loan (-)
Change in eating habits (-)

Chart Review Form

Beck Depression Inventory score at admission (-)
Beck Depression Inventory score at discharge (-)
Operation or major physical illness in past year (-)

SCALE Hs

Life Events Form

Total life events

Chart Review Form

Beck Depression Inventory score at admission

SCALE D

Biographical Information Form

History of treatment for emotional problems
Currently in psychological or psychiatric treatment

Life Events Form

Total life events
Change in number of arguments with family members

Chart Review Form

Beck Depression Inventory score at admission
Depression was a focus of treatment during program
Depression was a focus of treatment during follow-up
Rating of contribution of affective disorder to overall disability
History of treatment for pain problem with psychotherapy
History of suicidal ideation

SCALE Hy

No unique correlates.

SCALE Pd

Biographical Information Form

History of arrest for other than motor vehicle violation
History of treatment for emotional problem
Currently in psychological or psychiatric treatment
First-degree relative with history of alcohol or drug treatment

Life Events Form

Total life events
Sexual difficulties
Change to different line of work
Change in number of arguments with family members

Chart Review Form

Beck Depression Inventory score at admission
Depression was a focus of treatment during program
History of treatment for pain problem with psychotherapy

SCALE Mf

Biographical Information Form

History of treatment for emotional problems

Chart Review Form

Beck Depression Inventory score at admission

SCALE Pa

Biographical Information Form

Total family income (-)
Last time went to a physician (more recent)
History of treatment for emotional problem
Currently in psychological or psychiatric treatment
Second-degree relative with history of treatment for emotional problems

Life Events Form

Total life events
Change in number of arguments with family members
Change in eating habits

Chart Review Form

Beck Depression Inventory score at admission
Depression was a focus of treatment during program
Depression was a focus of treatment during follow-up
Rating of contribution of affective disorder to overall disability
History of affective disorder
History of suicidal ideation
Depression reduction was listed as specific treatment goal

SCALE Pt

Biographical Information Form

History of treatment for emotional problems
Currently in treatment for emotional problems

Life Events Form

Total life events
Sexual difficulties
Change in number of arguments with family members

Change in social activities
Change in number of family outings and holidays
Change in eating habits

Chart Review Form

Number of previous treatments for pain
Beck Depression Inventory score at admission
Beck Depression Inventory score at discharge
Depression was a focus of treatment during program
Depression was a focus of treatment during follow-up
Rating of contribution of affective disorder to overall disability
Rating of contribution of other psychiatric problem to overall disability
History of treatment for pain problem with psychotherapy
History of affective disorder
History of suicidal ideation

SCALE Sc

Biographical Information Form

History of treatment for emotional problems

Life Events Form

Total life events
Change in number of arguments with family members
Change in eating habits

Chart Review Form

Beck Depression Inventory score at admission
Beck Depression Inventory score at discharge
Depression was a focus of treatment during program
Depression was a focus of treatment during follow-up
Rating of contribution of affective disorder to overall disability
Rating of contribution of other psychiatric problem to overall disability
History of affective disorder
History of suicidal ideation

SCALE Ma

Biographical Information Form

History of drug use (more use and problems)
History of arrest for other than motor vehicle violation

Life Events Form

Total life events

SCALE Si

Biographical Information Form

Currently in psychological or psychiatric treatment

Life Events Form

Total life events

Chart Review Form

Number of previous treatments for pain
Beck Depression Inventory score at admission
Depression was a focus of treatment during program
Depression was a focus of treatment during follow-up
Rating of contribution of affective disorder to overall disability
History of suicidal ideation

SCALE ANX (Anxiety)

Biographical Information Form

Last time visited a physician (more recent)
Currently in psychological or psychiatric treatment

Life Events Form

Total life events
Sexual difficulties
Change in number of arguments with family members
Change in eating habits

Chart Review Form

Beck Depression Inventory score at admission
Beck Depression Inventory score at discharge
Depression was a focus of treatment during program
Depression was a focus of treatment during follow-up
Rating of contribution of affective disorder to overall disability
History of treatment for pain problem with psychotherapy
History of suicidal ideation

SCALE FRS (Fears)

No unique correlates.

SCALE OBS (Obsessiveness)

Biographical Information Form

History of treatment for emotional problem

Life Events Form

Total life events
Change in number of arguments with family members

Chart Review Form

Beck Depression Inventory score at admission
Depression was a focus of treatment during program
Rating of contribution of other psychiatric disorder to overall disability

SCALE DEP (Depression)

Biographical Information Form

History of treatment for emotional problems
Currently in psychological or psychiatric treatment

Life Events Form

Total life events
Change in health of family member
Change in number of arguments with family members

Chart Review Form

Beck Depression Inventory score at admission
Depression was a focus of treatment during program
Depression was a focus of treatment during follow-up
Rating of contribution of affective disorder to overall disability
History of suicidal ideation

SCALE HEA (Health Concerns)

Biographical Information Form

History of receiving a ticket for speeding

Life Events Form

Total life events
Change in sleeping habits
Change in number of family outings or holidays

Chart Review Form

Beck Depression Inventory score at admission

SCALE BIZ (Bizarre Ideation)

Life Events Form

Total life events

Chart Review Form

Beck Depression Inventory score at admission

SCALE ANG (Anger)

Biographical Information Form

History of arrest for other than motor vehicle violation
History of treatment for an emotional problem
History of drug use

Life Events Form

Total life events
Change in financial status
Change in number of arguments with family members

Chart Review Form

Beck Depression Inventory score at admission

SCALE CYN (Cynicism)

Life Events Form

Total life events
Take out small loan

SCALE ASP (Antisocial Practices)

Biographical Information Form

History of drug use and/or problems
History of arrest for other than a motor vehicle violation

Life Events Form

Total life events

SCALE TPA (Type A)

Life Events Form

Total life events
Change of personal habits

SCALE LSE (Low Self-Esteem)

Biographical Information Form

Currently in psychological or psychiatric treatment

Life Events Form

Total life events

Chart Review Form

Beck Depression Inventory score at admission
Depression was a focus of treatment during program
History of suicidal ideation
History of suicide attempt(s)

SCALE SOD (Social Discomfort)

Life Events Form

Total life events

Chart Review Form

Number of previous treatments for pain problem
Beck Depression Inventory score at admission
Depression was a focus of treatment during program
History of treatment for pain problem with psychotherapy

SCALE FAM (Family Problems)

Biographical Information Form

History of arrest for other than a motor vehicle violation
History of treatment for an emotional problem
Currently in psychological or psychiatric treatment
Second-degree relative with history of treatment for emotional problems

Life Events Form

Total life events
Change to different line of work
Change in number of arguments with family
Change in eating habits

Chart Review Form

Beck Depression Inventory score at admission
History of suicidal ideation

SCALE WRK (Work Interference)

Biographical Information Form

History of treatment for an emotional problem

Life Events Form

Total life events
Change in health of family member
Change in number of arguments with family member

Chart Review Form

Beck Depression Inventory score at admission
Depression was a focus of treatment during program
Depression was a focus of treatment during follow-up
Rating of contribution of affective disorder to overall disability
History of suicidal ideation
History of suicide attempt(s)

SCALE TRT (Negative Treatment Indicators)

Biographical Information Form

Currently in psychological or psychiatric treatment

Life Events Form

Total life events
Change in health of family member
Sexual difficulties
Change in number of arguments with family members

Chart Review Form

Beck Depression Inventory score at admission
Depression was a focus of treatment during program
Depression was a focus of treatment during follow-up
Rating of contribution of affective disorder to overall disability
History of suicidal ideation
History of suicide attempt(s)

SCALE MAC (MacAndrew Alcoholism)

Biographical Information Form

History of drug use (more use and problems)
Total family income (-)
Have lived most of life in city as opposed to town or rural area
History of arrest for other than motor vehicle violation

Chart Review Form

History of alcohol abuse problem
History of assaultiveness or destruction of property

SCALE ES (Ego Strength)

Biographical Information Form

Describes self as having physical handicap (-)

Life Events Form

Total life events (-)
Personal injury or illness (-)
Change in living conditions (-)

Chart Review Form

Beck Depression Inventory score at admission (-)
Beck Depression Inventory score at discharge (-)
Depression was a focus of treatment during program (-)
Depression was a focus of treatment during follow-up (-)
Rating of contribution of affective disorder to overall disability (-)

SCALE A (Anxiety)

Biographical Information Form

History of treatment for emotional problems
Currently in psychological or psychiatric treatment

Life Events Form

Total life events
Change in number of arguments with family members

Chart Review Form

Beck Depression Inventory score at admission
Depression was a focus of treatment during program
Depression was a focus of treatment during follow-up
Rating of contribution of affective disorder to overall disability
History of treatment for pain problem with psychotherapy
History of suicidal ideation
History of suicide attempt(s)

SCALE R (Repression)

Life Events Form

Total life events (-)

Appendix M

Correlates of Top Quartiles of Validity, Clinical, Content, and Supplementary Scales for Chronic Pain Women

(Items are positively associated with upper quartile of scale unless followed by (-) notation.)

SCALE L

Biographical Information Form

Education (-)

Life Events Form

Change of personal habits (-)

SCALE F

Biographical Information Form

History of treatment for emotional problems

Life Events Form

Total life events
Change in living conditions

Chart Review Form

Beck Depression Inventory score at admission

SCALE K

Life Events Form

Total life events (-)

Chart Review Form

Beck Depression Inventory score at admission (-)
Depression was a focus of treatment during program (-)

SCALE HS

Life Events Form

Total life events
Change in health of family member

Chart Review Form

Beck Depression Inventory score at admission
Rating of contribution of all "functional" factors to overall disability
History of treatment with nerve blocks or trigger point injections (-)

SCALE D

Life Events Form

Sexual difficulties

Chart Review Form

Beck Depression Inventory score at admission
Depression was a focus of treatment during program
Rating of contribution of affective disorder to overall disability
Receiving private insurance compensation for pain problem
History of suicidal ideation
History of suicide attempt(s)

SCALE Hy

Life Events Form

Total life events
Sexual difficulties

Chart Review Form

Rating of contribution of all "functional" factors to overall disability

SCALE Pd

Biographical Information Form

Age (-)
History of drug use (more use and problems)
History of treatment for emotional problems
History of hospitalization for emotional problems

Life Events Form

Total life events
Unable to pay mortgage or loan

Chart Review Form

Beck Depression Inventory score at admission
Rating of contribution of affective disorder to overall disability
Rating of contribution of alcohol use/abuse to overall disability
History of being victim of physical abuse
History of affective disorder
History of psychiatric hospitalization
History of suicidal ideation
History of suicide attempt(s)

SCALE Mf

No unique correlates.

SCALE Pa

Life Events Form

Total life events
Change in number of arguments with family members
Trouble with in-laws

Chart Review Form

Beck Depression Inventory score at admission
Rating of contribution of affective disorder to overall disability

SCALE Pt

Biographical Information Form

History of treatment for emotional problems

Life Events Form

Total life events
Sexual difficulties
Change in number of arguments with family members

Chart Review Form

Number of siblings (-)
Number of children (-)
Beck Depression Inventory score at admission
Depression was a focus of treatment during program
Depression was a focus of treatment during follow-up
History of suicidal ideation
History of suicide attempt(s)

SCALE Sc

Biographical Information Form

History of treatment for emotional problems
Currently in psychological or psychiatric treatment

Life Events Form

Total life events
Change in health of family members
Sexual difficulties
Change in financial status
Change in number of arguments with family members
Change in personal habits
Change in social activities
Change in sleeping habits
Change in number of family outings and holidays
Change in eating habits

Chart Review Form

Number of siblings (-)
Number of children (-)
Beck Depression Inventory score at admission
Depression was a focus of treatment during program
Depression was a focus of treatment during follow-up
History of affective disorder
History of suicidal ideation

SCALE Ma

Life Events Form

Total life events
Business difficulties or loss
Outstanding personal achievement
Change in recreation
Change in social activities

SCALE Si

Chart Review Form

Beck Depression Inventory score at admission
Depression was a focus of treatment during program
History of suicide attempt(s)

SCALE ANX (Anxiety)

Biographical Information Form

History of treatment for emotional problems

Life Events Form

Total life events
Sexual difficulties
Business difficulties or loss
Change in financial status
Change in number of arguments with family members
Change in social activities

Chart Review Form

Beck Depression Inventory score at admission
Beck Depression Inventory score at discharge
Depression was a focus of treatment during program
Depression was a focus of treatment during follow-up
Rating of contribution of affective disorder to overall disability
Rating of contribution of all "functional" factors to overall disability
History of suicidal ideation
History of suicide attempt(s)

SCALE FRS (Fears)

Biographical Information Form

More likely to be married

Life Events Form

Death of close family member

SCALE OBS (Obsessiveness)

Life Events Form

Total life events
Change in sleeping habits
Change in eating habits

Chart Review Form

Beck Depression Inventory score at admission
Depression was a focus of treatment during program

SCALE DEP (Depression)

Life Events Form

Total life events
Change in number of arguments with family members

Chart Review Form

Number of siblings (-)
Beck Depression score at admission
Depression was a focus of treatment during program
Depression was a focus of treatment during follow-up
Rating of contribution of affective disorder to overall disability
History of affective disorder
History of suicidal ideation
History of suicide attempt(s)

SCALE HEA (Health Concerns)

Life Events Form

Total life events
Change in health of family member
Change in number of arguments with family members
Change in sleeping habits
Change in eating habits

Chart Review Form

Beck Depression Inventory score at admission
Rating of contribution of all "functional" factors to overall disability
History of suicide attempt(s)

SCALE BIZ (Bizarre Ideation)

Life Events Form

Total life events
Death of a close family member
Sexual difficulties
Outstanding personal achievement
Change in personal habits

SCALE ANG (Anger)

Biographical Information Form

Age (-)
History of treatment for an emotional problem

Life Events Form

Total life events
Change in financial status

Chart Review Form

Number of children (-)
Beck Depression Inventory score at admission
History of suicidal ideation
History of suicide attempt(s)

SCALE CYN (Cynicism)

Life Events Form

Total life events

SCALE ASP (Antisocial Practices)

Biographical Information Form

History of drug use and/or problems

Life Events Form

Total life events

SCALE TPA (Type A)

Life Events Form

Total life events
Sexual difficulties
Business difficulties or loss
Change in personal habits

Chart Review Form

Beck Depression Inventory score at admission

SCALE LSE (Low Self-Esteem)

Life Events Form

Total life events

Chart Review Form

Beck Depression Inventory score at admission
Depression was a focus of treatment during program
Depression was a focus of treatment during follow-up
History of suicide attempt(s)

SCALE SOD (Social Discomfort)

Chart Review Form

Depression was a focus of treatment during program
Depression was a focus of treatment during follow-up

SCALE FAM (Family Problems)

Biographical Information Form

Age (-)
History of drug use and/or problems

Life Events Form

Total life events
Change in number of arguments with family members
Change in residence

Chart Review Form

Beck Depression Inventory score at admission

SCALE WRK (Work Interference)

Life Events Form

Total life events

Chart Review Form

Beck Depression Inventory score at admission
Depression was a focus of treatment during program
Depression was a focus of treatment during follow-up
History of suicidal ideation
History of suicide attempt(s)

SCALE TRT (Negative Treatment Indicators)

Life Events Form

Total life events

Chart Review Form

Beck Depression Inventory score at admission
Depression was a focus of treatment during program
Depression was a focus of treatment during follow-up
Rating of contribution of affective disorder to overall disability
History of suicide attempt(s)

SCALE MAC (MacAndrew Alcoholism)

Biographical Information Form

History of drug use (more use and problems)

SCALE ES (Ego Strength)

Life Events Form

Total life events (-)
Change in sleeping habits (-)

Chart Review Form

Beck Depression Inventory score at admission (-)
Depression was a focus of treatment during program (-)
Depression was a focus of treatment during follow-up (-)
Rating of contribution of affective disorder to overall disability (-)

SCALE A (Anxiety)

Life Events Form

Total life events
Change in number of arguments with family members
Change in social activities

Chart Review Form

Number of siblings (-)
Number of children (-)
Beck Depression Inventory score at admission
Depression was a focus of treatment during program
Depression was a focus of treatment during follow-up
Rating of contribution of affective disorder to overall disability
History of suicidal ideation
History of suicide attempt(s)

SCALE R (Repression)

Life Events Form

Total life events (-)
Change in financial status (-)

Appendix N

Frequencies of Profile High Points (Any Elevation), MMPI-2 Norms vs. Hathaway-Briggs Norms

A. MEN

Highest Scale	MMPI-2 Freq.	MMPI Freq.	% Matching
Hs	95 (35%)	102 (38%)	74%
D	45 (17%)	85 (32%)	100%
Hy	83 (31%)	34 (13%)	35%
Pd	8 (3%)	15 (6%)	75%
Pa	10 (4%)	2 (1%)	20%
Pt	11 (4%)	7 (3%)	55%
Sc	10 (4%)	17 (6%)	90%
Ma	6 (2%)	6 (2%)	83%
		Overall total:	64%

B. WOMEN

Highest Scale	MMPI-2 Freq.	MMPI Freq.	% Matching
Hs	60 (26%)	47 (20%)	62%
D	45 (19%)	52 (22%)	91%
Hy	101 (43%)	87 (37%)	77%
Pd	10 (4%)	20 (9%)	100%
Pa	4 (2%)	3 (1%)	75%
Pt	4 (2%)	4 (2%)	75%
Sc	4 (2%)	8 (3%)	100%
Ma	6 (3%)	13 (6%)	100%
		Overall total:	78%

Note: Scales are K-corrected.

Appendix O

Frequencies of Spikes and Two-Point Codes for MMPI-2 Norms vs. Hathaway-Briggs Norms

A. MEN

Codetype	MMPI-2 Freq.	MMPI Freq.	% Matching
Normal Limits	18 (7%)	15 (6%)	83%
Spike 1	18 (7%)	9 (4%)	44%
Spike 2	7 (3%)	6 (2%)	86%
Spike 3	4 (2%)	2 (1%)	50%
Spike 4	0	3 (1%)	0%
Spike 6	1 (1%)	1 (1%)	100%
Spike 9	2 (1%)	2 (1%)	100%
1-2/2-1	27 (10%)	65 (25%)	85%
1-3/3-1	102 (38%)	58 (22%)	58%
1-4/4-1	5 (2%)	11 (4%)	100%
1-6/6-1	2 (1%)	1 (1%)	0%
1-7/7-1	4 (2%)	1 (1%)	25%
1-8/8-1	4 (2%)	8 (3%)	75%
1-9/9-1	3 (1%)	4 (2%)	67%
2-3/3-2	16 (6%)	13 (5%)	25%
2-4/4-2	2 (1%)	8 (3%)	50%
2-6/6-2	6 (2%)	4 (2%)	67%
2-7/7-2	7 (3%)	19 (7%)	86%
2-8/8-2	2 (1%)	16 (6%)	100%
3-4/4-3	10 (4%)	5 (2%)	20%
3-6/6-3	3 (1%)	0	0%
3-7/7-3	8 (3%)	4 (2%)	14%
4-6/6-4	1 (1%)	0	0%
4-7/7-4	1 (1%)	0	0%
4-8/8-4	1 (1%)	2 (1%)	0%
4-9/9-4	1 (1%)	1 (1%)	0%
6-8/8-6	4 (2%)	0	0%
7-8/8-7	7 (3%)	0	0%
8-9/9-8	2 (1%)	3 (1%)	50%
		Overall total:	56%

Codetype	MMPI-2 Freq.	MMPI Freq.	% Matching
B. WOMEN			
Codetype	MMPI-2 Freq.	MMPI Freq.	% Matching
Normal limits	14 (6%)	23 (10%)	93%
Spike 1	3 (1%)	2 (1%)	33%
Spike 2	1 (1%)	6 (3%)	100%
Spike 3	5 (2%)	11 (5%)	0%
Spike 4	2 (1%)	5 (2%)	100%
Spike 9	2 (1%)	2 (1%)	100%
1-2/2-1	19 (9%)	19 (9%)	63%
1-3/3-1	105 (45%)	66 (30%)	67%
1-4/4-1	3 (1%)	4 (2%)	67%
1-6/6-1	1 (1%)	1 (1%)	100%
1-7/7-1	3 (1%)	4 (2%)	67%
1-8/8-1	2 (1%)	2 (1%)	50%
1-9/9-1	0	2 (1%)	—
2-3/3-2	19 (8%)	14 (6%)	61%
2-4/4-2	2 (1%)	11 (5%)	100%
2-7/7-2	15 (6%)	11 (5%)	71%
2-8/8-2	1 (1%)	3 (1%)	0%
3-4/4-3	17 (7%)	16 (7%)	59%
3-6/6-3	3 (1%)	3 (1%)	100%
3-7/7-3	2 (1%)	2 (1%)	50%
3-8/8-3	3 (1%)	1 (1%)	0%
3-9/9-3	6 (3%)	7 (3%)	83%
4-6/6-4	1 (1%)	1 (1%)	100%
4-8/8-4	0	2 (1%)	0%
4-9/9-4	1 (1%)	1 (1%)	100%
6-8/8-6	1 (1%)	1 (1%)	100%
6-9/9-6	0	1 (1%)	0%
7-8/8-7	1 (1%)	0	0%
8-9/9-8	1 (1%)	2 (1%)	100%
		Overall total:	67%

Appendix P
Correlates of Common Codetypes for Men

(Items are positively associated with codetype membership unless followed by (-) notation.)

NORMAL-LIMITS CODETYPE

Biographical Information Form

Number of times married (-)

Life Events Form

Total life events (-)

Chart Review Form

Beck Depression Inventory score at admission (-)
Depression less likely to be a focus of treatment during program
Depression less likely to be a focus of treatment during follow-up
Depression reduction less likely to be listed as goal for patient

Content Scales

LSE (-) Low Self-Esteem
OBS (-) Obsessiveness
HEA (-) Health Concerns
DEP (-) Depression
ANX (-) Anxiety
WRK(-) Work Interference
TRT (-) Negative Treatment Indicators

SPIKE 1 CODETYPE

Content Scales

FAM (-) Family Problems
DEP (-) Depression
ANX (-) Anxiety
WRK(-) Work Interference

1-2/2-1 CODETYPE

Content Scales

ASP   Antisocial Practices
SOD   Social Discomfort

CONVERSION-V CODETYPE

Life Events Form

Total life events (-)

Chart Review Form

Total number of pain complaints

Content Scales

LSE (-) Low Self-Esteem
ANG (-) Anger
OBS (-) Obsessiveness
ASP (-) Antisocial Practices
SOD (-) Social Discomfort
FAM (-) Family Problems
TPA (-) Type A
HEA   Health Concerns
DEP (-) Depression
ANX (-) Anxiety
WRK(-) Work Interference
TRT (-) Negative Treatment Indicators
CYN (-) Cynicism

NEUROTIC-TRIAD CODETYPE

No unique correlates.

SC CODETYPES

Chart Review Form

Rating of contribution of other psychiatric problem to disability
History of schizophrenia or unspecified psychosis

Content Scales

LSE   Low Self-Esteem
ANG   Anger
OBS   Obsessiveness
ASP   Antisocial Practices
FAM   Family Problems
BIZ   Bizarre Ideation
DEP   Depression
ANX   Anxiety
WRK   Work Interference
TRT   Negative Treatment Indicators
CYN   Cynicism

Appendix Q

Correlates of
Common Codetypes
for Women

(Items are positively associated with codetype membership unless followed by (-) notation.)

NORMAL-LIMITS CODETYPE

Life Events Form

Total life events (-)
Pregnancy

Chart Review Form

Beck Depression Inventory score at admission (-)
Rating of contribution of affective disorder to disability (-)

Content Scales

HEA (-) Health Concerns
DEP (-) Depression
ANX (-) Anxiety
WRK (-) Work Interference

CONVERSION-V CODETYPE

Chart Review Form

Beck Depression Inventory score at admission (-)
History of suicidal ideation (-)

Content Scales

LSE (-) Low Self-Esteem
ANG (-) Anger
OBS (-) Obsessiveness
ASP (-) Antisocial Practices
SOD (-) Social Discomfort
FAM (-) Family Problems
DEP (-) Depression
ANX (-) Anxiety
WRK (-) Work Interference
TRT (-) Negative Treatment Indicators
CYN (-) Cynicism

NEUROTIC-TRIAD CODETYPE

No unique correlates.

2-7/7-2 CODETYPE

Content Scales

LSE	Low Self-Esteem
OBS	Obsessiveness
SOD	Social Discomfort
DEP	Depression
ANX	Anxiety
WRK	Work Interference
TRT	Negative Treatment Indicators

3-4/4-3 CODETYPE

Life Events Form

Divorce
Business difficulties or loss

Content Scales

DEP	Depression

Appendix R

Mean MMPI-2 Profiles for Cluster Groups by Sex and Cohort

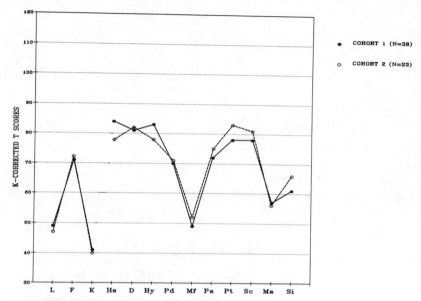

Mean MMPI-2 Profiles for First Male Cluster by Cohort

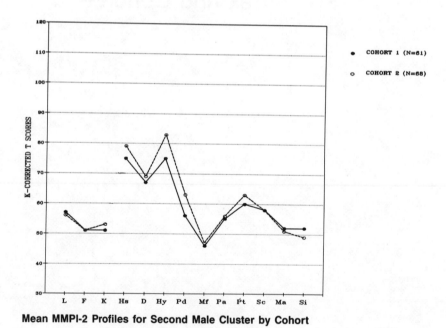

Mean MMPI-2 Profiles for Second Male Cluster by Cohort

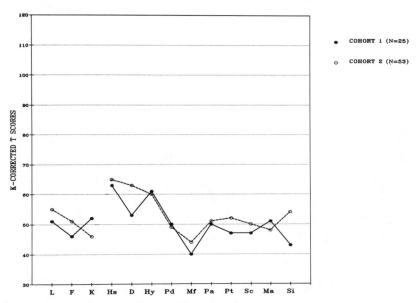

Mean MMPI-2 Profiles for Third Male Cluster by Cohort

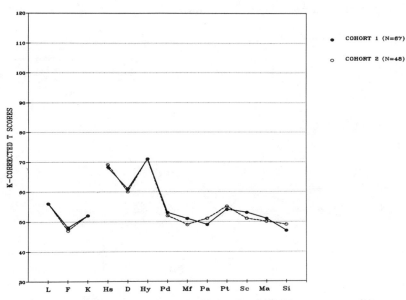

Mean MMPI-2 Profiles for First Female Cluster by Cohort

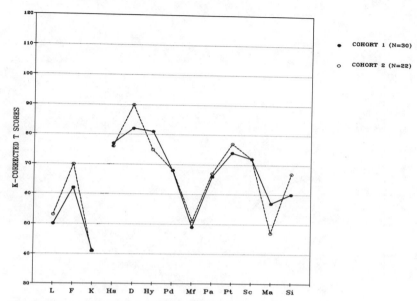

Mean MMPI-2 Profiles for Second Female Cluster by Cohort

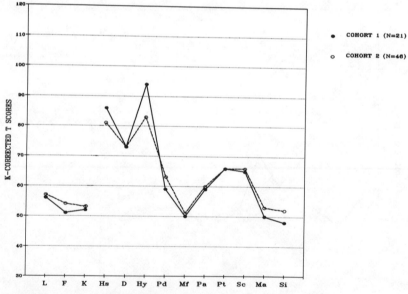

Mean MMPI-2 Profiles for Third Female Cluster by Cohort

Appendix S
Correlates of Cluster Types for Men

(Items are positively associated with cluster membership unless followed by (-) notation.)

CLUSTER 1 (General Elevation)

Life Events Form

Total life events
Change in number of arguments with family members

Chart Review Form

Beck Depression Inventory score at admission
Rating of contribution of other psychiatric problems to disability
Rating of contribution of street drug use to disability
History of suicidal ideation

Content Scales

LSE	Low Self-Esteem
ANG	Anger
OBS	Obsessiveness
ASP	Antisocial Practices
SOD	Social Discomfort
FAM	Family Problems
TPA	Type A
HEA	Health Concerns
BIZ	Bizarre Ideation
DEP	Depression
ANX	Anxiety
FRS	Fears
WRK	Work Interference
TRT	Negative Treatment Indicators
CYN	Cynicism

CLUSTER 2 (Neurotic Triad)

Content Scales

LSE (-) Low Self-Esteem
OBS (-) Obsessiveness
ASP (-) Antisocial Practices
FAM (-) Family Problems
TPA (-) Type A
BIZ (-) Bizarre Ideation
DEP (-) Depression
TRT (-) Negative Treatment Indicators
CYN (-) Cynicism

CLUSTER 3 (Normal Limits)

Life Events Form

Total life events (-)
Change in number of arguments with family members (-)

Chart Review Form

Beck Depression Inventory score at admission (-)
Beck Depression Inventory score at discharge (-)
Depression less likely to be a focus of treatment during program
Depression less likely to be a focus of treatment during follow-up
Rating of contribution of affective disorder to disability (-)

Content Scales

LSE (-) Low Self-Esteem
ANG (-) Anger
OBS (-) Obsessiveness
SOD (-) Social Discomfort
FAM (-) Family Problems
TPA (-) Type A
HEA (-) Health Concerns
BIZ (-) Bizarre Ideation
DEP (-) Depression
ANX (-) Anxiety
FRS (-) Fears
WRK(-) Work Interference
TRT (-) Negative Treatment Indicators

Appendix T
Correlates of Cluster Types for Women

(Items are positively associated with cluster membership unless followed by (-) notation.)

CLUSTER 1 (Neurotic Triad)

Life Events Form

Total life events (-)

Content Scales

ANG (-) Anger
ASP (-) Antisocial Practices
SOD   Social Discomfort
FAM (-) Family Problems

CLUSTER 2 (General Elevation)

Life Events Form

Total life events
Change in health of family member
Sexual difficulties
Change in number of arguments with family members
Change in church activities

Chart Review Form

Beck Depression Inventory score at admission
Depression more likely to be a focus of follow-up treatment
Rating of contribution of affective disorder to overall disability
History of suicidal ideation

Content Scales

LSE   Low Self-Esteem
ANG   Anger
OBS   Obsessiveness
FAM   Family Problems
TPA   Type A
HEA   Health Concerns
BIZ   Bizarre Ideation
DEP   Depression
ANX   Anxiety
WRK   Work Interference
TRT   Negative Treatment Indicators

CLUSTER 3 (Conversion V)

Chart Review Form

Beck Depression Inventory Score at admission (-)
Depression less likely to be a focus of treatment during program

Depression less likely to be a focus of treatment during follow-up
Rating of contribution of affective disorder to disability (-)

Content Scales

LSE (-) Low Self Esteem
OBS (-) Obsessiveness
SOD (-) Social Discomfort
FAM (-) Family Problems
HEA (-) Health Concerns
DEP (-) Depression
ANX (-) Anxiety
FRS (-) Fears
WRK (-) Work Interference
TRT (-) Negative Treatment Indicators

Index

Compiled by Eileen Quam and Theresa Wolner

Laura S. Keller is staff psychologist for the adult outpatient program in the mental health division of Human Services, Inc. in Washington County, Minnesota. In 1988 she received her Ph.D. from the University of Minnesota Clinical Psychology Training Program. Keller interned at the University of Washington School of Medicine in 1985–1986, including a rotation on the chronic pain service. She was a consultant to National Computer Systems in 1988, working with Dr. James Butcher on the revised adult clinical and personnel interpretive reports for the MMPI-2. Throughout her graduate school years, Keller served as a research assistant on various aspects of the MMPI Restandardization Project as well as working with Assessment Systems Corporation and National Computer Systems on computerized psychological assessment systems. Her work on objective personality assessment and computerized assessment has appeared in several book collections as well as the *Journal of Consulting and Clinical Psychology*.

James N. Butcher is a professor of psychology at the University of Minnesota, having taught at the University since 1964. He was a member of the MMPI Restandardization Project and is the author of numerous books, including *Development and Use of the MMPI-2 Content Scales,* co-authored with John R. Graham, Carolyn L. Williams, and Yossef S. Ben-Porath (Minnesota, 1989), *A Handbook of Cross-National MMPI Research,* with Paolo Pancheri (Minnesota, 1976), *New Developments in the Use of the MMPI* (Minnesota, 1979), and *Abnormal Psychology and Modern Life* (1988). Butcher is the editor of *Personality Assessment: A Journal of Consulting and Clinical Psychology* and contributes to the *Journal of Personality and Social Psychology* and the *International Journal of Applied Psychology.*